ENT
HEAD & NECK
EMERGENCIES

A **LOGAN TURNER** COMPANION

ENT
HEAD & NECK
EMERGENCIES
A **LOGAN TURNER** COMPANION

EDITED BY

S. MUSHEER HUSSAIN, MBBS, MSc(Manc), FRCS(Ed & Eng), FRCS(ORL-HNS), FRCP(Ed)
Consultant ENT surgeon and honorary professor of otolaryngology at Ninewells Hospital and the University of Dundee School of Medicine, UK

SECTION EDITORS

PAUL WHITE, FRCS Ed, FRACS
Consultant ENT surgeon at Ninewells Hospital and the University of Dundee School of Medicine, UK

KIM W AH-SEE, MD, FRCS (ORLHNS)
Consultant ENT and Head and Neck Surgeon at Aberdeen Royal Infirmary, Aberdeen, UK

PATRICK SPIELMANN, MBChB, FRCS (ORL-HNS)
Consultant Otolaryngologist at Ninewells Hospital and the University of Dundee School of Medicine, UK

MARY-LOUISE MONTAGUE, MBChB (Hon), PG, Dip Clin Ed, FRCS (ORL-HNS)
Consultant Paediatric Otolayngologist at the Royal Hospital for Sick Children and Honorary Senior Clinical Lecturer at the University of Edinburgh, Edinburgh, UK

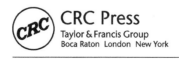

CRC Press
Taylor & Francis Group
Boca Raton London New York

CRC Press is an imprint of the
Taylor & Francis Group, an **informa** business

CRC Press
Taylor & Francis Group
6000 Broken Sound Parkway NW, Suite 300
Boca Raton, FL 33487-2742

© 2019 by Taylor & Francis Group, LLC
CRC Press is an imprint of Taylor & Francis Group, an Informa business

International Standard Book Number-13: 978-1-138-61653-0 (Hardback)
International Standard Book Number-13: 978-1-138-62642-3 (Paperback)

Library of Congress Cataloging-in-Publication Data

Names: Hussain, Musheer, editor.
Title: ENT, Head & Neck Emergencies : a Logan Turner companion / [edited by] Musheer Hussain.
Other titles: ENT and head and neck emergencies
Description: Boca Raton : CRC Press, [2019]
Identifiers: LCCN 2017058919 (print) | LCCN 2017059323 (ebook) | ISBN 9781315228624 (General eBook) | ISBN 9781138626423 (paperback : alk. paper)
Subjects: | MESH: Otorhinolaryngologic Diseases | Emergency Treatment--methods | Craniocerebral Trauma | Neck Injuries
Classification: LCC RF56 (ebook) | LCC RF56 (print) | NLM WV 140 | DDC 617.5/1--dc23
LC record available at https://lccn.loc.gov/2017058919

Visit the Taylor & Francis Web site at
http://www.taylorandfrancis.com

and the CRC Press Web site at
http://www.crcpress.com

Contents

Contributors

Richard Adamson, MB BS, FRCSEd (ORL-HNS), MSc, DMI
Consultant Otolaryngologist, Head and Neck Surgeon
Ear, Nose and Throat Department
University of Edinburgh
Edinburgh, UK

Kim W Ah-See, MD, FRCS (ORL-HNS)
Consultant ENT Head and Neck Surgeon
Department of Otolaryngology Head and Neck Surgery
Aberdeen Royal Infirmary
Aberdeen, UK

Panagiotis Asimakopoulos, BA, MBChB, MSc, FRCS (ORL-HNS)
ENT Specialist Registrar
Department of Otolaryngology
University of Edinburgh
Edinburgh, UK

Adonye Banigo, FRCS (ORL-HNS)
ENT Specialist Registrar
Aberdeen Royal Infirmary
Aberdeen, UK

Paramita Baruah, PhD, FRCS (ORL-HNS)
Consultant ENT Surgeon
University of Leicester NHS Trust
Leicester, UK

Neil Bateman, BMedSci, BM, BS, FRCS (ORL-HNS)
Consultant Paediatric Otolaryngologist
Royal Manchester Children's Hopsital
Manchester, UK

Alex Bennett, MBBS, DLO, FRCS (ORL-HNS), MEd, DIC
Consultant ENT Surgeon and
Honorary Senior Lecturer
Ear, Nose and Throat Department
University of Edinburgh
Edinburgh, UK

Brian Bingham, FRCS (ORL-HNS)
ENT Consultant
Department of ENT
Queen Elizabeth University Hospital
Glasgow, UK

Duncan Bowyer, FRCS (ORL-HNS)
Consultant ENT Surgeon
Department of Otolaryngology
Shrewsbury and Telford Hospital NHS Trust
Shrewsbury, UK

Iain Bruce, MD, FRCS (ORL-HNS)
Consultant Paediatric Otolaryngologist
Department of Paediatric Otolaryngology (ENT)
Royal Manchester Children's Hospital
Manchester, UK

John Crowther, FRCS
Consultant Otolaryngologist and Skull Base
Surgeon
Institute of Neurological Sciences
Queen Elizabeth University Hospital
Glasgow, UK

Jaime Doody, MB, BCh, BAO, BA, MD, MRCS, FRCS (ORL-HNS)
Specialist Registrar in Otolaryngology
Temple Street Children's University Hospital
Dublin, Republic of Ireland

Catriona M Douglas, MD, FRCS (ORL-HNS)
ENT Registrar
Department of ENT
Queen Elizabeth University Hospital
Glasgow, UK

Quentin Gardiner, FRCS (Eng & Edin), FRCS (ORL)
Consultant Rhinologist and Honorary Senior
Lecturer
Ear, Nose and Throat Department
Ninewells Hospital and Medical School
Dundee, UK

Rohit Gohil, BMedSci (Hons), BM BS, MRCS, DOHNS
Specialty Registrar in Otolaryngology
Department of Otolaryngology
University of Edinburgh
Edinburgh, UK

Richard Green, MBBS, DOHNS
ENT Registrar
Ear, Nose and Throat Department
Ninewells Hospital and Medical School
Dundee, UK

Iain Hathorn, BSc (Hons), MBChB, DOHNS, PGCME, FRCSEd (ORL-HNS)
Consultant ENT Surgeon
Royal Infirmary of Edinburgh
and
Honorary Clinical Senior Lecturer
University of Edinburgh
Edinburgh, UK

Bridget Hemmant, MD FCROphth, MB ChB, B Med Sci, PGCert
Consultant Ophthalmologist
James Paget University Hospital
Norfolk, UK
and
Honorary Senior Lecturer
Norwich Medical School
University of East Anglia
Norwich, UK

Omar Hilmi, FRCS (ORL-HNS), FRCS (Edin)
Honorary Senior Lecturer
University of Glasgow
and
Consultant Otolaryngologist
Glasgow Royal Infirmary
Glasgow, UK

Richard M Irving, MD, FRCS (ORL-HNS)
Consultant Otologist, Neurotologist and Skull
Base Surgeon
Department of Neurotology and Skullbase
Surgery
Queen Elizabeth University Hospitals
Birmingham, UK

Faisal Javed, MBBS, FCRS-ORL, FCPS-ORL, DO-HNS
Cochlear Implant and Lateral Skull Base Fellow
Ear, Nose and Throat Department
Queen Elizabeth University Hospital
Glasgow, UK
and
University Hospital Crosshouse
Kilmarnock, UK

Stephen Jones, FRCS (ORL-HNS)
Consultant ENT Surgeon
Ninewells Hospital and Medical School
Dundee, UK

Rahul Kanegaonkar, FRCS (ORL-HNS)
Consultant ENT Surgeon
Medway NHS Foundation Trust
Professor of Medical Innovation
Visiting Professor in Otorhinolaryngology
Medway Campus
Canterbury Christ Church University
Canterbury, UK

Raghu Nandhan Sampath Kumar, PhD, FRCS (ORL-HNS)
Neurotology and Skullbase Fellow
Department of Neurotology & Skullbase Surgery
Queen Elizabeth University Hospitals
Birmingham, UK

Simon A McKean, MBChB, BSc, DOHNS, FRCS (ORL-HNS), Glasgow
Consultant ENT Surgeon
Ear, Nose and Throat Department
Raigmore Hospital
Inverness, UK

AE Louise McMurran, MBChB, MRCS (Glasg), DOHNS
Specialty Trainee in Otolaryngology – Head and Neck Surgery
Department of Otolaryngology
Aberdeen Royal Infirmary
Aberdeen, UK

Mary-Louise Montague, MBChB (Hons), PG Dip Clin Ed, FRCS (ORL-HNS)
Consultant Paediatric Otolaryngologist
The Royal Hospital for Sick Children
and
Honorary Clinical Senior Lecturer
Department of Otolaryngology
University of Edinburgh
Edinburgh, UK

Salil Nair, MD, FRCS
Rhinologist
Department of Otolaryngology, Head and Neck Surgery
Auckland City Hospital
Auckland, New Zealand

Carl Philpott, MD, ChB, DLO, FRCS (ORL-HNS), MD, PGCME
Professor of Rhinology & Olfactology and Head of Rhinology Research Group
Norwich Medical School
University of East Anglia
Norwich, UK
and
Honorary Consultant Rhinologist and ENT Surgeon
James Paget University and Norfolk & Norwich Hospitals
Norfolk, UK

Catherine Rennie, PhD, FRCS
Consultant Rhinologist
Imperial College Healthcare NHS Trust
Imperial College London
London, UK

Peter J Robb, BSc (Hons), MB, BS, FRCS, FRCSEd
Emeritus Consultant ENT Surgeon
Epsom & St Helier University Hospitals
Epsom, Surrey, UK

Peter Ross, MBChB, FRCS (ORL) Glasgow, FRCS (Edin)
ENT Consultant
Ear, Nose and Throat Department
Ninewells Hospital and Medical School
Dundee, UK

Helena Rowley, MB, FRCSI, FRCSI (ENT), FRCSI (ORL-HNS), MD
Consultant Paediatric Otolaryngologist
Children's University Hospital
and
Consultant Otolaryngologist, Mater University Hospital
Dublin, Republic of Ireland

Simone Schaefer, MD
Consultant Paediatric Otolaryngologist
Royal Manchester Children's Hospital
Manchester, UK

David K Selvadurai, MD, FRCS, FACS
Director, Auditory Implant Service
Department of Otolaryngology, Head and Neck
Surgery
St George's Hospital
London, UK

Muhammad Shakeel, FRCSED (ORL-HNS)
Consultant ENT/Thyroid Surgeon
Aberdeen Royal Infirmary
Aberdeen, UK

**Ravi Sharma, FRCS (ORL-HNS), FRCS
(Otolaryngology), DLO, MPhil**
Consultant Paediatric Otolaryngologist
Department of Otolaryngology, Head and Neck
Surgery
Alder Hey Children's Hospital Trust
Liverpool, UK

Salil Sood, FRCS (ORL-HNS), MRCS, MS
Paediatric ENT Clinical Fellow
Ear, Nose and Throat Department
Alder Hey Children's Hospital Trust
Liverpool, UK

**Kate Stephenson, FRCS (ORL-HNS), FCORL (SA),
MMed**
Consultant Paediatric Otorhinolaryngologist
Ear, Nose and Throat Department
Birmingham Children's Hospital
Birmingham, UK

Andrew C Swift, FRCS, FRCS(Ed)
Honorary Senior Lecturer
University of Liverpool
and
Edge Hill University
Liverpool, UK

**Kim To, BSc (Hons), MBBS, DCH, MRCS (Eng),
DO-HNS (Eng)**
Specialist Registrar in ENT Surgery
Ear, Nose and Throat Department
University of Edinburgh
Edinburgh, UK

T Tikka, MRCS (Eng)
Glasgow Royal Infirmary
Glasgow, UK

Max Whittaker, FRCS (ORL-HNS), DO-HNS, MSc
Skull Base Fellow
Guy's & St Thomas Hospital NHS Trust
London, UK

Wai Keat Wong, MBChB
Specialty Registrar in ENT
Department of Otolaryngology, Head and Neck
Surgery
Auckland City Hospital
Auckland, New Zealand

SECTION 1

Emergencies in Rhinology

Epistaxis

IAIN HATHORN

INTRODUCTION

Epistaxis is defined as bleeding from the nose and is one of the commonest emergencies dealt with by the otolaryngologist. The overall incidence of epistaxis in the general population is difficult to determine because most cases are unreported, minor, self-limiting episodes or those controlled with simple first-aid measures. Fewer than 10% of patients seek medical attention for epistaxis and fewer than 10% of those requiring hospitalisation require surgical intervention for control of bleeding.

Due to the fact that many cases involve the elderly population, epistaxis is a significant cause of morbidity and even mortality in general otolaryngology practice. In England there were 22,671 admissions in 2014/2015, with a mean stay of two days.

The nose has an excellent blood supply from both the internal and external carotid arteries, which anastomose extensively within the lateral wall of the nose and septum. The external carotid artery supplies the nose via the facial and maxillary branches. The maxillary artery supply is via the sphenopalatine and greater palatine branches and the facial artery supply is mainly via the superior labial artery. The sphenopalatine artery is the most important blood supply to the nose and it enters the nose via the sphenopalatine foramen before dividing into the posterior septal artery, which runs medially across the face of the sphenoid to the posterior septum and subsequently Little's area, and the posterior lateral division, which supplies the inferior and middle turbinate. The internal carotid artery contributes the anterior and posterior ethmoid arteries via the ophthalmic artery, and supplies the superior part of the nasal septum and lateral wall.

Epistaxis can be classified anatomically into anterior (Kiesselbach's plexus) (Figure 1.1) and posterior (Woodruff's plexus) (Figure 1.2). Kiesselbach's plexus (or Little's area) is an arterial plexus on the anterior nasal septum and is a frequent site of bleeding. Woodruff's plexus is an area of prominent blood vessels lying just inferior to the posterior end of the inferior turbinate. This is a common site of epistaxis in adults. Perhaps a more useful classification, which has the advantage of guiding management, is based on aetiology and whether the epistaxis is primary (80%) or secondary (Table 1.1). Twenty percent of cases will be classified as secondary epistaxis with a local or systemic cause identified. There are also aetiological associations with epistaxis. These include septal deviations and spurs that disrupt normal airflow, causing dessication, increased mucosal

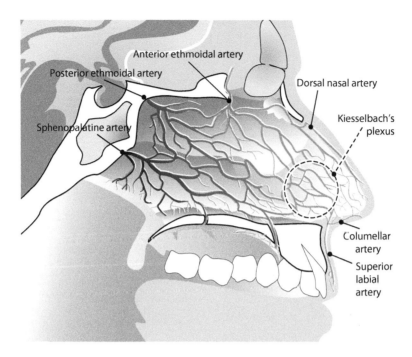

Figure 1.1 The vascular supply of the nasal septum and locus Kiesselbach's plexus.

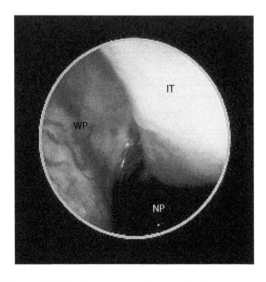

Figure 1.2 Endoscopic photograph of Woodruff's plexus. WP-Woodruff's Plexus, NP-Nasopharynx, IT-Inferior Turbinate.

Table 1.1 Aetiology of epistaxis

Idiopathic	80% of cases
Trauma	Digital, external, nasal trauma, iatrogenic
Coagulopathy	Idiopathic thrombocytopaenia (ITP) Disseminated intravascular coagulopathy (DIC)
Drugs	Warfarin, aspirin, clopidogrel, apixaban, dabigatran, rivaroxiban
Chronic granulomatous disease	Granulomatosis with polyangiitis, sarcoidosis
Neoplastic	Angiofibroma, inverted papilloma, squamous cell cancer
Hereditary	Hereditary haemorrhagic telangiectasia (HHT), haemophilia, von Willebrand's factor deficiency

fragility and epistaxis. Septal perforations often result in the formation of granulation tissue and crusting, due to the lack of epithelium covering the margins, which can result in epistaxis. Alcohol can affect bleeding time, even when platelet counts and coagulation factors are normal. Epistaxis patients are more likely to consume alcohol than matched control patients and are also more likely to have hypertension. Long-standing hypertension may result in vascular fragility from long-standing disease; however, it is rarely a direct cause of epistaxis.

MANAGEMENT

PRIMARY EPISTAXIS

Assessment and resuscitation

The patient presenting with epistaxis should be assessed as per Acute Life Support guidelines (Airway, Breathing, Circulation). They should be sitting up and leaning forward, with pressure applied to the anterior part of the nose by pinching continuously for 10 minutes. In patients with significant ongoing epistaxis, intravenous access should be obtained and a full blood count, coagulation screen and group and save sample taken. If there are signs of shock (tachycardia, hypotension, cool peripheries, prolonged capillary refill time >2 seconds) fluid resuscitation should be implemented with an initial 500 mL bolus of crystalloid (0.9% sodium chloride or Hartmann's solution) over less than 15 minutes. Smaller volumes (e.g. 250 mL) should be used for patients with known cardiac failure and they should be monitored closely for signs of fluid overload (crackles in the chest). In severe epistaxis, blood transfusion can be considered at haemaglobin thresholds of 7–9 g/dL, depending on symptoms and whether there is a history of ischaemic heart disease.

A targeted history should be taken to identify the severity of bleeding and the side and site of bleeding (anterior/posterior), and to identify any underlying aetiological factors, such as known coagulopathies, anticoagulant medications or recent trauma. Effective management of this condition should follow a logical sequence (Figure 1.3).

Direct therapy

The nose should be prepared with a topical vasoconstrictor (such as 1:1000 adrenaline, 0.5% phenylephrine hydrochloride or 0.05% oxymetazoline) to enable control of the bleeding and identify the bleeding point.

Ideally, the bleeding point is identified using rigid nasendoscopy and dealt with directly using either chemical cautery (silver nitrate) or electrocautery (bipolar diathermy). This allows rapid treatment and prompt discharge from hospital. If there are packs present that were inserted by the emergency department, these should be removed, allowing the bleeding point to be identified with a nasendoscope. Direct therapy to the bleeding point is the optimum management in adult epistaxis in dealing with both anterior and posterior epistaxis. Appropriate equipment is required to successfully identify the bleeding point and deal with it (Figure 1.4).

NASAL CAUTERY

1. Suction clots from the nose.
2. Prepare the nose with topical vasoconstrictor solution, either as a spray or applied on cotton wool.
3. Perform anterior rhinoscopy with a headlight and thudicum nasal speculum to identify an anterior bleeding point.
4. Apply a silver nitrate stick/bipolar diathermy to coagulate the bleeding point.
5. If no anterior source is visualised, rigid nasendoscopy should be performed to try to identify a more posterior bleeding point.
6. Use electrocautery to coagulate the posterior bleeding point if it is identified.
7. An absorbable haemostatic agent, such as Surgicel, can be used to apply direct pressure to a bleeding point not amenable to cautery.
8. Rigid nasendoscopy should always be performed, even following identification of anterior bleeding points, to exclude other more posterior sources or underlying sinister pathology.

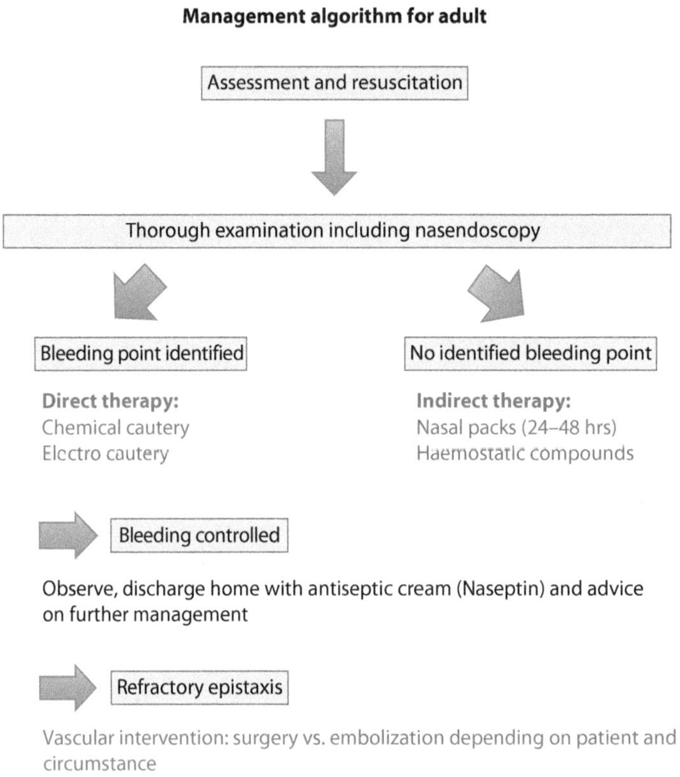

Management algorithm for adult

Assessment and resuscitation

↓

Thorough examination including nasendoscopy

Bleeding point identified

Direct therapy:
Chemical cautery
Electro cautery

No identified bleeding point

Indirect therapy:
Nasal packs (24–48 hrs)
Haemostatic compounds

Bleeding controlled

Observe, discharge home with antiseptic cream (Naseptin) and advice on further management

Refractory epistaxis

Vascular intervention: surgery vs. embolization depending on patient and circumstance

Figure 1.3 Management algorithm for adult acute idiopathic epistaxis.

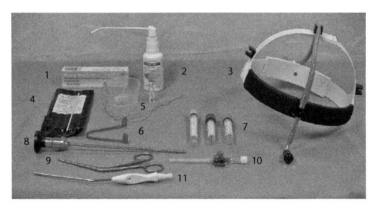

Figure 1.4 Epistaxis management: equipment and medicines. (1) Nasal cream (Naseptin); (2) Topical anaesthetic + decongestant (Co-phenylcaine); (3) Head light; (4) Silver nitrate cautery sticks; (5) Adrenaline vial + patties for application; (6) Nasal speculum (7) Blood bottles: full blood count, congulation, group and save; (8) Rigid nasal endoscope; (9) Tiley's dressing forceps; (10) Large bore cannula; (11) Suction.

Indirect therapy

If no bleeding point is identified, indirect therapies are employed to control the epistaxis. Nasal packs are the most commonly used indirect techniques, but others such as hot water irrigation and topical haemostatic agents can be used (e.g. tranexamic acid or Floseal). Anterior nasal packing includes nasal tampons (Figure 1.5), ribbon gauze and inflatable packs (Rapid Rhino™, Figure 1.6). If

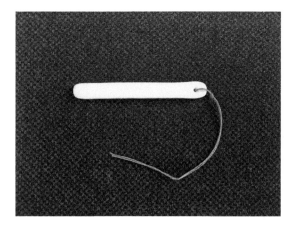

Figure 1.5 Nasal tampon.

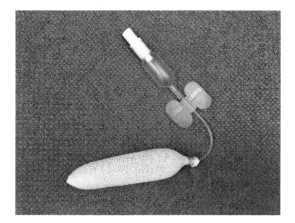

Figure 1.6 Rapid Rhino™ inflatable pack.

bleeding persists despite anterior packing, posterior packs may be required. Once in place, nasal packing should be left *in situ* for 24–48 hours. Antibiotic cover should be considered, particularly in patients with prosthetic heart valves. Local complications of nasal packs include sinusitis, septal perforation and alar necrosis.

NASAL PACKING

1. Suction clots.
2. Prepare the nose with a topical vasoconstrictor.
3. **Ribbon gauze** – Use gauze coated in Mupirocin, bismuth iodoform paraffin paste (BIPP) or petroleum jelly. Use bayonet forceps to layer the gauze horizontally along the floor of the nose and superiorly to fill the nose.

Nasal tampon – Inspect the nose for septal deviation, which can impair insertion. Coat with lubricant and slide posteriorly along the floor of the nose. Soak with saline to expand the nasal tampon.

Posterior packing – A Foley catheter can be advanced past the posterior choanae of the nasal cavity in the nasopharynx. Ribbon gauze packing can then be placed anteriorly.

Topical haemostatic compounds are an alternative indirect treatment option for epistaxis. Floseal, a compound consisting of gelatin granules and human thrombin, is a haemostatic agent that is effective in cases refractory to nasal packing. These are easy to use and are associated with low morbidity, although they are more costly when compared to simple chemical cautery. However, they are much more cost effective when compared to surgical intervention.

Refractory epistaxis

If the methods previously described fail to control the bleeding, then there are several options available, including surgical intervention and embolisation. A general anaesthetic may allow adequate nasal packing (anterior or posterior) in an uncooperative patient. This may also allow endoscopic examination and effective cauterisation. Correction of a deviated septum is also possible under general anaesthesia, allowing access to the bleeding site and permitting cautery. The option of surgical arterial ligation, including sphenopalatine artery and anterior ethmoid artery ligation, should be considered. Arterial ligation should be performed at the most distal (nasal) point, with a progression to more proximal ligation if the initial procedure is unsuccessful.

Endoscopic sphenopalatine artery ligation (ESPAL) is the most commonly employed surgical procedure to control refractory epistaxis and is successful in over 90% of cases, with a low complication rate. Internal maxillary artery and, thereafter, external carotid artery ligation are infrequently used. Anterior ethmoidal artery ligation is used in traumatic epistaxis (particularly nasal ethmoid fracture). It can also be combined with ESPAL in refractory epistaxis.

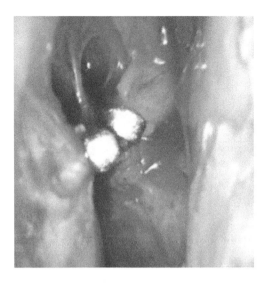

Figure 1.7 Haemostatic clips applied to spheno palatine artery during ESPAL.

ENDOSCOPIC SPHENOPALATINE ARTERY LIGATION (FIGURE 1.7)

1. Under general or local anaesthesia, prepare the nose with topical vasoconstrictor.
2. A rigid nasendoscope is used and an incision made approximately 1 cm anterior to the posterior end of the middle turbinate in the middle meatus.
3. The incision is onto the vertical plate of the palatine bone and a mucosal flap is elevated. An inferior/posterior uncinectomy and middle meatal antrostomy can be useful to identify the posterior wall of the maxillary sinus and identify where to raise the mucosal flap.
4. The crista ethmoidalis is identified as the flap is elevated. The flap tents at this point.
5. The sphenopalatine artery (SPA) is identified posterior to the crista ethmoidalis and the crista can be curetted to improve access.
6. The SPA is ligated using clips or coagulated using bipolar diathermy and then divided.
7. Once the SPA is divided, the dissection should be continued to identify any posterior branches, which should also be dealt with.

ANTERIOR ETHMOID ARTERY LIGATION

1. Make a gull-wing, medial canthal incision.
2. The incision is extended down through the periosteum and onto the bone.

3. Periosteal elevators are used to elevate the periosteum and the anterior lacrimal crest is identified. The orbital contents are retracted laterally as this plane is developed posteriorly. Once this plane is identified and opened broadly, an endoscope can be used to improve visualisation.
4. The dissection is continued posteriorly and the anterior ethmoid artery (AEA) is identified approximately 24 mm from the anterior lacrimal crest.
5. The AEA is clipped and divided.
6. Dissection can be continued to identify the posterior ethmoid artery approximately 12 mm behind the AEA. This can also be ligated and divided.

EMBOLISATION

Embolisation can be very effective for severe epistaxis and preoperatively for vascular tumours causing epistaxis (Figure 1.8). However, its usage

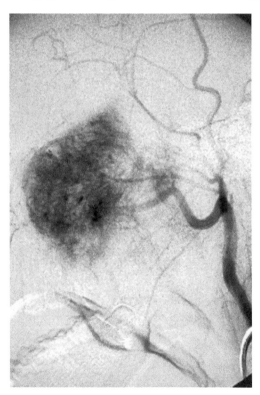

Figure 1.8 Angiogram of a juvenile angiofibroma demonstrating its blood supply from the internal maxillary artery, which can be embolised.

depends on the availability of an experienced interventional radiologist. This is indicated either after failure of ligation techniques or in patients who are deemed not suitable for surgery due to anaesthetic concerns. The bleeding point can be demonstrated using transfemoral angiography with subsequent embolisation of the maxillary or facial arteries with materials such as Gelfoam® or microcoils. Complications from embolisation are unusual, but are more common than following surgical ligation, and include facial skin necrosis, facial paraesthesia, cerebrovascular accident and groin haematoma. It is important that any BIPP packing is removed from the nose prior to embolisation, as the iodine will interfere with visualisation during angiography.

SECONDARY EPISTAXIS

Coagulopathies

Coagulopathies, including idiopathic thrombocytopaenia (ITP), disseminated intravascular coagulopathy (DIC), haemophilia and clotting factor deficiencies, pose a particular challenge. In these cases bleeding can arise from multiple sites and instrumentation can result in further mucosal trauma and exacerbate the bleeding. Therefore, indirect therapies may be indicated in preference to direct measures. Nasal packing and haemostatic compounds form the mainstay of treatment. Close communication with the haematology services is important to guide the use of clotting factor replacement and blood products.

Antiplatelets

Antiplatelet medications, such as aspirin or clopidogrel, are commonly used in the elderly population and can complicate epistaxis management. They have a prolonged effect on platelet function; therefore, there is little short-term benefit in stopping these agents. Local treatment with limited cautery can be attempted but is often ineffective, and nasal packing may be preferred. In uncontrolled, significant haemorrhage, platelet transfusions may be necessary.

Anticoagulants

Warfarin is used in the management of atrial fibrillation, venous thromboembolism and prosthetic heart valves. The therapeutic level can be measured using the International Normalised Ratio (INR). This group of patients can be challenging to manage as they are often older and have more comorbidities and their epistaxis can be difficult to control. They may present with an increased INR outside the therapeutic range. Whether the warfarin is stopped depends on the indication, the INR level, the severity of epistaxis and whether it is controlled with packing. If the INR is within the therapeutic range and the epistaxis is controlled with nasal packing, the warfarin can be continued at the normal dose. If the bleeding is controlled, with either direct or indirect management, but the INR is above the target range, warfarin should be omitted, the INR monitored and warfarin restarted once the INR is in the therapeutic range. If bleeding is controlled but the INR is very high (>8), or bleeding is not controlled, then vitamin K 0.5–2 mg IV (or 5 mg orally) should be considered. If, despite this bleeding continues, the haematology team should be contacted and factor VII, factor IX or fresh frozen plasma considered.

Newer anticoagulants, such as apixaban, rivaroxaban and dabigatran, are becoming more frequently used for stroke prevention in patients with atrial fibrillation. They have the advantage of rapid onset and short half-life and do not require routine monitoring. However, currently there are no antidotes available to reverse their effects, unlike the use of vitamin K with warfarin. This, therefore, makes managing significant epistaxis in these patients difficult. Close discussion with the haematologist is required and factor Xa (for apixaban, rivaroxaban) or tranexamic acid can be considered.

Septal perforation

Crusting and bleeding from a septal perforation can be troublesome and may be managed with topical chlorhexidine and neomycin cream (naseptin), followed by regular application of Vaseline. If bleeding continues, the bleeding point and granulation tissue, often at the posterior edge of the perforation, can be cauterised. In chronic bleeding a septal button can be inserted to allow re-epithelialisation of the margin or the perforation can be enlarged to remove bare/granular cartilage and re-epithelialise the margin with a local flap. Closure of the perforation is also an option, depending on the size and cause of the perforation.

Trauma

Epistaxis following trauma or surgery may require nasal packing, direct cautery or arterial ligation techniques. Anterior ethmoid artery ligation may sometimes be necessary when significant epistaxis has resulted from a nasal ethmoidal fracture.

Hereditary haemorrhagic telangectasia

Hereditary haemorrhagic telangectasia (HHT) is an autosomal dominant condition associated with recurrent bleeding from vascular anomalies. This results in the formation of telangectasia, arteriovenous malformations and aneurysms. Mild cases can be managed with topical emollients and oestrogens with interval laser/cautery of nasal telangectasia. In more severe cases other measures can be considered, including septodermoplasty, arterial ligation and arterial embolisation. Surgical closure of the nostrils (Young's procedure) is an option in the most severe cases. This can be effective in reducing the need for blood transfusions.

Tumours

Nasal tumours rarely present with isolated epistaxis, but blood-stained discharge in adults, along with unilateral obstruction, pain and swelling, raises the possibility of carcinoma. Juvenile nasopharyngeal angiofibroma (JNA) is a rare benign vascular tumour in adolescent males that can present with recurrent or severe epistaxis in association with nasal obstruction (Figure 1.9). In adults, benign (e.g. inverting papilloma, Figure 1.10) and malignant (e.g. squamous cell carcinoma) tumours can also cause epistaxis as well as unilateral nasal obstruction. It is important to examine the nose in epistaxis using a nasendoscope to ensure there is no underlying tumour.

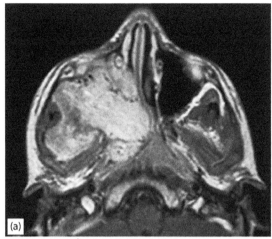
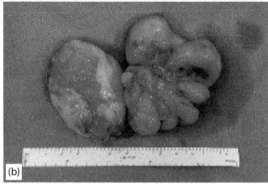

(a)

(b)

Figure 1.9 **(a)** MRI of a right-sided juvenile angiofibroma invading the infratemporal fossa. **(b)** The operative angiofibroma specimen.

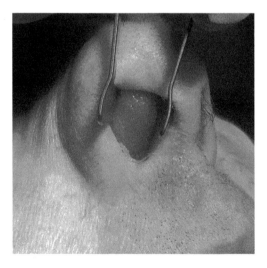

Figure 1.10 Inverting papilloma presenting in right nostril.

KEY LEARNING POINTS

- Epistaxis is a common ENT emergency that can be challenging to treat.
- Primary idiopathic epistaxis is ideally managed with direct therapy to the bleeding point.
- In refractory cases, surgery or embolisation may be required to control the bleeding.
- Endoscopic ligation of the sphenopalatine artery is successful in 90% of cases of posterior epistaxis and has a low complication rate.
- Management of secondary epistaxis requires treatment of the underlying cause and avoiding instrumentation of the nose as much as possible, as this can exacerbate the problem.

FURTHER READING

Ellinas A, Jervis P, Kenyon G, Flood LM. Endoscopic sphenopalatine artery ligation for acute idiopathic epistaxis. Do anatomical variation and a limited evidence base raise questions regarding its place in management? *J. Laryngol. Otol.* 2017 Apr;131(4):290–297.

Kunanandam T and Bingham B. Epistaxis in *Logan Turner's Diseases of the Nose, Throat and Ear: Head and Neck Surgery*, 11th Edition, 2016, Chapter 3, pp 23–29.

McGarry G. Epistaxis in *Scott-Brown's Otorhinolaryngology, Head and Neck Surgery*, 7th Edition, 2008, Vol 2, Chapter 126, pp 1596–1608.

Musgrave KM and Powell J. A systematic review of anti-thrombotic therapy in epistaxis. *Rhinology* 2016 Dec 1;54(4):292–391.

Spielmann PM, Barnes ML, White PS. Controversies in the specialist management of adult epistaxis: An evidence-based review. *Clin. Otolaryngol.* 2012, 37, 382–389.

2

Acute severe rhinological infection

WAI KEAT WONG AND SALIL NAIR

INTRODUCTION

Rhinosinusitis denotes an infection of the nasal cavities and paranasal sinuses. Infective agents such as viruses, bacteria and fungi are thought to play a direct role in causing acute rhinological infections. Acute rhinosinusitis is very common, and prevalence rates vary from 6–15%.

Fungal rhinosinusitis represents a heterogenous group of disorders where the spectrum of sinonasal manifestations is based on the patient's immune status. In immunosuppressed individuals, acute (fulminant) invasive fungal sinusitis has a high mortality rate and should be recognised early and treated aggressively. The lack of an effective neutrophilic host defence allows ubiquitous, opportunistic fungi to progress unchecked. Mucormycosis is a general term used to describe acute invasive fungal sinusitis caused by the class Zygomycetes, which includes *Mucor* and *Rhizopus*. Other potential opportunistic species include *Aspergillus*.

This should be differentiated from other severe manifestations of fungal infections such as chronic invasive fungal sinusitis and granulomatous invasive fungal sinusitis. The former is caused by *Aspergillus fumigatus* and classically has a chronic course and frequent association with immunosuppression. Importantly, vascular invasion by fungal elements and sparse inflammatory reaction is demonstrated histologically. Granulomatous invasive fungal sinusitis is common in North Africa and is caused by *Aspergillus flavus*. This infection is typified by histopathologic findings of non-caseating granuloma formation and fibrosis. Affected individuals are generally immunocompetent and usually present with proptosis.

Rhinoscleroma represents a chronic granulomatous condition of the nasal cavity and upper airway structures. It is transmitted by direct inhalation of droplets containing the pathogen. It starts in the vestibule of the nose (areas of epithelial transition). It is endemic to tropical regions of Africa and Asia as well as Central and South America. It tends to have a chronic and relapsing course.

Specific bacterial infection can involve the so-called 'danger triangle', which is essentially an area from the corners of the mouth to the nasal bridge. Infections include cellulitis or erysipelas affecting the face as well as vestibulitis. If left unchecked, infection in the 'danger triangle' can spread in a retrograde fashion along the facial venous system, resulting in cavernous sinus thrombosis, a condition associated with significant mortality.

Table 2.1 Potential causative organisms for rhinological infection

Pathogen category	Example
Virus	Rhinoviruses, coronaviruses, parainfluenza viruses, adenoviruses, influenza viruses, respiratory syncytial viruses
Bacteria	*Haemophilus influenza, Streptococcus pneumonia, Moraxella catarrhalis* and *Staphylococcus aureus*, anaerobes (odontogenic infections), *Klebsiella rhinoscleromatosis* (rhinoscleroma)
Fungi	*Mucoraceae* family (*Mucor, Rhizopus, Absidia*), *Aspergillus fumigatus, Aspergillus flavus Fusarium, Alternaria, Cryptococcus neoformans, Candida*

Table 2.1 lists the potential causative organisms for rhinological infection.

DIAGNOSIS

HISTORY AND EXAMINATION

A careful history will elicit complaints such as nasal congestion or obstruction, hyposmia, rhinorrhea and facial pain/pressure. A high fever (39°C) and a purulent nasal discharge or facial pain may help identify patients with acute bacterial rhinosinusitis.

'Red flags' such as severe headaches, change in mental status, periorbital or facial swelling and visual complaints are harbingers of a more serious pathology and require further investigations.

Anterior rhinoscopy is performed using a headlight and nasal speculum. However, the gold standard is an endoscopic examination. One should examine the middle meatus, inferior and middle turbinates, the nasal septum, lateral nasal wall and postnasal space. It is important to document inflamed, unhealthy or discoloured mucosa, the presence of mucopurulence and the absence or presence of polyps.

A more aggressive diagnostic approach is needed when assessing an immunosuppressed individual with sinonasal complaints. Immunocompromise may be as a result of leukaemia, bone marrow or solid organ transplant, diabetes mellitus or HIV. Patients with acute invasive fungal sinusitis tend to be very unwell, often with pyrexia of unknown origin, new-onset nasal congestion or discharge, severe headaches, facial numbness and altered mental status. The disease may rapidly progress over a matter of hours or days (Figure 2.1). Diplopia, decreased visual acuity or proptosis suggest orbital involvement. The presence of eschars on the nasal septum, turbinates or lateral nasal wall indicate active, advanced disease. Pale, insensate mucosa suggest tissue ischaemia. One should remember to examine the palate for signs of tissue necrosis, as the infection may spread to involve the oropharynx. A high index of suspicion for early diagnosis and prompt treatment is paramount. Figure 2.2 highlights the potential pathway of spread for acute invasive fungal sinusitis.

If left unchecked, acute invasive fungal sinusitis can invade the orbit and brain as well as cause carotid artery or cavernous sinus thrombosis,

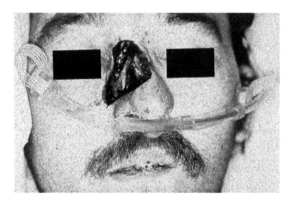

Figure 2.1 Mucormycosis in an immunosuppressed patient resulted in an erosive nasal cavity mass with nasal septal perforation, black necrotic crusts and gangrenous change. (From Wenig, BM (2016) *Atlas of Head and Neck Pathology*, 3rd Edition. Copyright © 2016 by Elsevier, Inc ISBN: 978-1-4557-3382-8.)

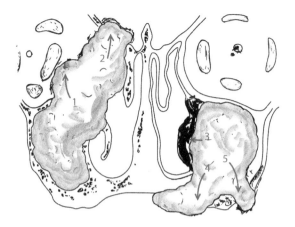

Figure 2.2 Illustration highlighting the different pathways of spread of acute invasive fungal sinusitis. (1) Orbital extension; (2) Intracranial extension; (3) Intranasal spread causing necrosis of turbinate and nasal mucosa; (4) Transpalatal spread; (5) Extension into soft tissue of face. (Illustrated by WK Wong.)

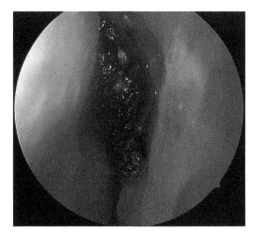

Figure 2.3 Endoscopic view of left middle turbinate demonstrating necrotic mucosa in a patient with acute invasive fungal sinusitis. (From Roxbury CR, Smith DF, Higgins TS et al. (2017) Complete surgical resection and short-term survival in acute invasive fungal rhinosinusitis. *Am J Rhinol Allergy* 31:109–116. doi:10.2500/ajra.2017.31.4420.)

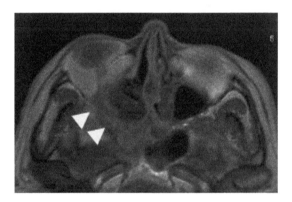

Figure 2.4 Axial T2-weighted MRI showing fungal invasion into the orbital apex (arrows) in a patient with progressive visual disturbance and a severe headache in the right temporal region. (From Takahashi H et al. (2011) Clinical features and outcomes of four patients with invasive fungal sinusitis. *Auris Nasus Larynx* 38(2):289–294. Copyright © 2010 Elsevier Ireland Ltd.)

cerebral infarction from fungal thrombosis of blood vessels and spread into the soft tissues of the pharynx and face. The spores invade the nasal mucosa and are not phagocytised as they would be in an immunocompetent individual. The spores germinate, forming angioinvasive hyphae that cause infarction of the involved tissue, resulting in a 'dry' gangrene appearance (Figure 2.3).

Patients with chronic invasive fungal sinusitis are often immunosuppressed from diabetes mellitus or prolonged treatment with steroids. Although it has an indolent course, it can be quite extensive at the time of presentation, occasionally with involvement of the cavernous sinus and cerebral infarcts. Typical symptoms include unilateral nasal obstruction and discoloured nasal discharge. Not uncommonly, it can manifest as orbital apex syndrome when the fungal mass has eroded into the orbital apex (Figure 2.4). Optic neuropathy presenting as diminished visual acuity, as well as ophthalmoplegia from multiple cranial nerves palsies, are the hallmarks of orbital apex syndrome.

Immunocompetency is generally preserved in patients with granulomatous invasive fungal sinusitis. Patients often present with a fever, nasal crusting and bleeding, headache, and altered mental status, as well as facial swelling and proptosis. The condition usually develops over months.

Orbital and intracranial complications from sinusitis carry significant morbidity and are covered in Chapter 6. Bony complications can complicate acute sinusitis, causing osteomyelitis. The frontal bones, and less commonly, the maxillary bones, are most likely to be affected. This can present as a Pott's puffy tumour when the anterior table of the frontal sinus is affected (Figure 2.5).

There are three distinct clinical phases with rhinoscleroma. The initial stage is characterized by nasal discharge and congestion. The discharge may be purulent and substantial crusting of the vestibule is observed. The proliferative phase is typified by a mass arising from the nose, often with involvement of the upper lip, palate and loss of maxillary dentition. Destruction of the nasal cartilage and epistaxis is sometimes observed (Figure 2.6). The disease has a slowly progressive clinical course (years). The granulation mass turns into fibrotic tissue which can obliterate the anterior nares.

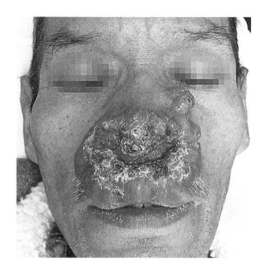

Figure 2.6 Rhinoscleroma. An otherwise well man with an extensive mass occupying the central region of his face and obliterating both anterior nares with upper lip extension. (From Castanedo Cázares JP, Martinez Rosales KI (2015) Rhinoscleroma. *N Engl J Med* 372:e33. doi:10.1056/NEJMicm1411602.)

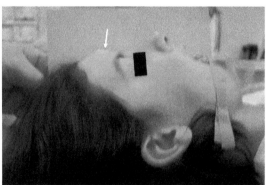

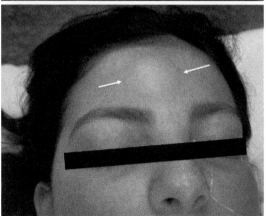

Figure 2.5 Pott's puffy tumour. A subperiosteal abscess (white arrows) associated with osteomyelitis secondary to acute frontal sinusitis. The spread of infection may be either direct or through haematogenic extension. This is obvious on the side profile but may be very subtle, only demonstrating a slight shiny swelling over the forehead. (Photos by S Nair.)

With central facial cellulitis, physical examination may reveal redness, tenderness and swelling in the affected area. Vestibulitis may sometimes develop into a localised abscess in the nasal vestibule. A patient with the above condition needs to be assessed promptly for potential cavernous sinus thrombosis if headache, visual symptoms or signs of raised intracranial pressure are reported. Apart from periorbital oedema and ptosis, signs such as ophthalmoplegia, mydriasis and altered sensation along V1 and V2 branches of the trigeminal nerve may be elicited.

INVESTIGATION

Diagnostic testing (sinus imaging or culture) is not routinely requested for uncomplicated sinusitis. Blind nasal swabs are generally unrepresentative and unreliable. Culture directed antibiotics are recommended in complicated rhinosinusitis. Specimens should be obtained under endoscopic guidance from the middle meatus. Sinus aspirate traps are another option, but are less readily available and generally less well tolerated.

Imaging is indicated when complications of rhinosinusitis are suspected. Multiplanar computed tomography (CT) scans without contrast are the workhorse for radiological assessment of the sinuses. However, in complicated sinusitis the use of contrast is essential, as this can help determine the patency of the dural and cavernous sinuses. In addition, it can help to assess the extent of disease and involvement of extrasinus structures such as the orbit and brain (Figure 2.7). In addition, CT imaging is mandatory if any surgery is contemplated, as it aids planning. CT scans may demonstrate pockets of air in the orbit and cranium, heightening the suspicion of direct involvement of these areas. In acute fungal sinusitis, bony destruction may range from subtle demineralization to extensive lytic changes.

Magnetic resonance imaging (MRI) is a useful adjunct and provides complementary soft tissue detail when extrasinus involvement or a sinonasal tumour is suspected, but lacks bony detail

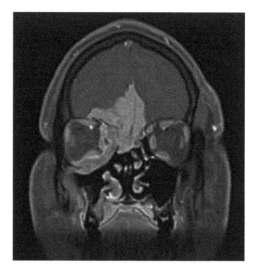

Figure 2.8 T1 coronal postgadolinium image showing displacement of orbital contents and intracranial spread in a patient with chronic granulomatous invasive fungal sinusitis. (From Halderman A, Shrestha R and Sindwani R (2014) Chronic granulomatous invasive fungal sinusitis: an evolving approach to management. *Int Forum Allergy Rhinol* 4:280–283.)

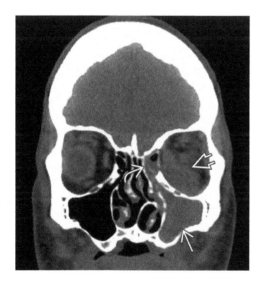

Figure 2.7 CT in a patient with diabetes, renal failure and orbital pain shows opacification of the left maxillary sinus (⇨) and ethmoid air cells (⇗) with extensive extra- and intraconal retroorbital soft tissue (⬗) encasing and displacing the medial and inferior rectus muscles. (From Koch BL, Hamilton BE, Hudgins PA, Harnsberger HR (2016) *Diagnostic Imaging: Head and Neck*, 3rd Edition, Chapter 225. ISBN: 978-0-323-44301-2. Inkling ISBN: 978-0-323-44315-9. Copyright © 2017 by Elsevier. All rights reserved.)

(Figure 2.8). It is also the preferred imaging for evaluation of infections involving the orbital apex. MR venogram may be useful if cavernous sinus thrombosis is suspected, because CT scans may miss up to 70% of cases of cavernous sinus thrombosis. Imaging characteristics of mucormycosis infection may initially be nonspecific, demonstrating a rim of soft-tissue thickness along the paranasal sinuses. On MR imaging, variable intensity within the sinuses on T1- and T2-weighted images is usually seen. Fungal elements usually cause a low signal intensity on T2 sequences. In acute fulminant disease, the affected tissue is prone to necrosis and devitalization, which in turn leads to a lack of enhancement seen on MR imaging – 'the black turbinate sign', a feature that it is thought may aid earlier detection of the disease (Figure 2.9).

If acute invasive fungal rhinosinusitis is suspected, affected tissue should be urgently biopsied and submitted fresh for immediate frozen section analysis, and a methenamine silver stain should be performed to confirm the diagnosis (Figure 2.10). Mucor and *Aspergillus* can be

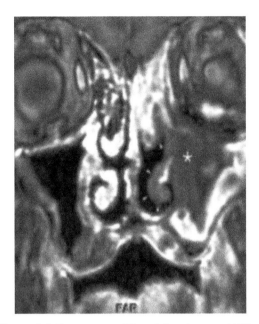

Figure 2.9 Postcontrast T1-weighted coronal MR image shows nonenhancing soft tissue, 'black turbinate sign', within the left maxillary sinus (asterisk). The mucosa of the inferior turbinate and a portion of the left middle turbinate demonstrate focal lack of the enhancement (arrowheads). (From Safder S, Carpenter JS, Roberts TD and Bailey N (2010) The 'black turbinate' sign: an early MR imaging finding of nasal mucormycosis. *Am J Neuroradiol* 31(4):771–774. doi:doi.org/10.3174/ajnr.A1808.)

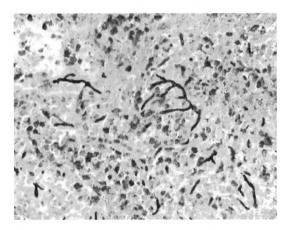

Figure 2.10 Grocott's methenamine silver stain showing a dense infiltrate of branching hyphae invasive into the surrounding tissues. (From D'Anza B, Stokken S, Greene HS, Kennedy T, Woodard TD, Sindwani R (2016) Chronic invasive fungal sinusitis: characterization and shift in management of a rare disease. *Intl Forum Allergy Rhinol* 6:1294–1300.)

Table 2.2 Microscopic characteristics of mucor and *Aspergillus*

Mucor	Aspergillus
Large, irregularly shaped nonseptate hyphae	Smaller hyphae that are septate
Branch at 90° angles	Branch at 45° angles

differentiated by certain characteristics, summarised in Table 2.2. The results, however, may not be available immediately and should not delay treatment. Histologically, tissue necrosis, vascular occlusion, haemorrhage and scant inflammatory response are frequently observed. Definite diagnosis is often difficult, ideally demonstrating deep tissue invasion on histology and positive fungal cultures.

The type of immunodeficiency influences the type of fungal sinusitis. *Fusarium* is often seen in neutropaenic patients, while *Aspergillus*, *Alternaria* and *Cryptococcus* are commonly seen in patients with cell-mediated immunodeficiency, such as in AIDS.

Other useful investigations include a full blood count and coagulation studies, as some patients may be thrombocytopaenic or coagulopathic from their comorbidities, and the risk of profuse bleeding following biopsy should be anticipated. Renal function tests and blood glucose levels need to be checked, as acute invasive fungal sinusitis can occur in renal failure and poorly controlled diabetics.

Aspergillus galactomannan antigen test is approved by the FDA and allows detection of *Aspergillus* cell wall antigen serologically. Reports indicate that it can be detected up to 14 days before acute invasive fungal sinusitis is clinically apparent. Hence, it may have a role in prolonged immunosuppressed individuals. Its use is not widespread, and it has a reported 10% false positive rate.

The diagnosis of rhinoscleroma is confirmed by demonstrating *Klebsiella rhinoscleromatis* in either blood or MacConkey agar. Histological identification of Mikulicz cells (macrophages with intracellular bacteria) is a cardinal feature of this condition (Figure 2.11).

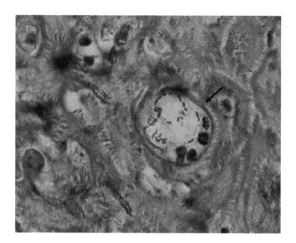

Figure 2.11 Mikulicz cells (arrow) with foamy cytoplasm and *Klebsiella rhinoscleromatis* (Warthin-Starry stain; x1000 original magnification). (From The Canadian Society of Otolaryngology Head and Neck Surgery, published by BC Decker in *Otolaryngol Head Neck Surg* April 2011 40(2):167–174.)

DIFFERENTIAL DIAGNOSIS

1. Autoimmune vasculitis, such as granulomatosis with polyangitis (GPA) and Churg-Strauss syndrome, or systemic granulomatous disorder, such as sarcoidosis.
2. Odontogenic infection – Infection spreading from dental sources, causing sinusitis, is a diagnostic consideration, especially when presented with unilateral sinonasal symptoms – usually maxillary sinusitis. Tooth pain may or may not be present. CT imaging may demonstrate an opaque maxillary sinus and a possible periapical lucency.
3. Sinonasal neoplasms – A complete discussion of sinonasal tumours is beyond the scope of this chapter. Dual modality imaging is recommended when investigating a suspected nasal tumour. MRI is useful to clarify whether changes seen on the CT are due to the underlying tumour or are inflammatory in origin. Inverting papilloma can cause secondary sinus obstruction, most commonly of the antrum.

MANAGEMENT

Acute invasive fungal sinusitis is a surgical emergency. The only contraindications to surgical management relate to the general condition of the patient or where extensive surgical debridement is likely to be futile. The management is generally multi-disciplinary and involves the ENT surgeon, intensivist and infectious disease specialist. With intraorbital and intracranial involvement, the ophthalmologist and neurosurgeon, respectively, should be consulted.

Apart from aggressive surgical debridement, patients would require high-dose antifungal therapy (amphotericin B, voriconazole, itraconazole) and correction of their immunosuppressed states. Diabetic patients would typically have ketoacidosis, which requires immediate treatment. Surgical debridement can usually be performed via an endoscopic approach. Exceptions included intracranial or orbital involvement, which may require a combined endoscopic and external craniotomy or orbital exenteration procedure. Prognosis is poor with intracranial extension.

Management of granulomatous invasive fungal sinusitis includes complete surgical removal of the fibrous fungal mass, which often extends into the orbit and intracranial spaces. Treatment with itraconazole (10 mg/kg/day) helps to prevent recurrence. Chronic invasive fungal sinusitis is managed with a combination of functional endoscopic sinus surgery and antifungal therapy. Surgery aims to remove the unhealthy diseased tissue and ventilate the sinuses.

The management of rhinoscleroma revolves around surgery and antibiotic therapy. Surgical excision is indicated for cicatrizing or obstructing nasal lesions. Third-generation cephalosporins or clindamycin are useful. Fibrotic lesions respond well to ciprofloxacin. Long-term treatment is needed to eradicate the infection.

In cavernous sinus thrombosis, apart from treating the infective cause with high-dose, broad-spectrum intravenous antibiotic, anticoagulants may be administered in certain cases, in consultation with the haematologists and infectious diseases teams.

KEY LEARNING POINTS

- Acute severe rhinological infections, although rare, carry significant morbidities and a high mortality rate.
- A heightened suspicion for acute invasive fungal sinusitis is required in patients with immunodeficiency.
- Investigation of severe rhinological infection involves several modalities, but CT and MR imaging are complementary.
- Underlying comorbidities, such as diabetes or renal failure, must be screened for and addressed.
- Surgery is needed for definitive diagnosis and debridement of affected tissue.
- Clinicians should have a high index of suspicion and act promptly, as early intervention is associated with a better prognosis.

FURTHER READING

Blackwell DL, Lucas JW, Clarke TC (2014) Summary health statistics for U.S. adults: National health interview survey, 2012. *Vital Health Stat* 10:1–161.

Chow AW, Benninger MS, Brook I, Brozek JL, Goldstein EJ, Hicks LA, Pankey GA, Seleznick M, Volturo G, Wald ER, File TM, Jr., Infectious Diseases Society of America (2012) IDSA clinical practice guideline for acute bacterial rhinosinusitis in children and adults. *Clin Infect Dis* 54:e72-e112. doi:10.1093/cid/cir1043.

Deshazo RD (2009) Syndromes of invasive fungal sinusitis. *Med Mycol* 47 Suppl 1:S309–314. doi:10.1080/13693780802213399.

Gallagher RM, Gross CW, Phillips CD (1998) Suppurative intracranial complications of sinusitis. *Laryngoscope* 108:1635–1642.

Herrmann BW, Forsen JW, Jr. (2004) Simultaneous intracranial and orbital complications of acute rhinosinusitis in children. *Int J Pediatr Otorhinolaryngol* 68:619–625. doi:10.1016/j.ijporl.2003.12.010.

Jones NS, Walker JL, Bassi S, Jones T, Punt J (2002) The intracranial complications of rhinosinusitis: Can they be prevented? *Laryngoscope* 112:59–63. doi:10.1097/00005537-200201000-00011.

Mukara BK, Munyarugamba P, Dazert S, Lohler J (2014) Rhinoscleroma: A case series report and review of the literature. *Eur Arch Otorhinolaryngol* 271:1851–1856. doi:10.1007/s00405-013-2649-z.

Puhakka T, Makela MJ, Alanen A, Kallio T, Korsoff L, Arstila P, Leinonen M, Pulkkinen M, Suonpaa J, Mertsola J, Ruuskanen O (1998) Sinusitis in the common cold. *J Allergy Clin Immunol* 102:403–408.

Safder S, Carpenter JS, Roberts TD, Bailey N (2010) The 'black turbinate' sign: An early MR imaging finding of nasal mucormycosis. *AJNR Am J Neuroradiol* 31:771–774. doi:10.3174/ajnr.A1808.

Yeh S, Foroozan R (2004) Orbital apex syndrome. *Curr Opin Ophthalmol* 15:490–498.

Zhong Q, Guo W, Chen X, Ni X, Fang J, Huang Z, Zhang S (2011) Rhinoscleroma: A retrospective study of pathologic and clinical features. *J Otolaryngol Head Neck Surg* 40:167–174.

3

Acute CSF rhinorrhoea

QUENTIN GARDINER

DEFINITION

Cerebrospinal fluid rhinorrhoea occurs when there is a communication between the nasal cavity and the intracranial space, usually the anterior fossa. For this to happen there must be a breach in the nasal mucosa *and* the bone of the skull base *and* the dura mater (except in the area of the cribriform plate where there is no dural layer). Occasionally, CSF comes from the middle or posterior fossa via the middle ear space and the Eustachian tube into the nose.

CAUSES

An acute leak may be spontaneous (often associated with idiopathic intracranial hypertension) or traumatic (either from accidents with associated head trauma, or iatrogenic during nasal or sinus surgery). Congenital, inflammatory and neoplastic processes may also cause CSF rhinorrhoea but generally do not present acutely.

SPONTANEOUS

With spontaneous leaks, the patient will usually complain of a unilateral, clear nasal discharge that may be intermittent and sometimes copious. They may have a salty taste when the leak is active. Occasionally an episode of meningitis occurs that triggers the search for an underlying cause. The leak is often from the lateral lamella of the cribriform plate (40%) (Figure 3.1), the frontal sinus (15%) or the sphenoid sinus (15%). It occurs more commonly in overweight women, as they appear to be more likely to have idiopathic intracranial hypertension, which is a causative factor. These leaks rarely resolve spontaneously.

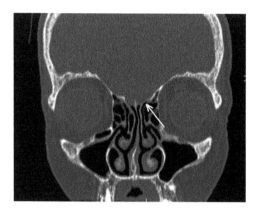

Figure 3.1 Lateral lamella of the cribriform plate.

HEAD TRAUMA

Cerebrospinal fluid rhinorrhoea in the acute phase after trauma has been reported in as many as 39% of patients with a skull base fracture (Figure 3.2). Most leaks start within 48 hours following trauma, and almost all will occur within three months of the injury. The majority (85%), however, will resolve spontaneously within seven days with conservative treatment such as bed rest or lumbar drain placement and will not require further surgical intervention. It is thought that nasal mucosal regrowth and fibrosis may facilitate leak

closure, as dura mater itself does not regenerate. Clearly the more severe the trauma and the larger the fracture, the less likely it will be to close spontaneously. Penetrating wounds and comminuted fractures also make spontaneous recovery less likely. Trauma to the area of the cribriform plate may be more problematic as the bone is fragile, and fractures may be more extensive. There is also no dural layer in this area to help prevent a breach; leaks here therefore tend to be more profuse and less likely to stop without intervention. The risk of meningitis is high in patients who continue to leak: there is a reported 30.6% risk of meningitis before surgical repair and a risk of 1.3% per day in the first 2 weeks after injury, 7.4% per week in the first month after injury, and a cumulative risk of 85% at 10-year follow-up in patients with ongoing CSF leak. The use of prophylactic antibiotics is usually discouraged, as they do not eradicate the bacteria in the upper respiratory tract and may lead to resistance. Any sign of infection, however, would necessitate their use. As an example, intravenous ceftriaxone and amoxicillin may be used, but this will depend upon local antibiotic policies.

IATROGENIC

Any surgery involving manipulation on or near the anterior skull base has the risk of causing a CSF leak (Figures 3.3 and 3.4). Even mobilisation

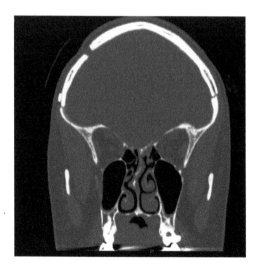

Figure 3.2 Fracture of the skull base at the left ethmoidal roof following trauma (note previous craniotomy for subdural haematoma evacuation).

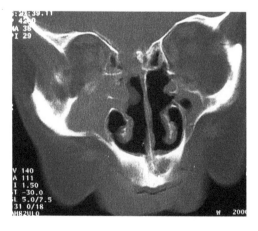

Figure 3.3 Coronal CT for CSF leak following nasal polyp removal with breach of the right cribriform plate.

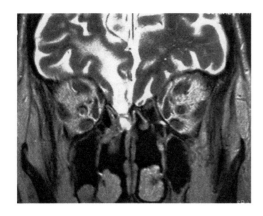

Figure 3.4 Coronal T2 weighted MRI of the same patient as in Figure 3.3 with right cribriform plate breach.

of the vomer or middle turbinate can cause a fracture of the cribriform plate. The risk of CSF leak during endoscopic sinus surgery (ESS) can be as high as 1%, and the surgical management of CSF leaks is an important element of competency for surgeons performing ESS. The areas where a leak is most likely to be caused are the lateral lamella of the cribriform plate (Figure 3.1) and the posterior ethmoid roof near the antero-medial sphenoid wall (Figure 3.5). Trauma to the lateral lamella occurs more commonly with inexperienced surgeons where it may not be obvious when operating how thin the bone is at this point. When operating lateral to the vertical attachment of the middle turbinate, the surgeon may feel the location is 'safe'

when it is not. The bone fractures easily and the lack of a dural layer means that CSF leak may occur with minimal trauma. Trauma to the posterior ethmoid roof is more common with experienced surgeons who are performing more extensive sinus surgery. The orientation of the skull base changes slightly in its most posterior aspect (Figure 3.5) and may lead to penetration.

DIAGNOSIS

The cornerstones for the definitive diagnosis of CSF rhinorrhoea are testing of the fluid for asialo-transferrin (β-transferrin) and high-resolution CT scanning of the skull base. T2-weighted MRI may also be useful if there is no clear bony defect (Figure 3.4) or if there is a suspected meningo- or encephalocoele (Figure 3.6).

Asialotransferrin is found abundantly in CSF but in minimal concentrations in nasal secretions and therefore has a reported sensitivity and specificity of up to 99% and 97%, respectively, in the diagnosis of CSF leak. It is confirmed by demonstrating the presence of the asialo band by electrophoresis and immunofixation. The test can be performed on a sample of 50 μl (two drops) collected in a plain, sterile container (white top) which should be kept cool and processed rapidly. A serum sample should also be sent (usually a yellow/gold

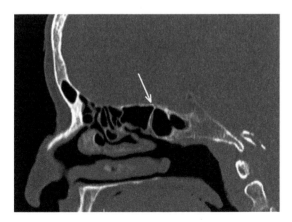

Figure 3.5 The change in slope of the posterior ethmoid roof where penetration may occur.

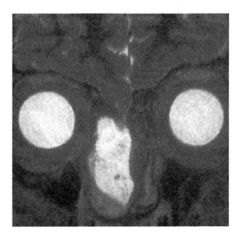

Figure 3.6 Coronal MRI showing an encephalocoele.

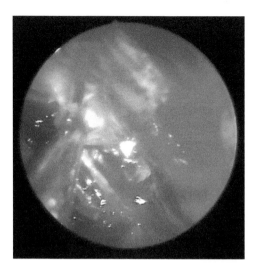

Figure 3.7 Fluorescein tracking from a leak in the posterior ethmoid roof.

top tube). Although the test is accurate, it usually takes several days to process and give a result.

CT scanning of the skull base may show direct evidence of a breach in the bone and allows an assessment of other injuries if the leak is traumatic. If the breach is small, it may not be directly visible, but fluid can sometimes be seen pooling within the sinuses nearby. MRI may allow better imaging of the soft tissue of the brain and meninges and will help delineate any prolapse of these through the skull base; it also shows fluid more clearly than CT.

When assessing spontaneous leaks, intrathecal injection of fluorescein may be useful to locate or confirm the defect (Figure 3.7); however, this is not generally used in the acute situation. If it is used, the patient should be consented and made aware that intrathecal injection is not a licensed use of fluorescein. As part of the work-up, a skin prick test using a drop of topical fluorescein (as used in ophthalmology) should be performed in case the patient has an allergy to the compound, and the patient should also be given IV chlorphenamine immediately prior to injection. It is important that the intrathecal injection is given prior to induction of anaesthesia in case a reaction occurs – if there is none, the patient may be anaesthetised and left head down for 30–60 minutes.

SPONTANEOUS

A patient presenting with a unilateral, clear nasal discharge should have a thorough endoscopic examination of the nose performed to see if the site of leak can be identified and to rule out other pathology. A sample of the fluid should be collected. The patient may need to take the sample container home with them, but if they do collect a sample this way, they must take it back to the hospital or their own doctor quickly, as the liquid degrades rapidly. In addition, a high-resolution CT of the sinuses and skull base should be requested to look for a bony defect. It is important to rule out a CSF leak because of the risk of meningitis. If the first test is negative for asialotransferrin, it should be repeated to ensure that a representative sample has been collected.

Many of the patients with a spontaneous leak have idiopathic intracranial hypertension. While the leak is active, the CSF pressure will be normal and there may be no signs or symptoms of raised intracranial pressure until the leak is closed. Severe headache or other signs of raised intracranial pressure post-operatively should prompt a neurosurgical referral, as these patients sometimes require a ventriculo-peritoneal shunt to normalise their intracranial pressure (and may require a shunt before closure of the leak can be achieved successfully).

Guidance with neuronavigation and intrathecal fluorescein are helpful in achieving closure, and most leaks in the area of the cribriform plate and sphenoid can be closed via an endonasal approach. Leaks into the frontal sinus may occasionally require an external approach to gain access.

HEAD TRAUMA

Patients with head trauma severe enough to cause a base of skull fracture may have other significant injuries that are immediately life-threatening, and the leak of CSF into the nose is not, of itself, a priority. It should be remembered, though, that there is a significant risk of meningitis when there is an active leak. CT scanning of the head is mandatory and may show the source of the leak. Eighty-five percent will cease spontaneously, so conservative management is appropriate unless contraindicated by symptoms. Some surgeons advocate lumbar drainage of CSF during this period, but this remains controversial. Antibiotics are not required unless meningitis is suspected. If the leak fails to stop within 7 days, surgical closure may be necessary using an endonasal, external or craniotomy approach, depending on the circumstances.

In some situations, such as open trauma, severe bony derangement and significant CSF discharge, urgent closure of the leak should be undertaken at the time of neurosurgical intervention.

IATROGENIC

If CSF is seen to be flowing during the procedure – often seen as a trickle of clear fluid in any blood or as a pulsatile clear discharge – the anaesthetist should be informed and the patient kept slightly head down on the table to prevent pneumocephalus. Repair should be undertaken at the time of surgery by the operating surgeon or by a colleague with specialist rhinology skills. If a leak is noted post-operatively, then a request for a CT scan of the sinuses and brain should be considered, as if a leak was not noted at surgery it is possible the surgeon may have caused more damage than a skull base breach alone. Small CSF leaks may close spontaneously and conservative management for a week is reasonable, with surgical closure if the leak persists. Antibiotics are not necessary unless the patient develops signs of meningitis.

SURGICAL APPROACHES FOR LEAK CLOSURE

ENDOSCOPIC

There are many methods of achieving closure of a leak, but the endonasal approach is successful in more than 95% of cases when chosen appropriately. Various grafts such as temporalis fascia, fascia lata,

nasal mucosa, septal cartilage, septal mucosal flaps, dural substitutes and many others are used. There are several glues that can also be used to hold grafts in position, including fibrin glue and other artificial substitutes. Techniques vary, placing the graft as an inlay (placed intracranially) and as an onlay (graft only on the nasal side of the defect), but the success rates of these procedures all seem similar. Lumbar drainage of CSF is advocated by some, but good results are achieved without it, and CSF diversion may cause complications.

EXTERNAL

External approaches may be required with more severe injuries – those that cannot be accessed endoscopically or with failure of the endoscopic technique. These include some fractures of the posterior wall of the frontal sinus (Figure 3.8), which can be approached through an osteoplastic flap, or transmastoid approaches to the tegmen and petrous temporal bone if the leak is into the middle ear.

INTRACRANIAL

Intracranial closure through a craniotomy approach may still be required in some cases but is now unusual. There is significant morbidity using this technique, with anosmia and epilepsy being just two possible complications.

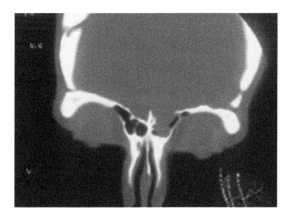

Figure 3.8 CSF leak through the posterior wall of the frontal sinus.

KEY LEARNING POINTS

- A clear, unilateral nasal discharge should be assumed to be CSF until proved otherwise.
- Asialotransferrin levels in the fluid from the nose and CT of the skull base are usually the most appropriate tests to request.
- Most traumatic CSF leaks resolve spontaneously within a week, but the patient is at risk of meningitis during this period.
- Iatrogenic leaks occurring during surgery should be repaired at the time they are noticed by the operating surgeon or a rhinology colleague.
- The endonasal approach has a high rate of successful closure and has few complications.

FURTHER READING

Marshall AH, Jones NS. Cerebrospinal fluid rhinorrhoea in *Scott-Brown's Otorhinolaryngology, Head and Neck Surgery*, 7th Edition. CRC Press; 2008, Vol 2, Chapter 129, pp 1636–1644.

Mirza S, Thaper A, McClelland L, Jones NS. Sinonasal cerebrospinal fluid leaks: Management of 97 patients over 10 years. *Laryngoscope*. 2005; 115(10): 1774–1777.

Prosser JD, Vender JR, Solares CA. Traumatic cerebrospinal fluid leaks. *Otolaryngol Clin N Am*. 2011; 44: 857–873.

Welch KC, Palmer JN. Intraoperative emergencies during endoscopic sinus surgery: CSF leak and orbital hematoma. *Otolaryngol Clin N Am*. 2008; 41: 581–596.

4

Management of acute nasal trauma

RICHARD GREEN AND PETER ROSS

INTRODUCTION

The nasal bones are a relatively brittle structure, with little force needed to cause a fracture (25–75 lb/in). Nasal trauma is most common in men aged 15–30 years, and is commonly seen as a result of assault, sports injuries and road traffic accidents. In cases of assault there may be police involvement or legal implications, this necessitates the attending clinician keeping a comprehensive medical record. Nasal skeletal injury is not normally limited to the external structures of the nose, as there is usually an associated septal deformity. Swelling and bruising becomes established rapidly, and this can make the accuracy of an early assessment difficult. Patients are encouraged to seek assessment within 48 hours to rule out a septal haematoma, and uncomplicated cases should be reviewed at 5–7 days after the injury. This will allow adequate assessment of any deformity once the swelling has subsided.

HISTORY AND EXAMINATION

REQUIRED HISTORY

The history begins with details of mechanism of injury. Though patient reports are often unreliable, it is important to assess the force and direction of the trauma to help predict the pattern and likelihood of other injuries. It is more common for fractures to be caused by a lateral force to the nasal pyramid. The nasal cartilages may act as a shock absorber to frontal injuries, to some extent. Detailing changes to the function of the nose

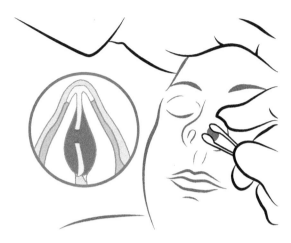

Figure 4.1 Diagram showing a septal haematoma during assessment of a nasal fracture.

(nasal airflow and sense of smell) is important. In most injuries there is an element of restriction of function due to oedema; however, functional asymmetry may point to a permanent structural change. Complete nasal obstruction should raise the level of suspicion of a septal haematoma (Figure 4.1).

Changes in appearance are commonly seen in nasal trauma. This can be difficult to assess given that significant swelling following the injury may still be present the first time the patient presents for assessment. Subsequent reviews may be necessary to allow an adequate evaluation to be made once the oedema has settled. Requests for pre-injury photographs of the face can help to assess any change, especially if this is not the first time the patient has had trauma to their nose. Change in vision (diplopia, epiphora, visual acuity) can indicate orbital involvement with or without a fracture, and this necessitates discussion/referral to ophthalmology or the maxillofacial surgeons. Assessment of the patient's teeth and bite and evidence of trismus may indicate mandibular injury.

Most nasal trauma patients will report epistaxis at the time of initial injury. If they have had ongoing issues with bleeding, further questions regarding the side, frequency and severity may indicate the need for admission and surgical management. If there is a history of watery rhinorrhoea or anosmia, this may indicate the presence of a skull base fracture.

EXAMINATION

There should be clear documentation of the following:

- Condition of skin
- External deformity
  - Bony alignment
  - Dorsal projection (dorsal hump or collapse of nasal profile)
  - Septal and cartilage alignment
  - Nasal length (significant loss of length is indicative of telescoping of the bony or cartilaginous fragments and increases the nasolabial angle)
  - Tip support

- Palpable fractures of the bones and cartilages of the nose (Figure 4.2)
- Integrity of orbital rim
- Internal
  - Septal alignment
  - Septal haematoma (present or not)

- Nasal function/air entry
- Eye movements
- Infraorbital nerve sensation

When recording the clinical findings with a nasal injury, to standardise the description, some clinicians will employ one of the two classification systems:

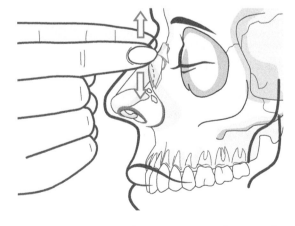

Figure 4.2 Diagram demonstrating palpation of the nasal fracture.

CLASSIFICATION

Extent of the deformity

0 - Straight nasal bones
1 - Bones deviated, displaced less than half the width of the nasal bridge
2 - Bones deviated, displaced half to one full width of the width of the nasal bridge
3 - Bones deviated, displaced more than one full width of the width of the nasal bridge
4 - Bones almost in contact with cheek

Patterns of nasal fractures

Class 1: A blow to the anterior nose, causing depression or displacement of the distal portion of the nasal bone. A fracture of the cartilaginous septum, running from the dorsum towards the bony septum, may also occur (Chevallet fracture) (Figure 4.3).

Class 2: Lateral trauma to the nose, resulting in lateral deviation of the bony nasal pyramid, and a horizontal or C-shaped fracture of the nasal septum (Figure 4.4).

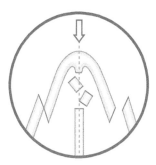

Figure 4.3 Diagram showing a class 1 nasal fracture.

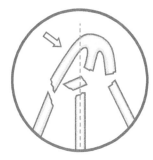

Figure 4.4 Diagram showing a class 2 nasal fracture.

Class 3: A high-energy injury to the nose, which leads to a complex fracture which extends into the ethmoid bone. The bony septum at the perpendicular plate of the ethmoid rotates backwards, taking the septum with it into the face. The nasal tip is also rotated upwards, giving greater show of the nostrils. There will be a saddle type deformity, and the nose will have a 'pig-like' appearance. Due to the disruption of the medial canthal ligament attachments, there may be telecanthus. This may be further complicated by dural tears, CSF leak and pneumocranium.

INVESTIGATION

In simple cases of nasal fracture, there is not normally any requirement for further investigation. Patients (or the police) will often ask if the nose is broken; this decision is a clinical one, and plain radiographs are *not used* to diagnose a simple nasal bone fracture. However, if there is concern of facial or skull fracture, plain radiographs will assist in identifying such fractures. CT scanning may be indicated in significant trauma, such as a class 3 fracture.

MANAGEMENT

A stepwise approach to management of nasal trauma is advised. As with all trauma, an ABC type of approach may be required if there is ongoing haemorrhage or evidence of significant airway compromise.

SOFT TISSUE

Wounds to the nose should be cleaned and closed at the first opportunity after the injury. Wounds should be closed appropriately, approximating the skin to its original location. Significant skin loss may require the use of flaps or grafting to close the defects, and if cartilage is visible, this should be discussed with the facial trauma team in the first instance. Tetanus immunisation status should be checked in open wounds. Swelling and bruising can be reduced with the use of ice.

THE NASAL BONES

Timing

Once assessment is made and deformity of the bones identified, there is a limited window of opportunity to manipulate the fracture to improve position. This is ideally 7–10 days post injury, but can be attempted at up to 3 weeks. Longer delays after the injury allow time for more callus to form, and there is less likelihood of successful manipulation. The narrow time window is more significant in children, where more rapid healing reduces the time available to manipulate fractures. Fractures can also be reduced immediately after the injury (within 1 hour), before the oedema has developed, and this approach is reasonable immediately following a sports injury, for example.

Many of the referrals with nasal trauma, once assessed, are often found not to have a nasal fracture and no further treatment is needed. Even in the event of a fracture, if the nasal bones are in a good position, i.e. not significantly displaced, and the patient is content, no treatment is the appropriate management. However, the patient should be made aware that once the period of the 'limited time window' is over, it will no longer be possible to perform a manipulation.

Anaesthesia

Either local anaesthesia or general anaesthesia is appropriate to assist with reduction of nasal fractures. There is conflicting evidence as to which method gives the best results. The choice is therefore determined by patient choice, service design and local expertise. Local anaesthetic can be injected into the dorsum of the nose, along the fracture sites, over the nasal bridge and to the infraorbital foramen to give a field block to the nose. Additional injection of local anaesthetic into the nasal septum is advised if Walsham's forceps are deemed necessary for the elevation of a depressed nasal bone fracture. Prior to injection it is best to apply topical local anaesthetic to the nasal cavities by spray or patties soaked in the chosen preparation.

Reduction techniques

Closed digital manipulation, with or without instruments, is the usual technique for reduction of nasal bone fractures. The first step is to disimpact the bones with force in the direction of the deviation, then to apply lateral force in the opposite direction to move the nasal bones to the midline. If there is infracture, or posterior displacement, a Walsham's forceps should be used to elevate the fragment. Following elevation, temporary packing under the previously depressed nasal bone may be required to maintain the position. External splinting or taping is advisable when the bones are very mobile and unstable following manipulation, as they are at risk from inadvertent displacement (Figures 4.5 and 4.6).

Open techniques are rarely necessary, but relative indications include:

- Infarction of the dorsum
- Profound fractures of the cartilaginous pyramid, with or without dislocation of the upper laterals

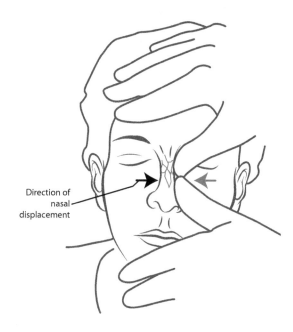

Direction of nasal displacement

Figure 4.5 Diagram demonstrating the digital manipulation of a nasal fracture.

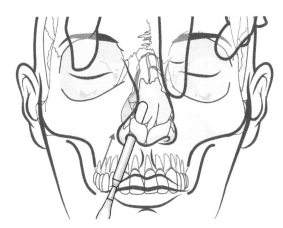

Figure 4.6 Diagram demonstrating the elevation of a depressed segment of nasal bone.

- Open fractures with significant bone or cartilage exposure or loss
- Bilateral fractures with dislocation of the dorsum and marked septal fracture and deformity

Care after the reduction

If absorbable packing has been used to support the fracture, then the patient will need to perform saline douching in order the help the pack dissolve over time. This tends to be started 48 hours after the reduction due to the discomfort in the initial post reduction period. If an external nasal splint has been used to support a mobile fracture, this will need to be removed in 7–10 days. The patient is given post reduction instructions to outline restrictions and aid healing. Patients should avoid activities that may result in further trauma for 6–8 weeks.

NASAL SEPTUM

Fifty percent of patients with a nasal fracture will have a septal fracture. Improvement of the septal deformity does not usually occur when managing acute nasal bone fractures. Digital manipulation or manipulation with Asch forceps may give the impression of improvement; however, the septum will usually return to its pre-intervention position, and septal manipulation is generally best avoided. The later assessment

of the septal deformity should be after about 6 months, once the swelling has resolved and healing is complete. At this stage it should be possible to determine if the septal deformity is significant and whether a septoplasty or septorhinoplasty may be required.

COMPLICATIONS

Poor result

Residual deformity is seen in 15–50% of cases. Factors contributing to this include the extent of the injury, time delay, septal fracture/dislocation, pre-existing deformity and postoperative trauma. Where appropriate, septorhinoplasty may be offered as a secondary procedure.

Epistaxis

Traumatic epistaxis usually settles once the tissue oedema is established and vessels tamponaded. However, patients who present with severe brisk bleeding episodes greater than 48 hours after a nasal fracture can prove challenging to manage and may require surgical intervention. As the bleeding is commonly from a fracture involving distal branches of the anterior ethmoidal artery, anterior ethmoidal artery ligation may be required.

CSF leak

A CSF leak may occur after nasal or facial trauma when the fracture involves the cribriform plate or the lateral lamella of the cribriform plate. These are the thinnest areas of the skull base, where the dura is very adherent to the bone and tears when the bone fractures. The most common presentation is unilateral watery rhinorrhea, which registers positive to Beta 2-transferrin (asialotransferrin) on testing. Beta 2-transferrin is a product of neuraminidase activity within the central nervous system, and is therefore only found within the CSF, perilymph and aqueous humor; it is therefore a highly sensitive test for the presence of CSF. The majority of traumatic CSF leaks resolve within 7–14 days with conservative management. This includes strict bed rest and elevation of the head, with avoidance of straining, retching or nose blowing. Antibiotics may mask meningitis, and discussion with the neurosurgeons is advised to check local policy. If the CSF leak does not settle, the location should be identified using high resolution CT scanning of the skull base, along with MRI if required. Endoscopic repair of the leak should be undertaken as soon as possible, as there is a significantly increased risk of meningitis (0.3–10% per year).

Septal haematoma

This is the presence of a haematoma under the perichondrium of the septum. The blood supply to the cartilage is disrupted when the perichondrium is elevated by bilateral haematoma. This will lead to ischaemia, and septal necrosis with perforation or septal collapse may ensue. Infection in the form of a septal abscess is within the danger area of the face and carries the risk of meningitis, brain abscess and cavernous sinus thrombosis. Care needs to be taken not to misdiagnose a septal haematoma as an anterior septal deformity. To differentiate, the area should be gently probed; a haematoma will be fluctuant and compressible, while a deviation of the septum will not. Aspiration will also confirm the presence of blood or pus.

Management involves drainage of the haematoma and securing the perichondrium back to the cartilage with quilting sutures, packing or nasal splinting. This can be achieved under local or general anaesthetic. The collection will often be too organised to aspirate and is best approached with formal incision and drainage. The patient will need to be reviewed 2–4 days after discharge to ensure that a reaccumulation has not occurred; if it has, this would require a further procedure (Figures 4.7 and 4.8).

Traumatic anosmia

The olfactory nerve fibres within the nose and cribriform plate may be damaged with nasal or head injuries. Up to 65% of patients with traumatic brain injury will have some form of olfactory disorder. This can be an indicator for the severity of

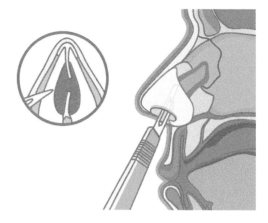

Figure 4.7 Diagrams demonstrating incision and drainage of a septal haematoma.

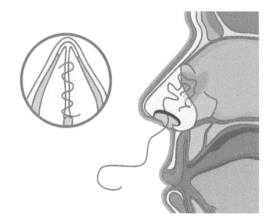

Figure 4.8 Diagrams demonstrating quilting suture to the perichondrium to prevent reaccumulation of haematoma.

the brain injury. This rarely fully recovers; assessment of the level of disability caused by the olfactory disorder and medical counselling/access to support are advised.

PAEDIATRIC NASAL FRACTURES

Nasal fractures in children are more difficult to diagnose and manage than in adults. The child's nose comprises a higher proportion of cartilage and is therefore more compliant.

There is reported to be a higher incidence of concurrent facial fractures in children. Nasal growth is mainly dependent on the septal cartilage growth centres, and trauma during early life risks damaging these growth centres, which are responsible for normal nasal development. In children under the age of 6 years, given the size of the nasal bones, fracture reduction is unlikely to result in a significant change unless there is gross deformity. Children are also more likely to undergo significant bone remodelling after trauma. Closed reduction of displaced fractures is considered safe, but secondary surgical techniques such as septorhinoplasty should be delayed until the nose is fully developed, i.e. normally around the age of 16.

If fracture reduction is deemed necessary, a closed technique under general anaesthetic is the preferred method of reduction. Open approaches are only occasionally used in severe trauma cases where open comminuted bony and cartilaginous fractures can't be reduced using closed techniques.

NASOORBITOETHMOIDAL (NOE) COMPLEX FRACTURES

Definition

These are fractures which involve the structures of the external nose and extend to involve the surrounding structures (orbits, frontals, ethmoids and skull base). They are important to identify, as simple nasal manipulation may not be the appropriate management and may worsen the situation, leading to epistaxis, CSF leak or orbital complications.

History and examination

NOE complex fractures are usually secondary to high-energy trauma (e.g. the face impacting a steering wheel in a road traffic accident). In such high-energy injuries, there should be a high index of suspicion for these complex fractures.

Classically, patients with fractures of the NOE complex are identified by the gross loss of nasal projection. The dorsal structures of the nose (upper laterals and nasal bones) are displaced inwards,

and the nasal tip is therefore rotated upwards. The nose will seem wide and flat. Other findings may include:

- Telecanthus from disruption to the medial canthal tendon, and lateral drift of the medial canthus. The normal intercanthal distance is approximately half the width of the interpupillary distance; an intercanthal width greater than this suggests a fracture. A distance of >35 mm is suggestive of a displaced fracture and >40 mm is considered diagnostic.
- Epiphora secondary to disruption of the lacrimal apparatus.
- CSF leak secondary to anterior skull base fracture, usually of the cribriform plate.

In patients with such findings, nasal endoscopy will help identify the internal injuries, and further investigation will be necessary.

Investigations

Plain film imaging is of little use for such injuries. Complex fractures may not be seen, and 3D imaging is required using CT initially, with 3D reconstructions (if available). This will inform the surgeon of the extent of the fractures and whether there are additional complications such as bony obstruction of the frontal sinuses. MRI may subsequently be required to investigate complications such as a CSF leak (Figure 4.9).

Management

Unlike simple nasal fractures, open surgery is usually required to reduce the fractures and try to restore the external nasal anatomy. Wide exposure with a bi-cornal incision is preferred, and miniplates are used to fix the fractures. Bone grafts may be needed if the fractures are highly comminuted and very unstable. In severe cases reconstruction of the medial orbital wall and nasal dorsum may be required; if a canthopexy is needed, this is usually performed with a transnasal wiring technique. Involving an ophthalmologist and a maxillofacial surgeon at an early stage is advisable. If there is bony obstruction of the

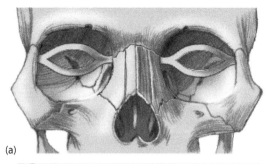

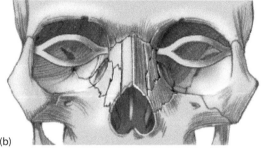

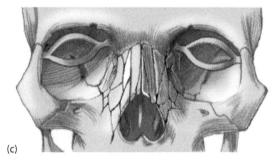

Figure 4.9 **(a)** Type I NOE fracture, single central fragment with the medial tendon attached. **(b)** Type II, comminution of the central fragment with the fracture external to the medial canthal tenton-bone insertion. **(c)** Type III comminution of the central fragment with the medial canthal tendon disrupted from its bony insertion. Image demonstrating the different classification of nasoorbitoethmoidal fractures.

drainage of the frontal sinuses, this may require planned management via either an open, endoscopic or combined approach. If there is damage to the nasolacrimal apparatus, advice from a lacrimal surgeon is best sought. They will advise whether lacrimal intubation and stenting will be needed. Management of CSF leaks, as mentioned on page 32, often settles with time.

KEY LEARNING POINTS

- The mechanism of injury may point to the type of fractures and whether other injuries have occurred.
- Early manipulation of nasal fractures (within an hour of injury) may be successful.
- The window to manipulate nasal fractures is 7–21 days; thereafter, the bones may have set.
- Cartilaginous nasal injuries tend not to respond to manipulation.
- Septal haematomas and other facial fractures should be excluded as part of the ENT assessment. Septal haematoma should be treated as a matter of urgency.
- Plain radiographs are not helpful in the assessment of nasal fractures and are not indicated unless other facial trauma is suspected.
- Traumatic epistaxis which persists may require surgical intervention (anterior ethmoid artery ligation +/– sphenopalatine artery ligation).

FURTHER READING

Basheeth N, Donnelly M, David S, Munish S. Acute nasal fracture management: A prospective study and literature review. *Laryngoscope.* 2015 Dec 1;125(12):2677–2684.

Cummings C, Haughey B, Thomas R. Cummings. *Otolaryngology-Head and Neck Surgery.* Elsevier Health Sciences; 2005.

Doerr TD. Evidence-based facial fracture management. *Facial Plastic Surgery Clinics of North America*. 2015 Aug 31;23(3): 335–345.

Gleeson MJ, Clarke RC, editors. *Scott-Brown's Otorhinolaryngology, Head and Neck Surgery*, 7th Edition: 3 volume set. CRC Press; 2008 Apr 25. Pages 1609–1617.

Papadopoulos H, Salib NK. Management of naso-orbital-ethmoidal fractures. *Oral and Maxillofacial Surgery Clinics of North America*. 2009 May 31;21(2):221–225.

Shibuya TY, Chen VY, Oh YS. Naso-orbito-ethmoid fracture management. *Operative Techniques in Otolaryngology-Head and Neck Surgery*. 2008;19(2):140–144.

5

Management of orbital injury and expanding orbital haematoma

BRIDGET HEMMANT AND CARL PHILPOTT

DEFINITION

Expanding orbital haematoma (or retrobulbar haemorrhage) is a rare, potentially sight-threatening complication which results from trauma to one of the orbital arteries – namely, the branches of the ophthalmic artery (anterior and posterior ethmoidal arteries) or orbital vein. Such an orbital injury can result from head trauma or can be iatrogenic (e.g. following injection into the orbit or surgery). Very rarely, it can occur spontaneously. Visual loss results either from central retinal artery occlusion, optic neuropathy from stretching of the optic nerve, or direct compression of the optic nerve venous drainage. As the haematoma expands within the confines of the bony orbit, the tense sheet of tissue that stretches across the anterior orbital opening – the orbital septum (Figures 5.1 and 5.2) – prevents the escape of blood. This leads to a rise in intraorbital pressure and visual loss. Prompt therapeutic intervention, including an emergency lateral canthotomy and cantholysis and/or orbital decompression, may restore vision.

CAUSES

Retrobulbar haemorrhage (RBH) can occur as a result of trauma, eyelid or orbital surgery, and other processes affecting the circulation within the orbit, such as arteriovenous malformations and lymphangiomas. The use of anticoagulant medication can increase the risk of RBH after relatively minor head trauma.

Although uncommon, there is an association between functional endoscopic sinus surgery (FESS) and orbital complications such as RBH, and if the orbit is inadvertently entered surgically, injury to other structures in the orbit can occur.

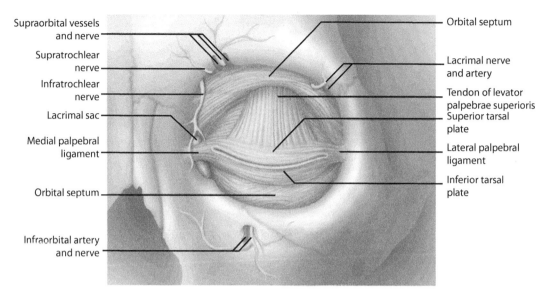

Figure 5.1 Anterior view of the orbit with orbital septum in place – dividing the anterior septal structures from the orbital contents.

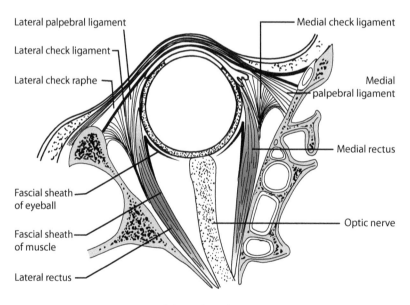

Figure 5.2 Anterior posterior cross section of the orbit, demonstrating the anatomy of the lateral canthal ligaments (lateral palpebral raphe, lateral check ligament and lateral palpebral ligament) attaching the orbital septum to the orbital rim.

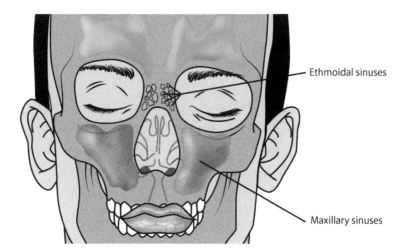

Figure 5.3 Demonstrates the anatomy of the orbit and the proximity of the ethmoid sinuses to the orbit – just separated by the thin lamina papyracae.

The other structures at risk from direct trauma are the optic nerve and the extraocular muscles, particularly the medial recti muscles. The rise in the popular use of microdebriders[1] has also seen a rise in debrider related injuries[2]; if the surgeon is not alert to the presence of peri-orbital fat in the field during FESS, then it can be very easy to quickly find both fat and muscle from the recti being removed by the debrider.[3–7] Damage to the optic nerve can lead to irreversible visual loss, and damage to the muscles can cause diplopia (double vision). There is also potential risk to the lacrimal drainage system during FESS surgery. This results in epiphora (watery eye); while this can transiently affect the vision, the tear duct obstruction can usually be corrected surgically with a dacryocystorhinostomy procedure (DCR) at a later date, should the watering not resolve (Figure 5.3).

SPONTANEOUS

With spontaneous retrobulbar haemorrhage (SRH), the patient will normally complain of a rapid acute onset proptosis (forward bulging of the globe), likely associated with some pain and loss of vision in the affected eye. There may also be an acute onset diplopia. If the haematoma is small, there may be mild optic neuropathy with a subtle change in the colour vision prior to any visual loss. SRH is more likely to occur in patients with pre-existing orbital vascular malformations, such as orbital lymphangioma, and arteriovenous malformations. Blood dyscrasias (e.g. sickle anaemia) are another rare cause of spontaneous RBH.

HEAD/FACIAL TRAUMA

Retrobulbar haemorrhage as a result of head or facial trauma may occur if there is trauma, either direct (via a penetrating orbital injury) or via a shearing action to the ophthalmic artery and/or the posterior and anterior ethmoidal arteries. The ethmoid arteries branch from the ophthalmic artery as it passes along the medial orbital wall at an angle of 90° and pass through fenestra in the lamina papyracae, placing them at risk from shearing forces. Patients on anti-coagulants are at greater risk from RBH, which can occur after relatively minor head trauma (Figure 5.4).

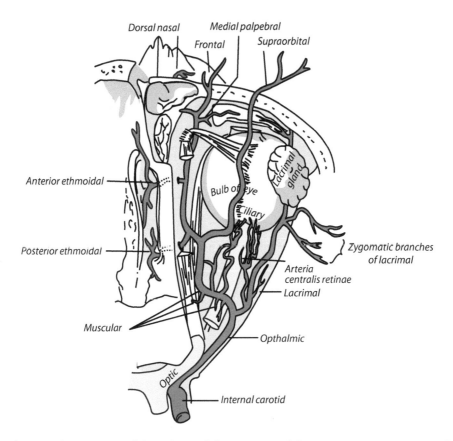

Figure 5.4 The vascular anatomy of the orbit and the passage of the anterior and posterior ethmoidal arteries through the lamina papyracae.

IATROGENIC

Any surgery (or injection) which encroaches on the orbit and its contents within the post-septal space (posterior to the orbital septum) has the risk of causing a retrobulbar haemorrhage. Retrobulbar injections were first introduced in the late nineteenth century and have commonly been given for cataract and other intraocular surgery (during the latter part of the twentieth century) with the attendant risk of RBH and trauma to the optic nerve. These injections were superseded by periorbital injections, and subsequently by topical anaesthesia, where there is no such risk. Surgery that penetrates the orbital septum anteriorly or the lamina papyracae medially carries the risk of damage to the orbital vessels. In ENT surgery and endoscopic sinus surgery, in particular, there is a risk that the thin lamina papyracae may be breached and the orbit entered. The risk of orbital injury

varies widely but is in the vicinity of 0.06–2.25%. The microdebrider is the instrument most likely to be associated with this type of surgical trauma. Pre-operative CT scans of the orbit and sinuses can aid the pre-operative plan by better visualisation of the ethmoidal anatomy. A pre-operative check of the scans should aim to identify the following areas for the risk of potential injury or complication[8]:

- Anterior and posterior ethmoid arteries – these can be seen in a coronal plane (Figure 5.5) and most often will lie within the skull base; however, in a minority of cases, the anterior ethmoid artery may lie within a bony 'mesentery' beneath the skull base, where it is at greater risk of injury from through-cutting instruments.
- Aerated posterior spheno-ethmoidal cells (Onodi cells) may lie alongside the optic nerve canal and may place a greater risk of injury

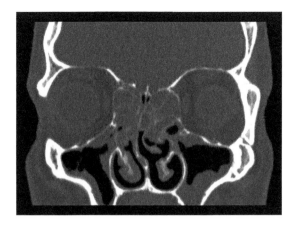

Figure 5.5 Showing the anterior ethmoid artery (also known as Kennedy's nipple) on a coronal CT scan slice and an infra-orbital ethmoid cell.

during ethmoidectomy/sphenoidotomy, especially if not recognised beforehand, as the bony covering of the nerve may be thin or even deficient (Figure 5.6). These anatomical variants are more common in some ethnic groups, e.g. South East Asians.

- Dehiscence of the lamina papryacea can be identified on coronal and axial CT sequences, and in cases of revision FESS, close attention should be paid to the possibility of this having occurred previously, especially where polyps are present in the ethmoidal areas.
- Hypoplasia of the maxillary sinus may affect the relative position of the lamina to the medial wall of the maxilla, with the possibility of the lamina lying more medial in the nose than the maxillary wall and leading the surgeon to believe they are entering the anterior ethmoids when in fact they are breaching the lamina.

- Infra-orbital ethmoid (Haller) cells are best identified on the coronal CT planes and should be identified if entry to the maxillary sinus and ethmoid infundibulum is anticipated during surgery (Figure 5.5).

DIAGNOSIS

Signs of a retrobulbar haemorrhage include peri-orbital swelling, bruising and oedema, conjunctival chemosis (fluid under the conjunctiva) and subconjunctival haemorrhage (Figure 5.7). The orbit may feel tense and there may be proptosis

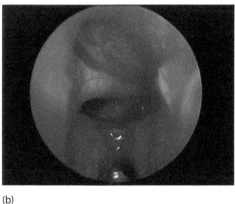

Figure 5.7 Clinical image of a patient's right eye with subconjunctival haemorrhage and chemosis.

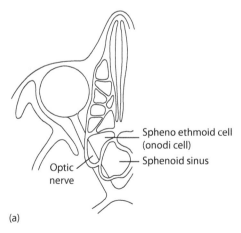

(a)

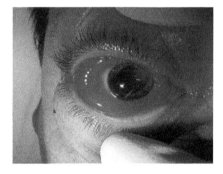

(b)

Spheno ethmoid cell (onodi cell)

Sphenoid sinus

Optic nerve

Figure 5.6 (a) Onodi cell. (b) Endoscopic view of optic nerve in Onodi cell.

(bulging forwards of the globe). Signs of optic nerve compromise include dilation of the pupil with a relative afferent pupillary defect (RAPD). If the patient is awake and cooperative, the visual function can be assessed further to check for optic neuropathy by assessing the colour vision and the visual field. Ocular motility can also be assessed to look for muscle restriction or weakness plus diplopia. During FESS it is advisable to keep the eyes uncovered to monitor them for any movement from traction on the orbital fat. Other indications of orbital penetration during the surgery are sudden swelling and bruising of the eyelids, conjunctival chemosis, subconjunctival haemorrhage and rapidly increasing proptosis. A more rapid onset follows an arterial bleed, which can result if a transected ethmoidal artery retracts into the orbit and continues to bleed. Injury to the optic nerve may be suspected if the pupil suddenly dilates during surgery or if, following surgery, there is visual loss and poorly reactive pupils with a relative afferent pupil defect. The dilation may be due to globe ischaemia or damage to the pupillomotor nerve fibres.

If an RBH is suspected, there is no time to order tests such as CT/MRI scans, as emergency treatment, either with a lateral canthotomy and cantholysis and/or with an orbital decompression, is required to drain the haematoma collection. However, if there is no RBH but direct damage to the optic nerve is suspected, an MRI of the orbit to visualise the soft tissues and bone is helpful with onward referral to an ophthalmic surgeon.

If there is diplopia following FESS surgery and there is a defect in the ocular motility that was not present prior to surgery, damage to the extraocular muscles should be assessed. Imaging with a CT or MRI can be helpful. If there is muscle or soft tissue entrapment in the orbital wall, this should be dealt with by an orbital surgeon before any strabismus surgery is considered. Patients may complain of epiphora following FESS surgery. This may be due to post-operative oedema in the area of the lacrimal drainage system, and this does often settle with reassurance and time. Radiology imaging may be helpful if the epiphora does not settle within 4–6 weeks.

MANAGEMENT

SPONTANEOUS

Whenever a retrobulbar haemorrhage is suspected, this is an ophthalmic emergency, and decompression of the orbit should be considered on an urgent basis. If there is a clotting disorder or blood dyscrasia clearly this needs to be addressed in addition to involvement of the haematology team. Depending on the optic nerve function, there may be time to consider an urgent radiology image (CT or MRI) to look for the source of the bleed.

HEAD/FACIAL TRAUMA

Patients with head and facial trauma significant enough to cause a retrobulbar haemorrhage may have other significant injuries that are immediately life-threatening. These need to be prioritised. There is, however, a significant risk of visual loss where there is an expanding orbital haematoma. If there is a rapidly progressive proptosis with visual loss and the history is suggestive of a retrobulbar haematoma, it may be necessary to perform an emergency lateral canthotomy and cantholysis, as delay can lead to permanent visual loss. If the diagnosis is less certain and where other injuries are suspected, then an urgent orbital CT or MRI should be performed. If an intraorbital foreign body is suspected, the nature of the material may dictate what type of imaging is ordered. This should be discussed with the radiologist. These patients should be referred to the ophthalmology department, preferably to a surgeon experienced in orbital surgery.

IATROGENIC

If a retrobulbar haemorrhage is suspected during a procedure, the surgery should cease immediately. If the haemorrhage occurs during FESS surgery, packing and suction should be removed from the site; the surgeon should not be tempted to continue to use the microdebrider to remove fat to 'decompress' the orbit. All ENT surgeons who undertake FESS should be familiar with the emergency procedure of lateral canthotomy and cantholysis, which can be practised in cadaveric sinus courses, but can also be observed in ophthalmology lists where entropion surgery is undertaken. Whilst the latter is an elective setting without the concern of a proptosing globe, it enables clear visualisation of the lateral canthal tendon that is superior to cadaveric specimens.

SURGICAL APPROACH FOR RETROBULBAR HAEMORRHAGE

Lateral canthotomy (Figures 5.8 and 5.9): A pair of sharp straight scissors are used to make a cut in the lateral canthal angle (canthotomy), and then the scissors are rotated 90° to cut through the lateral canthal tendon (lateral cantholysis) at its attachment to the bony orbital rim. The third cut is to cut deep to the skin, but through the orbital septum and conjunctiva below the tarsal plate in order to allow the haematoma to drain (Figure 5.9). In addition, the orbital pressure should be reduced. The patient should be given mannitol – 1 gm/kg IV over 30 minutes – plus acetazolamide – 500 mg IV. An urgent ophthalmology review should be arranged and an external (or endoscopic) orbital

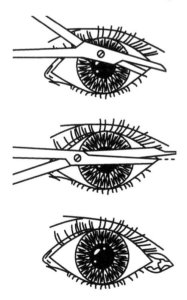

Figure 5.8 Lateral canthotomy to release the lateral canthal angle.

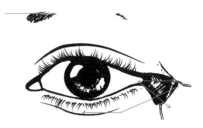

Figure 5.9 Diagram showing the incisions in blue to open the lateral canthal angle and to cut the lateral canthal tendon. The line in orange demonstrates the further incision – through the lid tissues posterior/deep to the skin below the lower border of the tarsal plate and through the orbital septum to release the septum and allow the haematoma to drain.

Table 5.1 Steps involved in managing a peroperative retrobulbar haemorrhage

Step	Management of retrobulbar haemorrhage in FES surgery
1	• Remove packing and suction at bleeding site if occurs during FESS
2	• Lateral canthotomy and cantholysis
3	• Mannitol – 1 gm/kg IV over 30 minutes
4	• Acetazolamide – 500 mg IV
5	• Urgent ophthalmology review
6	• Consider orbital decompression (externally or endoscopically)

decompression considered as the next immediate intervention, depending upon effectiveness of the canthotomy. As visual loss is the main risk with a retrobulbar haemorrhage, reducing the pressure in the orbit and allowing the haematoma to evacuate are the main concerns. Cosmesis is a secondary issue, as eyelid reconstruction is possible at a later date if required. Table 5.1 summaries these steps.

MANAGEMENT OF OTHER ORBITAL COMPLICATIONS OF IATROGENIC ORBITAL TRAUMA

FESS in inexperienced hands may be associated with RBH and with other complications, including direct trauma to the optic nerve, to the extraocular muscles and to the lacrimal drainage apparatus. If following FESS a patient complains of visual impairment, review by an ophthalmic surgeon is required. If direct damage to the optic nerve is suspected, an MRI of the orbit to visualise the soft tissues and bone is helpful.

If there is diplopia following FESS surgery, assessment by an ophthalmic surgeon is required. If there is a defect in the ocular motility that was not present prior to surgery, damage to the extraocular muscles should be considered. Imaging with a CT or MRI can be helpful. If there is muscle or soft tissue entrapment in the orbital wall or enophthalmos (sunken eye), this should be dealt with by an orbital surgeon before any strabismus surgery is considered.

Patients may complain of epiphora following FESS surgery. This may be due to post-operative oedema in the area of the lacrimal drainage system, and this does often settle with reassurance and time. Radiology imaging may be helpful if the epiphora does not settle within 4–6 weeks. If after 4–6 months the epiphora has not resolved and if there is a non-patent lacrimal drainage system, a lacrimal bypass procedure such as a dacryocystorhinostomy (DCR) can be considered.

- In an acute setting per-operatively (e.g. during FESS), surgery should immediately cease, and a lateral canthotomy and cantholysis should be performed and the haematoma encouraged to drain.
- Intravenous mannitol and acetazolamide should be administered to lower the orbital pressure osmotically.
- Emergency referral to ophthalmology should be made.
- The pupillary responses and vision should be monitored post canthotomy and a formal external orbital decompression considered.
- As visual loss is the main risk with a retrobulbar haemorrhage, reducing the pressure in the orbit and allowing the haematoma to evacuate are the main concerns. Cosmesis is secondary, with later reconstruction being possible if required.

KEY LEARNING POINTS

- Retrobulbar haemorrhage is an ophthalmic emergency. Visual loss is the main risk and may be permanent if timely treatment is not administered.
- FESS may be associated with orbital trauma, and RBH in particular, when the surgeon is inexperienced and is operating in the area of the ethmoid sinus.
- Progressive proptosis associated with periorbital bruising and swelling with a tense orbit should be assumed to be a retrobulbar haemorrhage until proven otherwise.

REFERENCES

1. Bruggers S, Sindwani R. Evolving trends in powered endoscopic sinus surgery. *Otolaryngol Clin North Am* 2009; 42(5): 789–98, viii.
2. Bhatti MT, Giannoni CM, Raynor E, Monshizadeh R, Levine LM. Ocular motility complications after endoscopic sinus surgery with powered cutting instruments. *Otolaryngol Head Neck Surg* 2001; 125(5): 501–9.
3. Demirayak B, Altintas O, Agir H, Alagoz S. Medial rectus muscle injuries after functional endoscopic sinus surgery. *Turk J Ophthalmol* 2015; 45(4): 175–8.
4. Huang CM, Meyer DR, Patrinely JR et al. Medial rectus muscle injuries associated with functional endoscopic sinus surgery: characterization and management. *Ophthal Plast Reconstr Surg* 2003; 19(1): 25–37.

5. Iieva K, Evens PA, Tassignon MJ, Salu P. Ophthalmic complications after functional endoscopic sinus surgery (FESS). *Bull Soc Belge Ophtalmol* 2008; (308): 9–13.

6. Martinez Del Pero M, Philpott C. A useful tool – systematic checklist for evaluating sinus scans. *Clin Otolaryngol* 2012; 37(1): 82–4.

7. Sohn JH, Hong SD, Kim JH et al. Extraocular muscle injury during endoscopic sinus surgery: a series of 10 cases at a single center. *Rhinology* 2014; 52(3): 238–45.

8. Thacker NM, Velez FG, Demer JL, Wang MB, Rosenbaum AL. Extraocular muscle damage associated with endoscopic sinus surgery: an ophthalmology perspective. *Am J Rhinol* 2005; 19(4): 400–5.

FURTHER READING

Alipanahi, Rakhshandeh; Sayyahmelli, Mirrahim; Sayyahmelli, Sima. Ocular complications of functional endoscopic sinus surgery. *JPMA. The Journal of the Pakistan Medical Association*; Jun 2011; vol. 61 (no. 6); p. 537–540.

Bhatti, M T; Schmalfuss, I M; Mancuso, A A. Orbital complications of functional endoscopic sinus surgery: MR and CT findings. *Clinical Radiology*; Aug 2005; vol. 60 (no. 8); p. 894–904.

Bleier, Benjamin S; Schlosser, Rodney J. Prevention and management of medial rectus injury. *Otolaryngologic Clinics of North America*; Aug 2010; vol. 43 (no. 4); p. 801–807.

Chu, Sau-Tung. Endoscopic sinus surgery under navigation system – analysis report of 79 cases. *Journal of the Chinese Medical Association: JCMA*; Nov 2006; vol. 69 (no. 11); p. 529–533.

Harkness, P; Brown, P; Fowler, S; Topham, J. A national audit of sinus surgery. Results of the Royal College of Surgeons of England comparative audit of ENT surgery. *Clinical Otolaryngology and Allied Sciences*; Apr 1997; vol. 22 (no. 2); p. 147–151.

Huang, Christine M; Meyer, Dale R; Patrinely, James R; Soparkar, Charles N S; Dailey, Roger A; Maus, Marlon; Rubin, Peter A D; Yeatts, R Patrick; Bersani, Thomas A; Karesh, James W; Harrison, Andrew R; Shovlin, Joseph P. Medial rectus muscle injuries associated with functional endoscopic sinus surgery: characterization and management. *Ophthalmic Plastic and Reconstructive Surgery*; Jan 2003; vol. 19 (no. 1); p. 25–37.

Jiang, Rong-San; Hsu, Chen-Yi. Revision functional endoscopic sinus surgery. *The Annals of Otology, Rhinology, and Laryngology*; Feb 2002; vol. 111 (no. 2); p. 155–159.

Krings, James G; Kallogjeri, Dorina; Wineland, Andre; Nepple, Kenneth G; Piccirillo, Jay F; Getz, Anne E. Complications of primary and revision functional endoscopic sinus surgery for chronic rhinosinusitis. *The Laryngoscope*; Apr 2014; vol. 124 (no. 4); p. 838–845.

Lee, Jonathan H; Sherris, David A; Moore, Eric J. Combined open septorhinoplasty and functional endoscopic sinus surgery. *Otolaryngology–Head and Neck Surgery: Official Journal of American Academy of Otolaryngology–Head and Neck Surgery*; Sep 2005; vol. 133 (no. 3); p. 436–440.

Lin, Xi; Lin, Chang; Zhang, Rong; Wu, Xihuang. Uncinectomy through the anterior nasal fontanelle in endoscopic sinus surgery. *The Journal of Craniofacial Surgery*; Nov 2011; vol. 22 (no. 6); p. 2220–2223.

McMains, K Christopher. Safety in endoscopic sinus surgery. *Current Opinion in Otolaryngology & Head and Neck Surgery*; Jun 2008; vol. 16 (no. 3); p. 247–251.

Mistry, S G; Strachan, D R; Loney, E L. Improving paranasal sinus computed tomography reporting prior to functional endoscopic sinus surgery – an ENT-UK panel perspective. *The Journal of Laryngology and Otology*; Oct 2016; vol. 130 (no. 10); p. 962–966.

O'Brien, William T; Hamelin, Stefan; Weitzel, Erik K. The preoperative sinus CT: avoiding a "CLOSE" call with surgical complications. *Radiology*; Oct 2016; vol. 281 (no. 1); p. 10–21.

Rodriguez, Michael J; Dave, Sandeep P; Astor, Frank C. Periorbital emphysema as a complication of functional endoscopic sinus surgery. *Ear, Nose, & Throat Journal*; Apr 2009; vol. 88 (no. 4); p. 888–889.

Suzuki, Sayaka; Yasunaga, Hideo; Matsui, Hiroki; Fushimi, Kiyohide; Kondo, Kenji; Yamasoba, Tatsuya. Complication rates after functional endoscopic sinus surgery: analysis of 50,734 Japanese patients. *The Laryngoscope*; Aug 2015; vol. 125 (no. 8); p. 1785–1791.

Tan, Bruce K; Chandra, Rakesh K. Postoperative prevention and treatment of complications after sinus surgery. *Otolaryngologic Clinics of North America*; Aug 2010; vol. 43 (no. 4); p. 769–779.

Trotter, W L; Kaw, P; Meyer, D R; Simon, J W. Treatment of subtotal medial rectus myectomy complicating functional endoscopic sinus surgery. *Journal of AAPOS: the Official Publication of the American Association for Pediatric Ophthalmology and Strabismus*; Aug 2000; vol. 4 (no. 4); p. 250–253.

Van Damme, D; Ingels, K; Van Cauwenberge, P. Per- and postoperative management of functional endoscopic sinus surgery. A questionnaire of otorhinolaryngologists in Flanders. *Acta oto-rhino-laryngologica Belgica*; 1998; vol. 52 (no. 3); p. 229–234.

Wolf, Jeffrey S; Malekzadeh, Sonya; Berry, Julie A; O'Malley, Bert W. Informed consent in functional endoscopic sinus surgery. *The Laryngoscope*; May 2002; vol. 112 (no. 5); p. 774–778.

6

Emergency management of the complications of infective sinusitis

ANDREW C SWIFT

INTRODUCTION

Infective sinusitis is a condition that many of us will have suffered from at some time in our lives during the course of a severe head cold. However, sometimes the infection may escalate to cause an acute complication. What is surprising is how quickly such events can occur. The rapidity of events reflects the pathogenicity of the infecting bacteria. However, these infections present infrequently and hands-on experience is not easily attained. Without an awareness of the serious nature of such an infection and the potential consequences, the outcome could become extremely poor and even lead to death.

The aim of this chapter is to highlight the key factors that need to be considered and to discuss the merits of the possible management options.

SPECIFIC COMPLICATIONS OF INFECTIVE SINUSITIS

The complications that we need to consider are those that affect the structures adjacent to the sinuses. These include the orbit, the intracranial cavity and the frontal bone. Occasionally, there may be a complication whereby infection occurs in more than one domain.

Complications of infective sinusitis occur in both children and adults, but children have always been much more prone to developing periorbital cellulitis.

The frontal sinus is probably the most frequent cause of complications, but infective purulent sinus infections typically include the ethmoid and maxillary sinuses as well.

Following an acute URTI, the sinus infection generally includes all or most of the paranasal

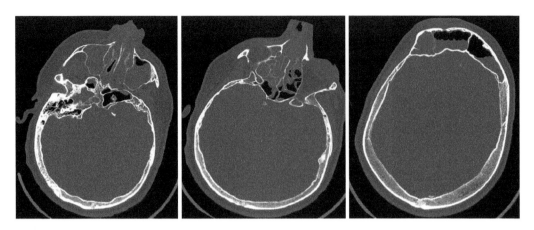

Figure 6.1 CT scan showing a patient with acute infective pan-sinusitis.

sinuses on both sides of the nose (Figure 6.1). In contrast, infection from a dental cause would usually affect the maxillary and ethmoid on one side only. Sinus infection is normally chronic, and complications are rare. However, occasionally infection can be severe, due to the combination of highly pathogenic aerobic and anaerobic bacteria, and serious intracranial and orbital complications leading to blindness have been described.

MICROBIOLOGY OF INFECTIVE SINUSITIS

The term 'infective sinusitis' in this context refers to bacterial purulent infection.

The infection may be polymicrobial but is more likely to be a single virulent bacterial species that is acting in a highly pathogenic way. Several bacterial species are capable of inducing such infection, but at the time of presentation, the organism will be unknown. However, upper respiratory aerobic bacteria such as *Streptococcus pneumoniae*, *Haemophilus influenzae*, *Moraxella catarrhalis*, *Streptococcus pyogenes* and *Staphylococcus aureus* are the most likely pathogens.

PREDISPOSING FACTORS

Most acute complications occur following a severe upper respiratory tract infection. However, this does not exclude patients with chronic rhinosinusitis as a complication of another condition such as an osteoma (Figure 6.2). The importance of the latter is very relevant when it comes to management of the patient once the acute infection has resolved.

As with all serious infection cases, predisposing conditions that affect the immune status should be considered. Relevant conditions include diabetes mellitus and recently administered systemic steroids. Immune deficiency and underlying haematological disorders are uncommon but should also be excluded.

In addition to these systemic disorders, there may be local sinus pathology, such as a mucocele, that predisposes to the development of a complication. A mucocele will cause expansion and thinning of bone over a period of time. When sited in the frontal sinus, it can cause dehiscence of the anterior and posterior bony walls of the sinus, and in the ethmoid sinus place the lamina papyracea is at risk. Mucoceles are prone to becoming infected and develop into a mucopyocele. Should the bony walls of a sinus be dehiscent, infection is more likely to spread (Figure 6.3).

Previous frontal trauma and comminuted skull fractures could also lead to susceptibility to purulent sinusitis, particularly if a head cold follows the injury.

PRINCIPLES OF EMERGENCY MANAGEMENT

Because of the potential for rapid progression of infection and pathogenic virulence, the principles of

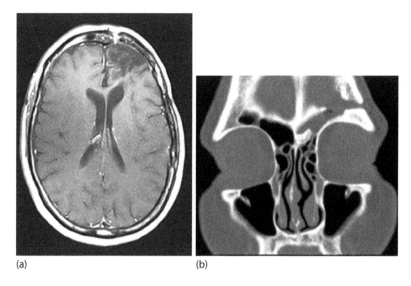

(a)   (b)

Figure 6.2 **(a)** MRI scan showing left frontal lobe scarring from a cerebral abscess secondary to acute frontal sinusitis. **(b)** CT scan 4 years later showing frontal osteoma blocking sinus drainage.

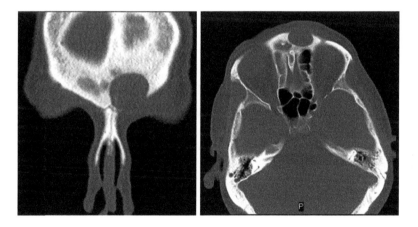

Figure 6.3 Dehiscence of the floor and anterior wall of left frontal sinus in a 25-year-old diabetic woman with pre-septal cellulitis and a mucopyocele. Note the soft tissue swelling.

management are to prevent progression of infection and the development of secondary complications.

All patients presenting with such complications should have regular assessment of their basic observations, including temperature, pulse and respiratory rate. Blood should be taken for culture as well as routine parameters such as full blood count, white cell count and renal function. Diabetes should be excluded.

IMAGING

Suitable and appropriate imaging should be considered. A multiplanar CT scan of the sinuses is likely to be required, but consideration should also be given to requesting simultaneous brain images with contrast. An MRI scan would be of value in any patient in whom infection is thought to have spread intracranially.

CULTURE AND SENSITIVITY

If pus is thought to be present within a sinus, the historical principle of early drainage should be strongly considered to prevent escalation of the infection and further complications. Any pus samples should be sent for culture and sensitivity. PCR (polymerase chain reaction) would facilitate rapid identification of pathogenic bacteria but is not generally available.

ANTIBIOTICS

Intravenous access should be established as soon as possible for both hydration and intravenous antibiotics. The antibiotic of choice should have a broad spectrum that will include the likely pathogens. Many hospitals will have an antibiotic policy for guidance, but discussion with a microbiologist is highly recommended. Antibiotic choice will vary between hospitals and is determined by expert microbiological opinion with regard to antibiotic resistance and prevention of antibiotic related complications.

ADDITIONAL MEDICAL THERAPY

Attention should be given to maintaining hydration, topical regular nasal decongestion to encourage drainage, adequate analgesia to optimise pain relief, and saline rinses to clear mucopus.

SURGICAL DRAINAGE

Surgical exploration should address the drainage of pus in all affected sinuses, and in frontal osteomyelitis, and other sinuses should be included in drainage procedures if the imaging investigations demonstrate they are also affected.

With the advent of widespread endoscopic sinus surgery and extended techniques to access the maxillary and frontal sinuses, consideration has to be given to the best surgical approach. This has led to a general reluctance to accept conventional drainage procedures such as antral washout and external approaches. However, the technique should be determined by the local expertise in sinus surgery, and the basic principle of adequate drainage of pus should be maintained.

It should be recognized that endoscopic surgery in an acutely inflamed, infected case is likely to be challenging and complicated by bleeding; if surgical expertise for an endoscopic approach is not available, then the safest option is to revert to an open approach. Any endoscopic surgery should proceed with extreme caution, and bony barriers of the orbit and skull base must not be breached. Consideration should also be given to combining endoscopic drainage with external drainage.

Open exploration is indicated in patients with a collection of pus over the forehead (Pott's puffy tumour). This may entail a frontal trephine via an incision hidden in the lower margin of the eyebrow(s) or an incision directly over abscess in a skin crease in the centre of the forehead. The latter affords excellent exposure to a bony defect in the anterior table and removal of necrotic bone. The scar should be well concealed with healing, but if bone necrosis occurs, this can leave a long-term depression in the forehead (Figure 6.4). Once pus has been cleared, it is helpful to leave a soft drain, such as a Penrose drain, in the frontal sinus to prevent recollection of pus (Figure 6.5).

With the advent of endoscopic surgery, external ethmoidectomy, particularly during the acute management of an infected patient, is not normally advocated, unless for some reason endoscopic equipment is not available.

The increased use of extended endoscopic surgery to access the frontal sinus endonasally may well facilitate draining an acutely infected frontal sinus. By identifying and enlarging the natural os, pus within the frontal sinus may be released or a mucopyocele opened and drained. Care must be

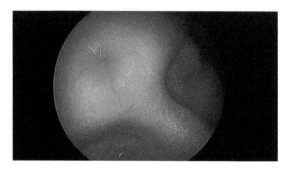

Figure 6.4 Frontal depression following acute frontal osteomyelitis and central bone necrosis.

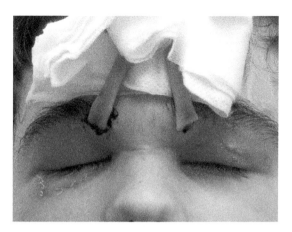

Figure 6.5 Penrose drains in a patient who had fronto-ethmoid fractures, subcutaneous pus, purulent sinusitis and a foreign body in the left frontal sinus.

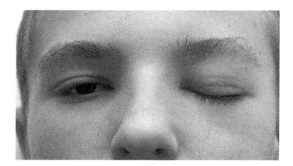

Figure 6.6 Periorbital cellulitis in a 10-year-old boy.

taken not to strip mucosa around the os and lead to stenosis and obstruction at a later date. However, if direct access via the os is not possible, then combining endoscopic surgery with external frontal sinus drainage may be the safest option.

SPECIFIC COMPLICATIONS

PERIORBITAL CELLULITIS

Periorbital cellulitis is a term used to encompass all infections within the orbit. The orbital septum is a fibrous sheet that effectively acts as a barrier to spread of infection, and infections are therefore categorised as pre-septal or post-septal. Infections included in the global term of periorbital cellulitis include pre-septal cellulitis, post-septal cellulitis, subperiosteal abscess and orbital abscess. Spread of infection into the orbit is either from the ethmoid or frontal sinuses, according to age, development and anatomy of the frontal sinus. Infection is often preceded by an upper respiratory infection, but underlying frontal or ethmoid sinus pathology may occasionally predispose to infection, especially in adults.

The condition is much more common in children, and most cases are pre-septal and may be unrelated to the sinuses[1] (Figure 6.6). As such, they often present to ophthalmologists and paediatricians, and are only referred to ENT surgeons in severe cases or when a subperiosteal abscess becomes evident.

Many hospitals now have agreed published guidelines on the management algorithm of periorbital cellulitis, and these will normally include advice on the choice of antibiotics.

The key factors to recognise in the clinical assessment are to determine whether the infection is pre- or post-septal, to identify a subperiosteal abscess and detect visual impairment at an early stage. Post-septal infection can cause proptosis, ophthalmoplegia and raised intraocular pressure. Visual acuity and colour vision should be assessed. The classification by Chandler is still widely quoted but does not necessarily reflect the severity of the condition[2] (see Table 6.1).

A subperiosteal abscess is most likely to affect the medial part of the orbit (Figure 6.7), but in older children and adults, it can occur in the superior aspect (Figure 6.8). This will cause proptosis and possible limitation of eye movement and should be clearly visible on MRI scan of the

Table 6.1 Chandler's classification of periorbital infection

	Group
I	Inflammatory oedema
II	Orbital cellulitis
III	Subperiosteal abscess
IV	Orbital abscess
V	Cavernous sinus thrombosis

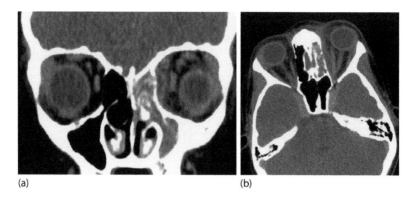

(a)   (b)

Figure 6.7 Coronal **(a)** and sagittal **(b)** CT scans showing a medial subperiosteal abscess in a 12-year-old boy.

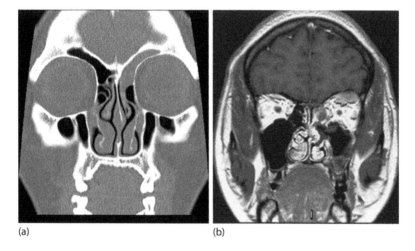

(a)   (b)

Figure 6.8 CT scan **(a)** and MRI scan **(b)** showing left-sided frontal sinusitis and a superior periorbital abscess in a 23-year-old woman.

sinuses (Figure 6.9). Subperiosteal abscesses are much more likely to occur in children than adults.[3] Again, it is important to emphasise that CT scans should include brain images to identify or exclude a concomitant intracranial complication.

The initial clinical management is to commence intravenous antibiotics as soon as possible and set up frequent monitoring of the eye, temperature, pulse and general well-being. Consideration should be given to seeking an ophthalmological opinion at an early stage.

Surgical intervention is indicated if there is a periosteal abscess, failure to improve or deterioration. Again, there is controversy about endoscopic versus conventional sinus surgery and external exploration and drainage should an abscess be present. The choice is determined by location and extent of the abscess, and the local surgical expertise. Whilst it may be possible to expose and remove the lamina papyracea to facilitate endoscopic drainage of a periosteal abscess, some abscesses will be multiloculated or extend above the orbit, making complete drainage more of a challenge. This is likely to be even more difficult in young children, particularly in the acute phase, when bleeding will be an issue. External drainage via a medial orbital incision and subperiosteal dissection should therefore be considered the safest

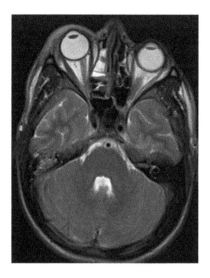

Figure 6.9 Sagittal T2 MRI scan showing right proptosis in a patient with a subperiosteal abscess and encephalitis.

option. Including a notch in the external incision will prevent late scar contracture and tenting, and careful attention to aesthetics with closure will minimise scarring. A transcaruncular incision offers an alternative approach to drainage of a subperiosteal abscess should there be a wish to avoid an external scar.

Clinically, it is important to determine if opacity in the medial orbit is subperiosteal cellulitis rather than an abscess before surgical exploration takes place. An abscess should display rim enhancement with contrast. However, if the abscess is small, this leads to a further clinical dilemma. Small abscesses will respond to therapy with intravenous antibiotics without the need for surgical intervention, providing certain criteria are observed.[4] Surgery is, however, much more likely to be necessary in children greater than 9 years old with orbital signs such as proptosis, limited ocular movement and elevated intraocular pressure.[5] The volume of the abscess, as assessed by CT, has been correlated to the need for surgery.[6] A volume of 3.8 mL was shown to be the ideal 'cut point' for the need for surgery. Should a small subperiosteal abscess be treated by antibiotics alone, it is imperative that close monitoring, with particular regard to vision, and monitoring by repeat scans take place.

OPTIC NEURITIS

Optic neuritis secondary to acute sinusitis is a rare event, but even so, knowledge of the potential association is helpful. Most cases of optic neuritis are in fact due to multiple sclerosis. Those cases associated with sinus disease may be due to an adjacent mucocele or mucopyocele or purulent acute sinusitis. The latter association may be predisposed by dehiscent bony barriers (Figure 6.10). The clinical signs suggesting optic neuritis include orbital pain, especially on eye movement, and blurring or loss of vision, especially centrally. The management should be multidisciplinary and should include ophthalmological advice, appropriate CT/MRI scans, microbiology and consideration for early decompression by sinus surgery.

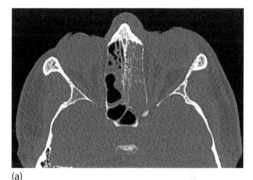

(a)

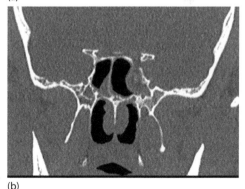

(b)

Figure 6.10 Left-sided acute sinusitis causing optic neuritis. Note the areas of dehiscence adjacent to the left optic nerve, in (a) axial view and in (b) coronal view.

FRONTAL BONE OSTEITIS AND SUBPERIOSTEAL ABSCESS/POTT'S PUFFY TUMOUR

Frontal bone osteitis is a complication of acute purulent frontal sinusitis. It presents with an acute onset of pain and swelling over the forehead, often after an upper respiratory infection. The swelling will be acutely tender and the overlying skin will be tense. It may be due to soft tissue cellulitis or a collection of frank pus according to the stage of presentation.

Intravenous antibiotics should be commenced as soon as possible after taking samples for blood culture. An urgent CT scan of sinuses and head with contrast should be obtained. This will often reveal a bony defect in the anterior wall of the frontal sinus, caused by bone necrosis (Figure 6.11). The scan will delineate which sinuses are affected, but in most cases, this will be a pan-sinusitis. The brain images will either confirm or exclude intracranial spread and avoid a delayed diagnosis of a more serious complication such as meningitis or an intracranial abscess.

The key clinical decisions are whether or not to manage the patient with intravenous antibiotics alone, whether to aspirate pus or whether to explore and drain the sinuses in theatre. These decisions will depend on clinical judgement for individual cases. Simple aspiration of a subcutaneous forehead collection or infected mucocele of the frontal sinus is tempting and may yield

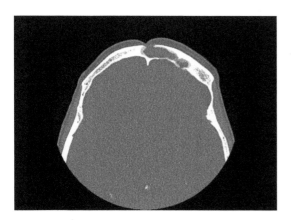

Figure 6.11 CT scan of the sinuses showing a bony dehiscence in a patient with frontal osteitis.

pus for culture, but risks inadequate clearance and rapid recurrence of the pus. Formal surgical drainage is therefore usually the best option recommended. If done at an early stage, recovery should be enhanced, and further complications should be prevented from developing (*vidra supra*).

INTRACRANIAL INFECTION

Intracranial infection from purulent sinusitis is a rare event, but it does occur, even with other complications, such as periorbital cellulitis and frontal osteomyelitis.[7] It should be considered and identified or excluded in all patients presenting with severe infective sinusitis. A delay in diagnosis could be life-threatening or lead to long-term disability.

Headache and general malaise will occur in all patients with acute infective sinusitis, but severe, incessant headache, vomiting and drowsiness are all suggestive of intracranial infection.

Infection can reach the intracranial cavity by direct spread through a breach in the bony sinus walls or by haematogenous spread. An infected frontal sinus is the most likely cause, but infection can also spread from the ethmoid sinuses.

Urgent MRI scans and CT scans with contrast and of the head should be obtained as soon as possible. The typical infective complications include an epidural abscess, subdural empyema, cerebral abscess and meningitis. The signs of intracranial infection can be subtle, and expert radiological advice is essential (Figure 6.12).

Intracranial infection due to infective sinusitis should be managed jointly with a neurosurgeon. Whilst the neurosurgeon will take the lead on the intracranial infection, he/she will look for guidance on the management of the sinus infection. The basic principle remains the same: that pus within the sinuses will need drainage. This will need to be coordinated with any neurosurgical intervention and, ideally, done under the same anaesthetic.

Broad-spectrum intravenous antibiotics are required and will be dictated by hospital policy and microbiological advice. Ceftriaxone and metronidazole are suitable, or vancomycin for MRSA infection.

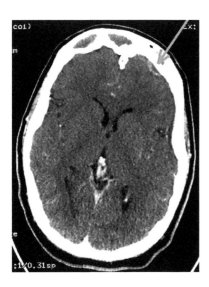

Figure 6.12 A subdural abscess in an 18-year-old patient with acute infective frontal sinusitis.

Cavernous sinus thrombosis

Cavernous sinus thrombosis is well known for its rapid onset, severe morbidity and risk of death but is fortunately very rare. It presents with swelling of both eyes in a seriously ill, pyrexial patient. The complication develops as septic thrombi pass along the afferent venous system to the cavernous sinuses. Infection typically originates from a furuncle in the mid-face, but it can also arise from sepsis of the ethmoid, maxillary and sphenoid sinuses.

MRI and CT brain with contrast should be obtained a soon as possible.

The principles of treatment include intravenous antibiotics with broad-spectrum cover and drainage of pus from the sinuses. Anticoagulants and fibrinolytics should be considered, but systemic steroids are generally not recommended.

Isolated acute sphenoiditis

Acute sphenoiditis is normally associated with pan-sinus infection. However, acute isolated sphenoiditis can occur, but is very rare. It is mentioned here because diagnosis is at risk of being delayed and the complications are serious. Providing a complication has not already occurred, it presents with headache in variable sites and facial and orbital pain.

Complications are due to spread of infection beyond the sphenoid sinus to include nearby intracranial structures and the orbit. These include the optic nerve and chiasm, cranial nerves (III, IV, V, VI), cavernous sinuses and pituitary gland. Complications include ophthalmoplegia, blindness, cranial nerve palsy, cerebral infarction, meningitis and intracranial infection.

Diagnosis relies on an early CT scan of the sinuses and treatment includes intravenous broad-spectrum antibiotics. Sphenoidectomy and drainage should be done should the patient fail to respond rapidly or should a complication have already occurred.

KEY LEARNING POINTS

- Complications of acute rhinosinusitis are uncommon but potentially serious.
- Acute sinus infection can rapidly escalate to lead to complications.
- The main complications are either orbital or intracranial, but remember that occasionally, both can occur together.
- Scans should ideally be obtained early in the course of events and should include settings for both sinuses and brain.
- The technique of surgical drainage is dependent on local expertise and philosophy, but the principle of draining pus effectively is of paramount importance.
- Consider early collaboration with neurosurgery and/or ophthalmology as deemed appropriate by the individual case.

REFERENCES

1. Upile NS, Munir N, Leong SC, Swift AC. Who should manage acute periorbital cellulitis in children? *International Journal of Pediatric Otorhinolaryngology*. 2012 Aug;76(8):1073–7.
2. Chandler JR, Langenbrunner DJ, Stevens ER. The pathogenesis of orbital complications in acute sinusitis. *Laryngoscope*. 1970; 80:1414–28.

3. Erikson BP, Lee WW. Orbital cellulitis and subperiosteal abscess: a 5-year outcomes analysis. *Orbit*. 2015 Jun;34(3):115–20.

4. Garcia GH, Harris GJ. Criteria for nonsurgical management of subperiosteal abscess of the orbit: analysis of outcomes 1988–1998. *Ophthalmology*. 2000 Aug;107(8):1454–6.

5. Smith JM, Bratton EM, DeWitt P, Davies BW, Hink EM, Durairaj VD. Predicting the need for surgical intervention in pediatric orbital cellulitis. *American Journal of Ophthalmology*. 2014 Aug;158(2):387–94.

6. Le TD, Liu ES, Adatia FA, Buncic JR, Blaser S. The effect of adding orbital computed tomography findings to the Chandler criteria for classifying pediatric orbital cellulitis in predicting which patients will require surgical intervention. *J AAPOS*. 2014 Jun;18(3):271–7.

7. Tandon S, Beasley N, Swift AC. Changing trends in intracranial abscesses secondary to ear and sinus disease. *Journal of Laryngology and Otology*. 2009; 123:283–8.

7

Nasal foreign bodies and rhinoliths

CATRIONA M DOUGLAS AND BRIAN BINGHAM

INTRODUCTION

It is common for young children to present to an accident and emergency department with an inserted foreign body inside the nose! It is estimated that this problem comprises 0.1% of paediatric accident and emergency visits. The peak childhood incidence is between 2 and 4 years, with the male to female ratio being equal. This young age is also the peak for otological and swallowed foreign bodies. Inserted nasal foreign bodies in adults are uncommon except in those patients with psychiatric disorders or very low intelligence.

Retained surgical foreign bodies can create significant medical and legal problems.

ANATOMY

Foreign bodies of the nose can be found in any area of the nasal cavity, but the most common sites of impaction are along the floor below the inferior turbinate or anterior to the middle turbinate. The nasal valve may be the narrowest part of the airway, but impacted foreign bodies in this area are easily removed before hospital attendance.

Table 7.1 Classification of nasal foreign bodies

Type of foreign body	Example
Inanimate	• solid (plastic beads, rubbers, pebbles, marbles, coins, broken needles) • soft (foam, lattice, cloth) • hygrophilic (vegetable matter, seed, popcorn)
Corrosive	Button battery
Animate	Fly maggot and screw worm

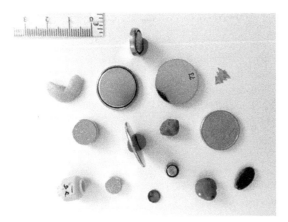

Figure 7.1 Different types and sizes of common nasal foreign bodies.

TYPES OF NASAL FOREIGN BODIES

Foreign bodies can be inanimate, animate or corrosive. Examples of nasal foreign bodies are listed in Table 7.1 and seen in Figure 7.1. Nasal foreign bodies can potentially cause a wide spectrum of damage, both locally and systemically.

INANIMATE OBJECTS

FIRM INANIMATE OBJECTS

Firm inanimate objects that are placed in the nose, such as beads, marbles, coins and pebbles, may

not cause harm to the patient while the object is in place. They may remain in the nose for years without causing mucosal abnormalities. However, if a patient presents with history of a foreign body insertion, then it is imperative to examine the nose and remove any object, if necessary.

SOFT INANIMATE OBJECTS/ HYGROPHILIC OBJECTS

Soft inanimate or hygrophilic objects made of foam, cloth or organic matter may be placed into the nose. These will absorb water from the surrounding tissue, causing swelling and an intense inflammatory reaction. Organic matter, particularly peanuts, often provokes a very brisk inflammatory reaction as it absorbs water and then starts to decompose. This local reaction in the nose causes retention of secretions and mucosal irritation. Bacterial invasion of this decomposing object will cause a foul odour. Such patients develop a unilateral vestibulitis and, in very rare circumstances, this bacterial laden foreign body may lead to toxic shock syndrome.

SURGICAL CONSUMABLES

The problem of retained surgical foreign bodies after surgery is a problem for the whole surgical team involved in the operation. The retention of a surgical object left in the nasal cavity has both potential medical and legal consequences; it is imperative, therefore, that systems are in place to ensure this risk is reduced. In nasal surgery, potential objects that could be retained after surgery include neurosurgical patties, sutures, internal nasal splints and nasal packing.

Good communication and completed documentation between the surgeon and the nursing team is essential to minimise risk. At the start of the operation a count of patties, temporary packing and sutures should be performed. The count is repeated when new additional items are added during the operation. A final count is undertaken before the surgeon completes the operation. It is mandatory practice that the scrub nurse informs the operating surgeon of any concerns regarding the count or informs that the 'count is correct'. If there is a concern about retained packing, then the surgeon must thoroughly inspect the nasal and sinus cavities. This may require the use of an endoscope. In the case of a broken needle, a surgeon should fully inspect the nasal cavity. Using an instrument, such as a small elevator, to 'stroke' soft tissue where a needle may be lost can help in identification. If, despite full nasal inspection and theatre staff checking all areas around the patient, there is still concern for a retained needle or surgical pattie, then an on-table x-ray should be undertaken. If, after the x-ray, there is no evidence of an intranasal foreign body, but there is still something missing on the count, then full documentation is required. Close observation of such a patient in the days and weeks after their surgery is important.

The operation notes and post-operative instructions must contain clear details about any intranasal splints or packing that are to be removed. It should be clear when, where and by whom any nasal splints or packing are to be removed. Dissolvable packing should be noted in the operative note. Most forms of nasal packing have the potential, albeit rarely, for a patient to develop toxic shock syndrome.

BUTTON BATTERIES

Inserted button batteries can, within hours, result in severe tissue damage in the nose. There are five types of batteries in common use, each with a different metal: manganese, mercury, silver, lithium and zinc. The most common design of button battery used is the alkaline variety. There are four different mechanisms of tissue injury that can arise from a button battery: direct electrical current effects on the nasal mucosa, producing mucosal burns; leakage of the battery contents, causing direct erosive damage; local toxic effect caused by absorption of battery substances (particularly mercuric oxide batteries); and, finally, pressure necrosis resulting from prolonged local pressure on the nasal tissue. When a burn injury occurs, it causes exudation of tissue fluids, creating a moist environment. In vitro studies have demonstrated that when alkaline batteries are exposed to moisture, spontaneous leakage of electrolyte solution occurs. This leaked alkaline solution penetrates deeply into surrounding tissue, causing a liquefying necrosis. The patient experiences extensive tissue damage, which can occur in a matter of hours.

It is important that a diagnosis of button battery impaction is reached quickly so that the object can be removed as soon as possible.

ANIMATE OBJECTS

Myiasis is a zoonotic infection, common in tropical climates and associated with low levels of hygiene. The most common infestation is from either the fly maggot or screw worm. In patients with animate nasal foreign bodies, the symptoms can be bilateral. There can be varying degrees of inflammatory reaction, from a mild localised infection to destruction of the nasal mucosa with necrosis of the septum and turbinates. Patients commonly present with nasal blockage, headaches, sneezing and a serosanguinous nasal discharge. On examination of the nasal cavity, there is usually extensive inflammation of the mucosa with contact bleeding. Constant motion of the worms is typically seen. These worms are firmly attached to the mucosa and difficult to extract. Due to the extent of local inflammation and bone destruction, produced by nasal infestation, secondary complications are not infrequent.

RHINOLITHS

A foreign body in the nose may act as a nidus for rhinolith development. Rhinoliths develop over many years. The foreign body, acting as a nidus, attracts and accumulates calcium, magnesium, iron and phosphorus salts around it. This calcified object grows with time.

Rhinoliths are more likely to present in an adult and are often asymptomatic. As they grow in size, a patient may present with unilateral nasal obstruction. The rhinolith nasal or paranasal sinus obstruction may cause mucus retention and a secondary inflammatory response. This may produce symptoms of headache, epistaxis and signs and symptoms of erosion into neighbouring structures, such as septal perforation. Surgical removal of the symptomatic rhinolith can usually be achieved with the aid of an endoscope.

Occasionally, a surgical drill is required to fragment a heavily calcified rhinolith.

HISTORY, SIGNS AND SYMPTOMS

The diagnosis of a foreign body in the nasal cavity can be difficult. A high index of suspicion is required.

Inanimate nasal foreign body – The child may be asymptomatic with a history of inserting a foreign body. The parent may have witnessed the insertion of the foreign body. Generally, inert nasal foreign bodies are painless. There have been case reports of inert nasal foreign bodies being present in the nasal cavity for years without causing any pain or problem.

Commonly, a child will present with a unilateral mucopurulent foul-smelling nasal discharge or a unilateral vestibulitis. This history is highly suggestive of a foam or cloth foreign body. Rarely, patients with a nasal foreign body can present with intermittent epistaxis and sneezing. Epistaxis, however, more commonly develops as the result of failed attempts at foreign body removal.

Animate nasal foreign body – In patients with animate nasal foreign bodies, symptoms are usually bilateral and include sneezing and serosanguinous discharge.

Button battery – A child may initially be asymptomatic, but very quickly they will develop pain, nasal obstruction and bloody discharge and potential signs of complication.

Rhinoliths – Patients are often asymptomatic when the rhinolith first develops. Symptoms of nasal obstruction may occur when the rhinolith enlarges.

INVESTIGATIONS

Any patient with a unilateral nasal discharge should raise concern about a retained nasal foreign body. In children with unilateral nasal discharge, a retained foreign body should be regarded as highly likely until proved otherwise. If the foreign object is easily seen on anterior rhinoscopy, then no further investigation is required. Endoscopic examination (usually flexible endoscopy) may be required if nothing is visualised on simple examination. Mucosal oedema or granulation tissue can make it difficult to see a foreign body. A vasoconstrictor or local anaesthetic solution can be helpful in those circumstances. Sometimes, however, where the index of suspicion is high, a general anaesthetic may be required to allow a thorough evaluation of the nasal cavity and to rule out the possibility of a retained foreign body.

If there is concern that a button battery has been inserted into the nasal cavity, but nothing is visible on anterior rhinoscopy, then an urgent plain film radiograph should be performed. Plain film radiographs have a low cost and are highly accurate at demonstrating a radio opaque object. Button batteries often have a very distinct appearance on a radiograph, as they have a bilaminar structure. This button battery bilaminar structure makes them appear to have a halo or double ring (double density) appearance on an anteroposterior view, with a step off at the separation between the cathode and anode on the lateral view. These features are seen in Figure 7.2. If the button battery is very small, these radiographic features may be hard to detect. If in doubt, a repeated radiographic view at a different angle may help achieve the diagnosis.

Coins, another common foreign body, can mimic the shape and size of a button battery, as shown in Figure 7.2. If a button battery is diagnosed as a coin on x-ray, then this could potentially delay the removal of the foreign object and increase local tissue damage. Coins do not have a

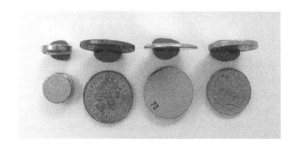

Figure 7.2 Button batteries and coins, demonstrating how a button battery could easily be mistaken for a coin on an x-ray.

'step off' on lateral view, and this fact highlights the benefit of obtaining two radiographic views in cases of doubt. If the nasal foreign body is a button battery, or could be a button battery, then urgent examination of the nose under general anaesthetic and removal of the foreign body is required.

If the history is suggestive of a rhinolith, then rigid endoscopic examination may be necessary. Examination of the nasal cavity will commonly show a grey irregular mass along the floor of the nose. This intranasal mass is very firm or hard on probing. If the examination is not conclusive and further evaluation is felt necessary, then a CT scan of the nasal cavity is recommended to assess the lesion.

MANAGEMENT

The greater the number of unsuccessful attempts at the removal of an intranasal foreign body, the greater the stress and trauma for patient, parents and hospital staff. Whoever undertakes the first removal procedure should be skilled in both intra-nasal procedures and managing children.

A cooperative patient is required in order to detect a foreign body and remove it with success. A child is best examined with their head tilting back slightly so that the ENT doctor is able to visualise the floor of the nose. Eversion of the nasal tip with a finger may be helpful. Careful thought should be given by the clinician before using a thudicums nasal retractor to open the nasal cavity of a child. The thudicums retractor can cause a young child great upset without a commensurate improvement in view! A young child may require to be swaddled in a blanket, with the head held steady. A paediatric nurse is very helpful in this circumstance. A good headlight is essential for the successful removal of a nasal foreign body. Fine suction, a range of blunt hooks, fine intranasal retrieval forceps and small artery clips (haemostats) should be available prior to the start of the examination.

MECHANICAL EXTRACTION

Some patients may require topical anaesthesia for pain control prior to removal of the foreign body.

Lidocaine applied topically, at a dose of 3 mg/kg, can be used and allowed 10 minutes to be effective. The routine use of a vasoconstrictor is not recom-mended. One side of the debate is the fact that the vasoconstrictor solution may reduce intranasal mucosal swelling and increase the chance of suc-cessful removal. On the other hand, there is a risk with mucosal vasoconstriction that a posteriorly placed foreign body will become loose and then dislodge into the airway, with the potential risk of aspiration.

Most inanimate foreign bodies in the nose, if seen easily, can be removed through the nostril using curved hooks, forceps, haemostats or suc-tion. Removal of spherical objects can be partic-ularly challenging due to the difficulty trying to grasp the object. A curved hook is best suited to attempting removal of a curved object. The hook is placed behind the object, with the object being advanced forward out through the nose. If the child becomes distressed, then there is a risk of marked epistaxis if the child moves while removal is attempted.

MOTHER'S KISS

In 1965, 'mother's kiss' was described by a New Jersey doctor, Vladimir Ctibor. The mother, or trusted adult, places her mouth over the child's open mouth while occluding the unaffected nos-tril. The adult blows until they feel resistance caused by closure of the child's glottis, at which point the adult gives a sharp exhalation to deliver a short puff of air into the child's mouth. This puff of air passes out through the non-occluded nostril and, if successful, causes expulsion of the foreign body from the nose. The technique has been shown to be successful in 60% of cases. A maximum of three attempts at this technique are recommended. There have been no reported adverse events using this technique.

GENERAL ANAESTHESIA

If a child becomes distressed at attempted removal of an intranasal foreign body, or it is not possible to remove the foreign body with the child awake, then a general anaesthetic may be necessary. In some circumstances, the only way to remove the foreign body is to push it posteriorly into the pharynx, and in that case endotracheal intubation or similar means of airway protection is required to prevent aspiration. If a button battery is present and attempted removal has failed, then the patient requires urgent general anaesthetic for removal. Button battery removal should not be delayed. Delay results in increased tissue damage and potential significant complication for the patient. It is important not to irrigate a nasal cavity that has had a button battery in place. Irrigation can spread the erosive alkaline content that may have leaked out from the battery. Use suction around the site of battery placement to aspirate any alkaline content.

If the patient has a rhinolith, then endoscopic removal under general anaesthetic may be required.

ANIMATE NASAL FOREIGN OBJECTS

If a patient is infested with intranasal screw worms or maggots, then a weak solution of 25% chloroform should be instilled into the nasal space to kill the larvae. This chloroform treatment may have to be repeated twice a week for about 6 weeks until all larvae are killed. After each treatment session, the patient blows their nose to expel the larvae. The larvae are aspirated out of the nose if the patient has required a general anaesthetic for the treatment.

After successful removal of the foreign object, careful examination of the nasal cavity is required to ensure no further foreign objects are present. If the patient has evidence of mucosal trauma as a result of the foreign body, then a course of antiseptic topical ointment is appropriate.

COMPLICATIONS

The complications that can arise from a nasal foreign body can be significant. The risk of complication is related to the time the foreign body has been present and the size, shape and nature of the foreign body. Epistaxis has been reported in around 6% of nasal foreign bodies and will most commonly occur with sharp or irregular objects. Unfortunately, epistaxis may occur when removal

of the foreign body is attempted, and it may be sensible to advise parents of this possibility.

The most serious complications arise from button batteries, particularly if their removal is delayed. Button batteries can cause nasal mucosal ulceration, nasal septal perforation and resultant saddle nose deformity. Other reported complications secondary to nasal foreign body include sinusitis, nasal septal perforation, periorbital cellulitis, meningitis and toxic shock syndrome.

One rare but potential complication from nasal foreign bodies is the risk of inhalation and lung aspiration. There have been cases of near fatal aspiration from a nasal foreign body dislodged while a child was being examined and foreign body removal attempted. Every clinician should consider the potential risk of inhalation with every nasal foreign body. A relative risk assessment should be taken for every case, considering age, nature of the foreign body and available clinical facilities.

KEY LEARNING POINTS

- Retained nasal foreign bodies are a common paediatric emergency.
- In patients presenting with unilateral nasal discharge, the presence of a foreign body must be excluded.
- Successful diagnosis requires a thorough and careful examination of the nasal cavity.
- Suspicion of the presence of a button battery foreign body necessitates urgent plane radiograph investigation.
- The confirmed presence of a button battery in the nasal cavity should be treated by urgent removal, without delay.

FURTHER READING

Brehmer D, Riemann R. The rhinolith – a possible differential diagnosis of a unilateral nasal obstruction. *Case Rep Med* 2010;2010: 845671. doi: 10.1155/2010/845671. Epub 2010 Jun 17.

Cook S, Burton M, Glasziou P. Efficacy and safety of the 'mother's kiss' technique: a systematic review of case reports and case series. *CMAJ* 2012;184(17):E904–12. doi: 10.1503/cmaj.111864. Epub 2012 Oct 15.

Dane S et al. A truly emergent problem: button battery in the nose. *Acad Emerg Med* 2000;7(2):204–6.

Endican S, Garap JP, Dubey SP. Ear, nose and throat foreign bodies in Melanesian children: an analysis of 1037 cases. *Int J Pediatr Otorhinolaryngol* 2006;70(9):1539–45. Epub 2006 May 16.

Kalan A, Tariq M. Foreign bodies in the nasal cavities: a comprehensive review of the aetiology, diagnostic pointers, and therapeutic measures. *Postgrad Med J* 2000;76:484–7.

Kiger JR, Brenkert TE, Losek JD. Nasal foreign body removal in children. *Pediatr Emerg Care* 2008;24(11):785–92.

Emergencies in Head and Neck

8

Head and neck infections

MUHAMMAD SHAKEEL AND AE LOUISE MCMURRAN

THROAT INFECTIONS

Common throat infections include:
1. Acute pharyngitis
2. Tonsillitis
3. Peritonsillar cellulitis
4. Peritonsillar abscess (Quinsy)
5. Glandular fever
6. Epiglottitis
7. Supraglottitis

ACUTE PHARYNGITIS

Acute pharyngitis refers to irritation/inflammation or infection of the pharynx and is commonly known as sore throat. Usually it is caused by viral infection but can also be a reflection of bacterial infection, most commonly by group A *Streptococci*. Other causes include allergy, trauma and toxins. Acute pharyngitis can occur as a part of a generalised upper respiratory tract infection or localised throat problem. On examination the posterior pharyngeal wall shows prominent lymphoid tissue along with generalised inflammation of the palate and tonsils with or without exudates (Figure 8.1). However, in the majority of the cases, the oropharynx has a normal appearance. Based on history and examination, it is difficult to distinguish between viral and bacterial causes of acute pharyngitis. However, few of these patients are referred for ENT assessment, as the condition is generally self-limiting with conservative management, including analgesia, fluids and rest. Oral antibiotic therapy may also be prescribed, though a recent Cochrane review shows that this shortens the duration of symptoms by only 16 hours compared to placebo, although the relatively small risk of associated complications is reduced.[1] Therefore, oral antibiotic therapy is not recommended for routine use in uncomplicated cases of acute pharyngitis.

ACUTE TONSILLITIS

Acute tonsillitis is an acute inflammation of the palatine tonsils commonly caused by group A beta-hemolytic *Streptococcus pyogenes*. Patients may present with sore throat, odynophagia, dysphagia, foul breath, tender cervical lymphadenopathy

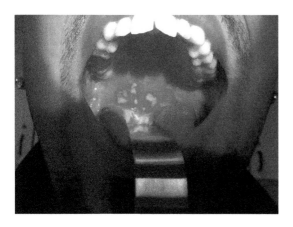

Figure 8.1 Sore throat secondary to fungal infection (Candida confirmed on throat swab).

and fever. On examination the patient may appear unwell, with fever, and has enlarged, inflamed tonsils with some exudates (Figure 8.2). The condition can be treated in the community with explanation, reassurance, improved oral hydration, regular adequate analgesia and oral antibiotics. If the patient is struggling at home with poor oral intake, then in-hospital treatment is required

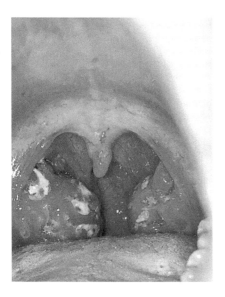

Figure 8.2 Acute bacterial tonsillitis. The tonsils are enlarged with infective exudates visible in the tonsillar crypts. The posterior pharyngeal wall shows inflamed lymphoid tissue (pharyngitis). Trismus is absent.

with intravenous hydration, analgesia and antibiotics. There is now some evidence of benefit from a single dose of steroid to ease pain in established cases. In general, antibiotics are indicated for all patients presenting to secondary care with sore throat symptoms.[2]

Complications from tonsillitis are rare, but there is some evidence that suppurative complications are increasing in incidence. Some have linked this trend to the rationalisation of routine antibiotic use in sore throat symptoms or the indications for tonsillectomy recommended in guidelines such as those produced by SIGN.[1,3,4] However, a recent prospective cohort study in a primary care population showed that roughly 1% of patients with sore throat developed suppurative complications regardless of whether they were given antibiotics, not given antibiotics or given delayed antibiotics.[5] In the same population of 14,610 patients, there were no non-suppurative complications.[5]

Non-suppurative complications of tonsillitis are extremely rare in the UK, and it is not considered necessary to provide antibiotic treatment in cases of sore throat to prevent these. Non-suppurative complications occur due to the effects of bacterial endotoxins and cross-reactive antibodies on other organ systems. For example, Scarlet fever may present with a rash, fever and widespread lymphadenopathy secondary to acute streptococcal tonsillitis and the bacterial endotoxins produced. The same endotoxins may affect the myocardium in rheumatic fever and the nephron in glomerulonephritis.

PERITONSILLAR CELLULITIS

Some patients present with marked symptoms of acute tonsillitis that may be worse on one side of the throat. They may have ipsilateral referred otalgia but usually have full mouth opening. On examination there is swelling of the tonsil and of the adjacent soft palate with marked redness (Figure 8.3). There is no fluctuation of the swelling on gentle palpation with tongue depressor, and no pus is found on needle aspiration. The patients are best managed with intravenous antibiotics, hydration, 2–3 doses of intravenous dexamethasone and adequate analgesia.

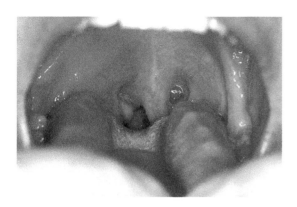

Figure 8.3 Right peritonsillar cellulitis. Note absence of trismus.

PERITONSILLAR ABSCESS (QUINSY)

Peritonsillar abscess is the collection of pus between the tonsil capsule and the superior pharyngeal constrictor muscle it lies upon. Peritonsillar abscess occurs in fewer than 2 in 1000 patients presenting with sore throat[6] but is a common reason for referral to ENT services. This complication usually presents unilaterally after acute tonsillitis, predominantly in adolescents and the young adult population.[7] However, there is some recent evidence to suggest peritonsillar abscess develops not from tonsil infection but from infection of minor salivary glands in that area.[8] Spread of infection to the peritonsillar area occurs due to highly functioning lymphatic drainage from the tonsil, and abscess formation may be preceded by peritonsillar cellulitis.[9]

The patients present with severe symptoms of acute tonsillitis but in addition may also have trismus, referred otlagia, drooling and 'hot potato' voice. They are often dehydrated, and on examination there is a bulge superior and lateral to the tonsil. The soft tissue swelling may be pointing and is the best area for needle aspiration or incision and drainage under local anaesthetic (Figure 8.4). Some centres have reported the use of 'hot tonsillectomy' for this patient group. However, as these infections generally settle with aspiration and IV antibiotic management, and because of the potential for increased post-tonsillectomy haemorrhage from the tonsil bed

secondary to the infection, this operation is not commonly performed in the UK.

After aspiration of pus, patients should stay in hospital for intravenous hydration, antibiotics, 2–3 doses of IV dexamethasone and adequate analgesia. Pus drained from a peritonsillar abscess may re-collect despite antibiotic therapy, and further aspiration or formal incision may be required. The resolution of trismus is a good indicator of improvement, at which stage the patient can continue with oral antibiotics and analgesia at home.

GLANDULAR FEVER

Epstein-Barr virus (EBV) causes acute pharyngitis as part of the infectious mononucleosis syndrome. Patients with glandular fever present with symptoms of acute bacterial tonsillitis but with a longer duration and often have marked lethargy. The clinical clues to the diagnosis of EBV infection include petechial haemorrhage of the palate, membranous exudate on the tonsils (Figure 8.5), extensive lymphadenopathy and slower resolution of clinical features with a relative lymphocytosis seen on full blood count. A monospot test on admission can confirm the presence of EBV infection. The treatment is largely supportive with adequate analgesia, hydration and corticosteroids. If added bacterial infection is evident, then antibiotics may be required, but it is important to avoid the use of beta-lactam antibiotics in these cases due to the known hypersensitivity reaction in this condition, which can cause an itchy maculopapular rash on extensor surfaces. The patient should be warned about the associated risk of hepatosplenomegaly and the need to avoid contact sports for 6 weeks to avoid splenic rupture.

EPIGLOTTITIS

Epiglottitis is an acute inflammation and oedema of the epiglottitis, generally caused by infection with Haemophilus influenza Type B (HIB). The incidence of this condition has decreased rapidly in the UK since the introduction in 1992 of the HIB vaccine to the vaccination schedule for children. In adults, the most common organism that causes acute epiglottitis is *Haemophilus influenzae* (25%),

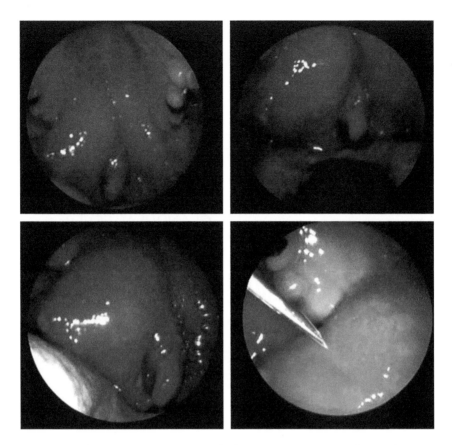

Figure 8.4 Right peritonsillar abscess (Quinsy). Marked trismus is present and therefore a zero degree rigid endoscope was used trans-orally for examination and further management.

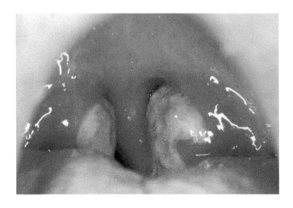

Figure 8.5 Symmetrically enlarged tonsils with thick exudates in glandular fever. The uvula is central and the soft palate appears normal.

followed by *H parainfluenzae*, *Streptococcus pneumoniae* and group A *Streptococci*. Noninfectious causes of epiglottitis include thermal damage, caustic ingestion, foreign body impaction and expulsion, and chemotherapy for head and neck cancer.[10]

Epiglottitis can cause a potentially life-threatening obstruction of the upper airway and presents with stridor, drooling and sepsis. The adults may also have symptoms of preceding upper respiratory infection and muffled voice. Children presenting with possible epiglottitis should be managed by an ENT surgeon and senior paediatric anaesthetist, with priority placed on securing the airway without causing distress to the child.

The management of this condition requires a careful systematic approach, avoiding any intervention that can cause agitation with resultant airway compromise. The patients need intravenous antibiotics, dexamethasone, hydration and adequate analgesia, along with humidified oxygen.

SUPRAGLOTTITIS

Supraglottitis is a generalised inflammation and oedema of the supraglottis that can lead to airway obstruction (Figure 8.6). This condition is generally seen in adults and may be of bacterial or viral in origin. Patients usually present with sore throat, fever, odynophagia and dysphagia and may have signs of developing airway obstruction including stridor.

Supraglottitis should be considered where a patient has symptoms in keeping with tonsillitis but relatively normal looking oropharynx with presence of anterior neck tenderness. These patients typically have markedly raised CRP along with high WBC count and neutrophilia.

Ensuring the airway is secure is crucial in supraglottitis, though unlike in children where it is imperative not to cause distress by examination, in adults it is generally safe to pass a flexible nasendoscope to assess the extent of supraglottic inflammation. Some patients will require discussion with the anaesthetic team and intubation, though most will settle with use of nebulised adrenaline, IV antibiotics (third-generation cephalosporins, with or without metronidazole), steroids and fluid.

NECK INFECTIONS

BACKGROUND

The neck infections are broadly discussed under the headings of superficial and deep infections (Figure 8.7). The superficial neck infections

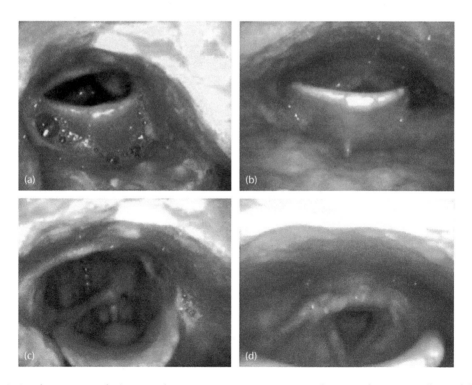

Figure 8.6 Awake transnasal pharyngolaryngoscopy in acute supraglottitis. There is swelling of the vallecula pushing the epiglottis posteriorly along with inflammatory secretions (a). The left hypopharynx including the left pyriform sinus, left aryepiglottic fold and left false cord are swollen (c). Complete resolution is evident in (b) and (d).

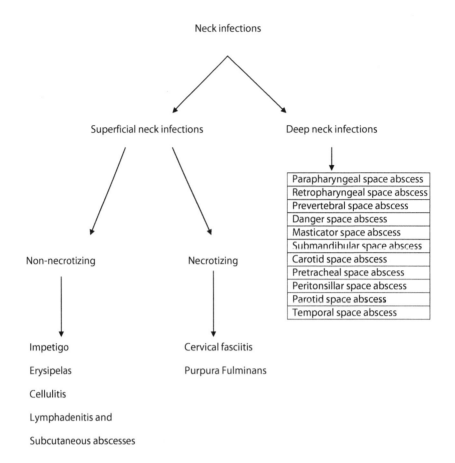

Figure 8.7 Flow chart of neck infections.

typically involve the skin and subcutaneous tissue, including the superficial fascia. These are further divided into non-necrotising and necrotising infections. The deep infections involve the deeper neck tissues, which are surrounded by multiple layers of fascia with potential spaces between them. It is crucial to have a clear idea of the deep cervical fascia and associated deep neck spaces to have a better understanding of the deep neck infections and abscesses.

LYMPHADENITIS AND SUBCUTANEOUS ABSCESSES

Superficial neck infections

Common examples of non-necrotising infections include impetigo, erysipelas, cellulitis, lymphadenitis and subcutaneous abscesses. It is

important to differentiate these from skin rashes and reactions.

Impetigo is a common superficial bacterial skin infection primarily caused by *Staphylococcus aureus* and is most frequently encountered in children. The lesions are mostly located in the head and neck region. There is good evidence that topical mupirocin and topical fusidic acid are equally, or more, effective than oral treatment. However, oral antibiotics may be required in patients with extensive impetigo.

Erysipelas and cellulitis are the most common skin and soft tissue infections requiring in-hospital treatment. Erysipelas is a superficial skin infection that does not involve the subcutaneous tissue. It has a typically raised, well demarcated and localised rash compared to cellulitis. Cellulitis involves both the dermis and the subcutaneous tissue. Clinically, it may be difficult to differentiate between these two conditions, and lately these are considered manifestations of the same condition. These are commonly caused by *Streptococci* and *Staphylococci* and are treated with antibiotics, but community-associated methicillin resistant *Staphylococcus aureus* is a growing problem. In diabetics and patients with suppressed immunity, a deep-seated infection should always be kept in the differential diagnosis of a superficial skin infection.

Non-tuberculous cervico-facial lymphadenitis is a relatively common condition in children and adults. The treatment options are varied – wait-and-see approach, medical therapy and surgical excision – and should be discussed with the patient and carers according to risks and benefits in each case. At times it is difficult to rule out superficial neck abscess, which is the second most common diagnosis after cellulitis in children. In children presenting to the emergency department with a neck infection, the factors predicting surgical drainage of an abscess included fluctuance, previous emergency department visit and age less than 4 years.[11]

Necrotising superficial neck infections

These include necrotising fasciitis and purpura fulminans. Both conditions have a high morbidity and mortality if not diagnosed and treated early.

Cervical necrotising fasciitis is a rare and rapidly progressive infection of the superficial fascia characterised by necrosis of the subcutaneous tissue. It has the potential to cause necrotising mediastinitis and can lead to progressive sepsis with toxic shock syndrome. Historically, group A beta-haemolytic *Streptococcus* has been identified as a major cause of this infection. However, these infections are now commonly found to be polymicrobial. Diagnosis should be made as soon as possible by looking at the skin inflammatory changes, and magnetic resonance imaging is carried out to detect the presence of air within the tissues. Percutaneous aspiration of the soft tissue infection followed by prompt Gram staining should be conducted. Intravenous antibiotic therapy and early surgical fasciotomy and debridement are required to treat this life-threatening skin infection. Non-operative

catheter drainage of cervical necrotising fasciitis has also been successfully employed. Hyperbaric oxygen therapy complemented by intravenous polyspecific immunoglobulin are useful adjunctive therapies.

Purpura fulminans is a rare syndrome of intravascular thrombosis and haemorrhagic infarction of the skin; it is rapidly progressive and accompanied by vascular collapse. Clinically it presents as septic shock, and the newest revolutionary advancement in the treatment of neonatal purpura fulminans is the use of activated protein C.

Deep neck infections

Deep neck infections (DNIs) involve the neck structures surrounded by multiple layers of the deep cervical fascia. The DNIs can result from the following processes: lymphatic system spreading the infection from the oral cavity, face and superficial neck compartment to deep neck spaces; cervical lymphadenopathy may lead to suppuration and localised abscess formation; and a penetrating trauma can introduce the infection in the deeper neck compartment. The infection spreads along the fascial planes and the resultant pus can expand the potential spaces between the different layers of the deep cervical fascia. The signs and symptoms of DNIs develop because of the mass effect of the inflamed tissues or abscess cavity on the surrounding structures and because of the direct involvement of the surrounding structures in the infectious process. The DNIs can happen in any age group but are historically associated with poor oral hygiene and lack of dental care. Depending upon the anatomical location, the DNIs can be named as listed in Table 8.1.

Clinical presentation

A high index of suspicion is required for early diagnosis of DNIs, as the patients may only have minimal symptoms and signs. However, some patients may present in distress and with life-threatening signs. Clinical features include fluctuant pyrexia, malaise, dehydration, sore throat, odynophagia, dysphagia, referred otalgia, drooling, respiratory distress, stridor, trismus, hoarseness, neck swelling, painful neck movements and

Table 8.1 Deep neck infections/abscesses[12]

Number	Name	Predictive descriptors on history and examination
1	Parapharyngeal space abscess	Anterior compartment infection/abscess causes: • Marked trismus; odynophagia and dysphagia • Induration at the angle of mandible • Medial displacement of the lateral pharyngeal wall and tonsil Posterior compartment infection/abscess causes: • Medial displacement of the posterior pillar of the tonsil and posterior pharyngeal wall • Thrombosis of internal jugular vein
2	Retropharyngeal space abscess	May present with airway occlusion at the pharynx level. Anterior displacement of one or both sides of the posterior pharyngeal wall. Torticollis and reduced neck movement. Asymmetry of neck and lymphadenopathy. Much more common in children under 5 years of age.
3	Prevertebral space abscess	Torticollis and reduced neck movement. Most common aetiology is iatrogenic trauma – instrumentation. Can cause vertebral osteomyelitis and spinal instability.
4	Danger space abscess	Extension of abscess from the mentioned three spaces. It can lead to mediastinitis, empyema and sepsis.
5	Masticator space abscess	Trismus. Originates from third mandibular molar infection. May spread to the parapharyngeal, parotid, or temporal space.
6	Submandibular space abscess	Ludwig angina refers to cellulitis or abscess in this space and may present with pain, trismus, drooling, odynophagia, dysphagia, neck swelling and worsening airway caused by displacement of tongue. Develops secondary to oral trauma, submaxillary or sublingual sialadenitis, or dental abscess of mandibular teeth. May spread to the parapharyngeal space or retropharyngeal space.
7	Carotid space abscess	Vocal cord paralysis Horner syndrome
8	Pretracheal space abscess	Dysphagia, odynophagia, pain, fever, hoarseness and airway obstruction. Mostly caused by perforation of the anterior oesophageal wall by endoscopic instrumentation, foreign bodies or trauma. Can involve the superior mediastinum.
9	Peritonsillar space abscess	Trismus, throat pain, referred otalgia, odynophagia, drooling, a 'hot potato' voice and fever. There is uvular deviation, palatal asymmetry and displacement of the tonsil medially. It may spread to the parapharyngeal space. It is the most common deep neck space abscess and represents a sequela of tonsillar infections.
10	Parotid space abscess	Pain, oedema and erythema in the region of the parotid. Trismus is a later finding. Risk factors include dehydration and elderly patients with poor oral hygiene who develop salivary duct obstruction. Can spread to parapharyngeal space.
11	Temporal space abscess	Pain and trismus with or without deviation of the mandible.

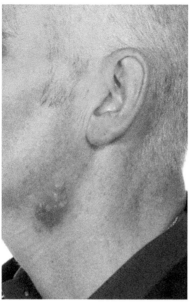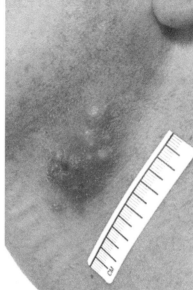

Figure 8.8 Superficial neck abscess.

torticollis. Predisposing factors for mediastinal extension in DNIs are older age, involvement of two or more spaces (especially including the retropharyngeal space) and presence of cardiovascular and pulmonary comorbidities. Some examples of the deep neck infections are given in Figures 8.8 through 8.17.

Aetiology

Today, tonsillitis remains the most common aetiology of deep neck space infections in children, whereas odontogenic origin is the most common aetiology of DNIs in adults. Further aetiological factors in DNI are listed in Table 8.2. The patients with a history of intravenous drug abuse and with human immunodeficiency virus are at risk of developing wound botulism and tubercular deep neck space infection and abscess.

Examination

Deep neck infections are difficult to palpate and impossible to visualise externally because of normal soft tissues covering the deeper neck spaces. However, Ludwig's angina is a rapidly progressing cellulitis involving the submandibular neck space.

It is characterised by induration of the submental region and floor of mouth. It is a clinical diagnosis, and close airway monitoring is essential as the upward and backward tongue elevation can result in a compromised airway.

Peritonsillar abscess (PTA) often presents with sore throat, dysphagia, peritonsillar bulge, uvular deviation, trismus and a muffled voice. The diagnosis of PTA can be made based on history and physical examination. In children the

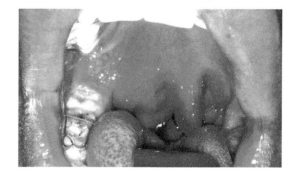

Figure 8.9 Right parapharyngeal space abscess pushing the normal-looking right tonsil medially. The oedematous uvula can be seen pushed to the left, and the patient had a mild degree of trismus.

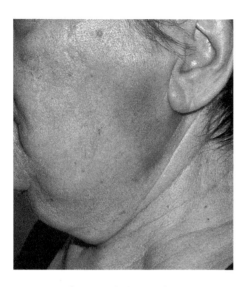

Figure 8.10 Left parotid gland infection (parotitis).

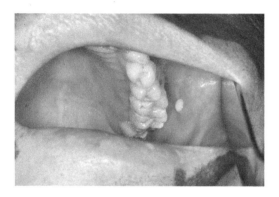

Figure 8.11 Left parotid gland abscess – pus can be seen at the opening of the left parotid duct.

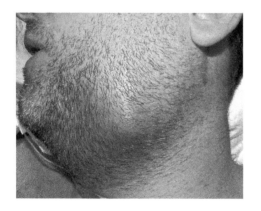

Figure 8.12 Left submandibular gland infection/abscess. The patient is intubated and ready to undergo incision and drainage of abscess.

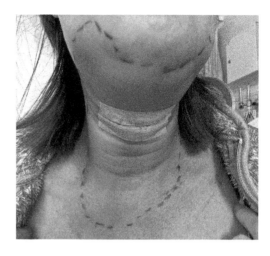

Figure 8.13 Submental abscess after post-operative wound infection.

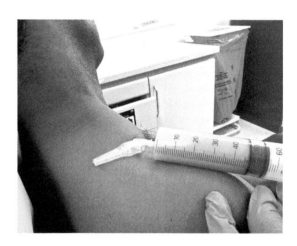

Figure 8.14 Right neck supraclavicular abscess secondary to tuberculosis.

situation might be complicated by a child who is not cooperating with allowing proper assessment of the condition.

Based on published evidence it would appear that often more than one deep neck space is involved in DNIs. The clinical evaluation underestimates the extent of deep neck infection in the majority of patients, which may lead to conservative treatment with worse prognosis.

On clinical examination, the patients with DNIs may exhibit signs mentioned in Table 8.1.

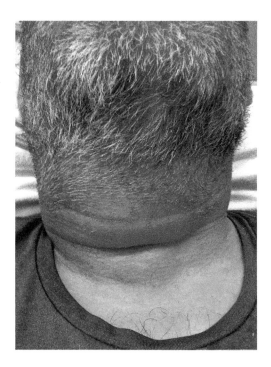

Figure 8.15 Large anterior neck abscess.

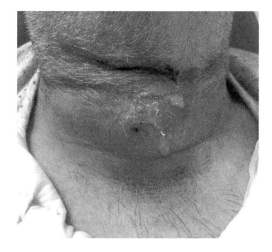

Figure 8.16 Thyroid abscess – incision and drainage under local anaesthetic.

Investigations

Because of the complex anatomy of the neck and deep-seated nature of the DNIs, precise localisation on clinical grounds is challenging and investigations are helpful in this situation. The patients should have laboratory tests to confirm

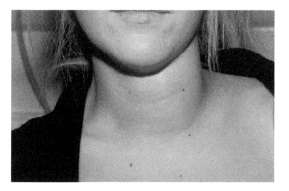

Figure 8.17 Acute bacterial thyroiditis – diffuse swelling of the left side of the neck with loss of normal anatomy associated with an extremely painful stiff neck.

Table 8.2 Aetiology of deep neck space infections/abscess[11]

1	Pharyngitis
2	Tonsillitis
3	Peritonsillar abscess
4	Odontogenic infection
5	Salivary gland infection
6	Penetrating oropharyngeal injury
7	Iatrogenic perforation of oesophagus
8	Fish bone ingestion
9	Foreign body inhalation
10	Suppurative lymph node
11	Branchial cleft anomalies
12	Thyroglossal duct cysts
13	Thyroiditis
14	Mastoiditis
15	Laryngopyocele
16	Intravenous drug abuse
17	Malignant necrotic lymph node

raised markers of infection, and blood cultures are required in septic patients. Radiological assessment may include lateral neck radiograph, ultrasound scan and computed tomography. It is important to note that a normal radiograph does not rule out DNIs in children. The CT scan with contrast is regarded as the gold standard investigation. The presence of air indicates abscess in all cases. The CT scan can be helpful in differentiating the retropharyngeal adenitis from abscess, thereby guiding the clinician to avoid unnecessary surgical intervention. However, a central necrotic cervical metastatic lymph node may sometimes also mimic a simple pyogenic deep neck abscess on both clinical pictures and CT images. Therefore, a routine biopsy of the tissue must be performed during surgical drainage. The MRI scan can yield better soft tissue delineation. The arteriography is chosen if major neck vasculature is suspected to be involved in the infectious process.

The ultrasound scan not only helps in diagnosing the DNIs but it can also be very useful for guided fine needle aspiration for microscopy, culture and sensitivities. The bacteriology of the deep neck space abscess is polymicrobial and it mostly reflects the oral flora. Both aerobic as well as anaerobic organisms are isolated and both gram positive and gram negative organisms are cultured. In one study, children younger than 16 months and/or with lateral neck abscesses were at a significantly increased risk of having a *Staphylococcus aureus* infection, the majority being MRSA.[11]

Management[11]

With advancements in laboratory testing, radiological investigations and broad spectrum antibiotics, the overall morbidity and mortality of DNIs have improved. The clinicians need to be aware of the principles of managing DNIs in an efficient and timely manner to avoid potentially life-threatening complications.

Some patients with DNIs can present in a moribund condition with impending airway compromise, and securing the airway must take priority for such patients. These patients should be kept in the resuscitation section of the accident and emergency department until the patients can be safely transferred by the airway management team to theatre for securing the airway. The anaesthetist should always be part of the team looking after these patients in a calm and controlled fashion. The standard orotracheal and nasotracheal intubation in patients with DNIs are difficult because of trismus, swollen pharyngeal walls and oedema of the supraglottis impairing the vocal cords visualisation, deviation of the larynx, external tracheal compression, restricted neck movement because of paraspinal muscles spasm, and laboured breathing. In such situations oropharyngeal instrumentation should be avoided, as it can aggravate the pharyngeal swelling. Ideally, when diagnostic flexible pharyngolaryngoscopy is carried out, it should be as atraumatic as possible and the procedure video recorded so the anaesthetists can have a better assessment of the airway without having to repeat the laryngoscopy. In compromised airway scenarios it is perhaps a better option to carry out tracheostomy under local anaesthetic, and equipment should be made available for cricothyroidotomy and crash tracheostomy along with good suction facility.

Stable patients suspected to have DNIs should ideally be nursed in a close monitoring area of the ward with facilities available for prompt intervention should a need arise. The patients need adequate analgesia, fluid resuscitation, and parenteral broad spectrum antibiotics which should be reviewed once the culture and sensitivity results are available. The choice of empiric therapy should be based on local protocols, taking into account the most likely source of DNIs. The duration of medical therapy depends upon the patient's progress. If the patient continues to improve and no abscess is located on initial investigations, then parenteral antibiotics can be switched to oral ones.

A trial of high dose intravenous antibiotics in stable children with close observation is warranted as first-line treatment, especially for small deep space neck infections. However, if medical therapy fails, timely surgical intervention in the form of incision and drainage is essential to prevent any adverse outcome. The decision to initiate surgical drainage depends on the patient's clinical status and the accessibility of the abscess. Most deep neck space abscesses are drained through the trans-cervical route, but retropharyngeal abscess is preferably drained trans-orally. Quinsy-tonsillectomy remains controversial but is an option to deal with the peritonsillar abscess. In patients unfit for the general anaesthetic, needle drainage under ultrasound and/or CT guidance is a viable option but requires a motivated, experienced radiologist.

Table 8.3 Complications of deep neck infections/abscesses[12]

1	External compression of trachea
2	Rupture of DNIs into the trachea
3	Internal jugular vein thrombosis
4	Carotid artery erosion
5	Mediastinitis/empyemea
6	Cranial nerve dysfunction
7	Brain and pulmonary abscesses
8	Osteomyelitis of the spine, mandible or skull base
9	Grisel syndrome (i.e., inflammatory torticollis causing cervical vertebral subluxation)
10	Septic shock

The incidence of life-threatening complications, including airway obstruction, sepsis, pneumonia and death, is significantly higher in patients with extension of DNIs into the mediastinum. Normally the patients do very well once the acute episode is settled and do not have any long-term sequelae. However, as outlined in Table 8.3, life-threatening complications can happen because of a delay in diagnosing the DNIs, or if there has been an inadequate treatment.

KEY LEARNING POINTS

- Neck infections can be divided into superficial and deep, depending on the anatomical region involved.
- The superficial and deep cervical fascial layers divide the neck into potential spaces which expand by pus when infection spreads along the fascial planes.
- The symptoms and signs of deep neck infections develop because of the mass effect of the inflamed tissues or abscess cavity on the surrounding structures.
- Clinically, the patients may only have minimal symptoms and signs but some may present distressed with compromised airway.

- The tonsillitis remains the most common aetiology of deep neck space infections in children, whereas odontogenic origin is the most common aetiology in adults.
- The CT scan with contrast is regarded as the gold standard investigation. The presence of air indicates abscess in all cases.
- The bacteriology of the deep neck space abscess is polymicrobial, mostly reflecting the oral flora, aerobic as well as anaerobic organisms are isolated.
- The incidence of life threatening complications is significantly higher in patients with extension of deep neck infection into the mediastinum.

REFERENCES

1. Spinks A, Glasziou PP, Del Mar CB. Antibiotics for sore throat. *Cochrane Database Syst Rev*, 2013; Issue 11.
2. Bird JH, Biggs TC, King EV. Controversies in the management of acute tonsillitis: an evidence-based review. *Clin Otolaryngol*, 2014; 39:368–374.
3. SIGN (2010) Management of sore throat and indications for tonsillectomy: a national clinical guideline. Scottish Intercollegiate Guidelines Network. www.sign.ac.uk
4. Lau AS, Upile NS, Wilkie MD, Leong SC, Swift AC. The rising rate of admissions for tonsillitis and neck space abscesses in England, 1991–2011. *Ann R Coll Surg Engl*, 2014; 96:307–310.
5. Little P, Stuart B, Hobbs FDR, Butler CC, Hay AD, Campbell J et al. Predictors of suppurative complications for acute sore throat in primary care: prospective clinical cohort study. *BMJ*, 2013; 347:f6867.
6. Little P, Watson L, Morgan S, Williamson I. Antibiotic prescribing and admissions with major suppurative complications of respiratory tract infections: a data linkage study. *Br J Gen Pract*, 2002; 52:187–90.

7. Mazur E, Czerwinska E, Korona-Glowniak I, Grochowalska A, Koziol-Montewka M. Epidemiology, clinical history and microbiology of peritonsillar abscess. *Eur J Clin Microbiol Infect Dis*, 2015; 34:549–544.

8. El-Saied S, Kaplan DM, Zlotnik A, Abu Tailakh M, Kordeluk S, Joshua BZ. A comparison between amylase levels from peritonsillar, dental and neck abscesses. *Clin Otolaryngol*, 2014; 39:359–361.

9. Blair AB, Booth R, Baugh R. A unifying theory of tonsillitis, intratonsillar abscess and peritonsillar abscess. *Am J Otolaryngol*, 2015; 36:517–520.

10. emedicine.medscape.com accessed on 17.04.2017.

11. Hussain SM, ed. *Logan Turner's Diseases of the Nose, Throat and Ear: Head and Neck Surgery*, 11th edition, 2016. Boca Raton, Florida: CRC Press.

9

Neck trauma

T TIKKA AND OMAR HILMI

INTRODUCTION

Neck injuries are a relatively uncommon presentation in the emergency departments, with variation across different geographical areas owing to differences in patient demographics. They account for 5–10% of all trauma. Their evaluation and management can be challenging, especially for the inexperienced doctor, because of the complexity of the neck anatomy, which includes vital structures in a confined space.

NECK TRAUMA CLASSIFICATION

There are different ways to classify neck trauma. They are based on the mechanism of injury, the region of the neck affected and the nature of the damage caused in the neck. These classifications are usually used in combination when assessing and describing neck trauma. They help understand the nature of injury and possible implications and help formulate a plan of management. This includes initial examination and treatment, investigations and an informed pathway of definitive care.

MECHANISM OF INJURY (LOW VELOCITY VS HIGH VELOCITY)

The history of the events that led to the injury is very important in obtaining an estimation of the energy that was exchanged within the neck. This allows for consideration of the specific problems that may arise following the trauma.

Depending on the speed involved in the trauma, the injury can be classified as low velocity or high velocity. Low velocity neck injuries are associated with less collateral trauma. When an object is used to cause the trauma, the injury is predictable by tracing the path of the weapon. As a result, low velocity injuries are associated with less cavitation. In contrast, high velocity injuries are associated with large cavitation and significant collateral damage.

PENETRATING VS BLUNT TRAUMA

Penetrating neck trauma includes all wounds violating the platysma. Depending on the speed involved during the trauma, a temporary or permanent cavitation may be formed. Other factors that affect trauma are: the profile of the objects used, their tumble (in the case of high velocity injuries) and whether object fragmentation is present. The most common mechanism of penetrating neck injury is a low velocity injury due to a stab wound (44%), followed by gunshot injuries (40%). Less common mechanisms of injury are from shotguns (4%) or other weapons (12%). Gunshot injuries are twice as likely to involve damage to vascular and aerodigestive structures compared to stab wounds. In firearms wounds, peripheral and cranial nerves injury are three times as likely to occur, whereas damage to the spinal cord is increased by more than a factor of ten.

Blunt neck trauma composes about 5% of all neck injuries. Two forces are involved in blunt trauma: shear and compression. These can affect the formation of the cavitation injury, which also depends on the type of collision. The most common mechanism of blunt trauma is road traffic accidents (75%). Cervical spine injuries are most commonly seen in this type of trauma. High velocity accidents can cause significant nerve injuries, which range from 0.7 to 1.3% in car accidents to more than 4% in motorcycle accidents. Vascular injuries are seen in less than 2% of reported blunt trauma cases. Aerodigestive tract injuries are rare (0.4%).

NECK ZONES

Depending on the level of the injury, the clinician must have a high suspicion of potential structures at risk (Table 9.1 and Figure 9.1). This will guide the evaluation of injury and the imaging investigations required. In penetrating neck trauma, zone II is most commonly affected (47%), followed by zones III (19%) and I (18%). In one-sixth of the cases, more than one neck zone is involved. More than two-thirds of stab wounds are on the left side of the neck, presumably reflecting the majority of assailants (including self-induced injuries) being right-handed.

OVERVIEW OF MANAGEMENT

Prompt assessment and management of neck trauma is crucial in reducing morbidity and mortality, with the latter being reported as high as 10%. Patients can present in a variety of states, from completely asymptomatic and haemodynamically stable at initial presentation to soft signs of injury to neck structures; they may have hard signs of internal organ injuries (Table 9.2) or be haemodynamically unstable.

In the last few decades the management of open neck injuries has moved away from the mandatory neck exploration of all neck injuries violating the platysma to a more selective surgical management guided by patient symptoms and anatomical area of injury (Table 9.1). The use of appropriate imaging modalities is now key to the decision-making process in defining treatment. This has reduced the number of unnecessary neck explorations, postoperative morbidity and mortality.

The first priority when assessing a patient with a neck injury is to identify the unstable patient requiring urgent surgical attention. Imminent airway compromise with audible stridor, breathlessness and low saturation levels despite medical treatment; wound air leak; presence of expanding pulsate neck haematoma or severe active

Table 9.1 Trauma neck zones

Zones	Anatomical landmarks	Structures at risk
Zone I	Clavicles/sternal notch to inferior border of cricoid cartilage	Branchiocephalic veins Innominate artery Subclavian arteries and veins Vertebral arteries Common carotid Aortic arch Jugular veins Trachea Oesophagus Cervical spine/cord/nerve roots Thyroid Lung apices
Zone II	Inferior border of cricoid cartilage to angle of mandible	Common carotid artery Internal and external carotid arteries Jugular veins Vertebral arteries Pharynx Larynx Trachea Oesophagus Cervical spine/cord
Zone III	Angle of mandible to skull base	Internal and external carotid arteries and their branches Jugular veins Oesophagus Trachea Salivary glands Spinal cord Vertebral bodies Branches of lower cranial nerves

haemorrhage; uncontrollable haematemesis or haemoptysis; and evidence of unresponsive hypovolemic shock require emergency surgical exploration (Table 9.2). Presence of focal neurological deficit requires urgent involvement of the neurosurgical team with immobilisation of the cervical spine as part of the primary trauma survey.

REDUCING SECONDARY INJURY

Secondary trauma is further injury that occurs subsequent to the initial insult as a result of interventions or by neglect. Examples of secondary injury are traumatic intubation injuries, preventable inflammation, secondary infection and poor tracheostomy tube care.

PRINCIPLES OF EMERGENCY DEPARTMENT MANAGEMENT

The patient must be evaluated in a systematic fashion using the Advanced Trauma Life Support 'ABCDE' approach and appropriate resuscitation initiated.

Attention to the airway, cervical spine and haemodynamic status will guide the decision for

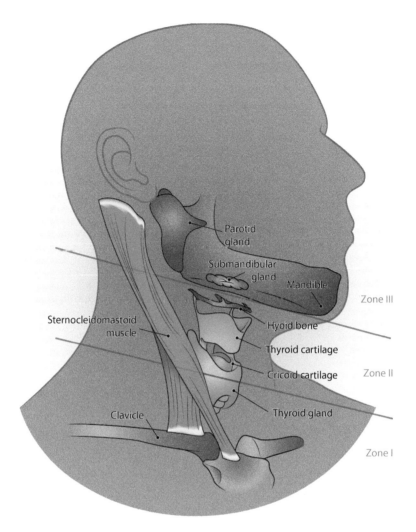

Figure 9.1 Neck zones.

Table 9.2 Neck trauma signs

Hard signs	Soft signs
Airway obstruction (stridor, low saturation level, respiratory distress)	Hoarseness/ cysphonia
	Dyspnoea
Wound air leak (blowing or sucking wound)	Dysphagia/ odynophagia
Unresponsive shock	Haemoptysis/ haematemesis
Severe active bleeding	
Expanding haematoma	Subcutaneous emphysema
Decreased/absent radial pulse	Mediastinal air
Uncontrollable haematemesis/ haemoptysis	Non-expanding haematoma
	Active bleeding
Vascular bruit/thrill	Focal neurological deficit
Cerebral ischaemia	

urgent surgical neck exploration. During the primary survey, patients must be screened for the following life-threatening conditions:

- Airway obstruction (laryngotracheal trauma/ external compression)
- Tension pneumothorax
- Major active bleeding
- Spinal cord injury
- Ischaemic brain damage (carotid artery occlusion)

CERVICAL SPINE AND AIRWAY ASSESSMENT AND MANAGEMENT (FIGURE 9.2)

Regardless of the type of injury and mechanism of trauma, the first priority is attention to the airway. This is performed while maintaining alignment of the cervical spine. The spinal cord must be protected until injury is excluded by clinical assessment guided by radiography where appropriate.

Cervical spine injuries are reported to be less than 0.2% in penetrating neck trauma. It is proposed that cervical spine immobilisation should be performed only in patients with presence of obvious neurological deficit at initial presentation

or for the unconscious patient. Blunt high velocity neck trauma is associated with higher risk of cervical spine injuries. Studies have shown that patients who have immobilisation of the cervical spine in the emergency setting suffer increased mortality rates. It has been suggested that this might be due to delayed prehospital care and transfer; missed identification of signs of instability due to the presence of the hard collar; suboptimal placement of a definite airway; and the fear of collar removal for management of critical injuries.

The 'Look – Listen – Feel' approach helps in identifying signs of airway obstruction.

- Look: – Observe the patient's behaviour. Are they agitated or obtunded (suggesting hypoxia and hypercarbia, respectively)? Detect low oxygenation using pulse oximetry and check the respiratory rate. Look for the presence of cyanosis, use of accessory muscles and tracheal tug that indicate laboured breathing. Inspect the airway for the presence of foreign bodies. Observe for the presence of facial, mandibular or tracheal/laryngeal fractures causing airway compromise.
- Listen: – Listen for abnormal breathing sounds (stertor, stridor, gurgling). Evaluate voice quality for hoarseness or dysphonia.
- Feel: – Feel the location of the trachea and check for palpable fractures and the presence of surgical emphysema or haematoma compromising the airway.

When the airway is not critical, then give priority to dealing with massive haemorrhage in preference to a slightly compromised airway.

Injuries to the larynx and trachea occur in up to 7% of neck traumas. They can manifest with acute stridor, breathing difficulty, cyanosis or acute onset of hoarse voice. In the unconscious patient, desaturation and difficulty intubating, distorted anatomy on direct laryngoscopy or flexible nasal endoscopy are signs of laryngotracheal trauma. In a previously intubated patient, inability to safely extubate is another potential sign of trauma. Bubbling of air through an open wound is pathognomonic of laryngotracheal damage; urgent airway management is summarised here. This is performed in a

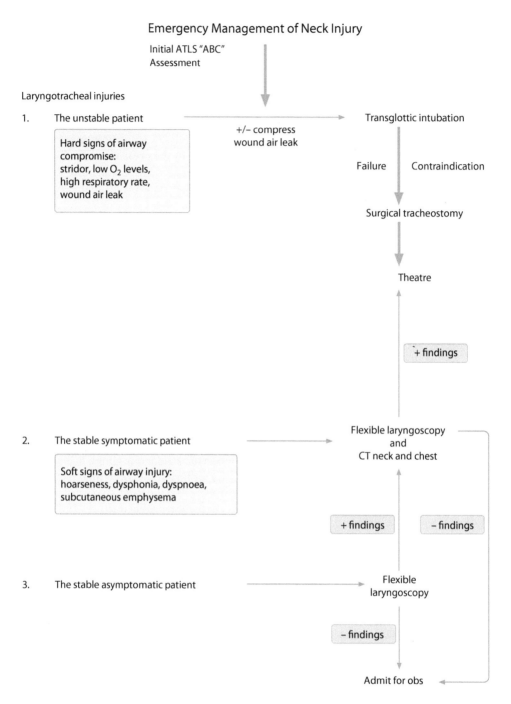

Figure 9.2 Managing laryngotracheal injuries.

stepwise manner, re-assessing airway patency after each step.

- Suction blood and secretions from the airway.
- Administer high flow oxygen (15 L/min).
- Improve airway patency with simple manoeuvres (chin-lift, jaw-thrust).
- Use simple airway adjuncts (orotracheal, nasopharyngeal airway).
- Secure the airway (GCS score 8 or less, hard signs of airway obstruction), performing endotracheal intubation or establishing a surgical airway.

THE UNSTABLE PATIENT

In unstable patients with signs of significant imminent airway compromise, the first priority is to secure a definitive airway; repair of the injuries that caused airway compromise can be dealt with subsequently. Thirty percent of laryngotracheal injuries require emergency department airway establishment. This can be achieved either with transglottic intubation or by performing an emergency surgical front of neck access. Standard intubation is a blind procedure after the initial visualisation of the larynx. This can be a significant problem in patients with laryngeal trauma, as the passage of the tube through the glottis can cause further laryngeal disruption and, in the presence of severe trauma, it can enter the surrounding structure of the neck, rendering a compromised airway critical. Fibre-optic intubation is similarly contraindicated, as the tube can still get caught in the larynx prior to entering the trachea. Needle cricothyroidotomy is also not recommended. As a definitive, safe procedure requiring very basic equipment, tracheostomy may therefore be the primary choice of airway management in the presence of airway damage. Air bubbling through an open neck wound requires firm pressure, which will improve oxygenation and reduce air leak.

THE STABLE PATIENT

In the stable but symptomatic patient, flexible nasal endoscopy can guide management by evaluating the extent of laryngeal damage. The laryngeal mobility can be assessed and the presence of oedema, mucosa tear, fresh blood or haematoma noted. Formal investigations include neck and chest x-rays to assess for the presence of surgical emphysema or pneumothorax. A computed tomography (CT) scan of the neck and chest is the investigation of choice for identifying laryngeal or lower airway trauma and plan for surgical management. For the stable, asymptomatic patient with negative flexible nasal endoscopy findings, admission to the ward for a period of observation may be appropriate to ensure that secondary oedema of the airway does not occur.

DEFINITIVE MANAGEMENT OF LARYNGOTRACHEAL INJURIES

Stable patients with minor airway symptoms and evidence of minor haematoma or laryngeal fracture can be treated conservatively with humidified oxygen and close observations. Stable or unstable patients with evidence of airway compromise and signs of oedema and laryngeal contour disruption may require surgical intervention. The initial surgical management of laryngotracheal injuries may be a surgical tracheostomy to secure the airway – when transglottic intubation has failed or it is contraindicated – followed by exploration of the neck and repair as required. The timing of any necessary laryngeal repair depends on the type of injury. In most cases, a delayed repair is preferred, allowing time for reduction of tissue oedema and inflammation. Nevertheless, grossly contaminated wounds or the presence of major uncontrolled bleeding will necessitate emergent exploration. Laryngotracheal discontinuity mandates urgent reconstruction to avoid tracheal retraction into the mediastinum. Surgical procedures include both endotracheal and open approaches, depending on local expertise. Depending on the traumatised area, different surgical techniques have been proposed (Table 9.3).

The structures at risk include: the airway mucosa; the muscular apparatus; the cricoarytenoid joint; the cartilaginous framework, including damage to the thyroid and cricoid cartilage, the epiglottis or the tracheal rings; and neural injury, including damage to the vagus or recurrent laryngeal nerve. Most mucosa trauma will heal by adopting a conservative approach, but damage to sensitive mucosal areas – anterior commissure, free edge

Table 9.3 Surgical modalities, depending on the injured laryngeal structure

Mucosal trauma	• Conservative management • Surgical closure or resection of ragged sensitive mucosal areas • Mucosal cover of damaged cartilage
Muscular trauma	• Conservative management • Repair of disrupted anterior attachment of vocalis muscle at anterior commissure (sutures/transglottic keel support)
Cricoarytenoid joint trauma	• Manipulation back to anatomic position • May require wire support

Framework damage	• Elevation and support of cartilage:
	  • Internal laryngeal stents
	  • Plating and/or fixation of cartilages

Neural injury	• Careful exploration and tension free anastomosis of recurrent laryngeal nerve

of the vocal cords, junction between the vocalis muscle, and the vocal process of the arytenoids – may require surgical intervention (Table 9.3).

While further repair is awaited, prompt wound care is necessary to avoid secondary damage. Patients with endotracheal tubes should remain heavily sedated, hence avoiding laryngeal movements during swallowing. Cuff pressure should be regularly monitored to prevent mucosal damage. The inhaled oxygen should be warmed and humidified and tracheal secretions regularly aspirated with minimal trauma. Steroids have been shown to improve and expedite the healing process, especially when surgical reconstruction is planned.

CIRCULATION AND BLEEDING CONTROL (FIGURE 9.3)

Control of bleeding and appropriate replacement of intravascular volume is essential during primary trauma assessment guided by the ATLS protocol. Fluid resuscitation must be initiated to restore tissue perfusion and oxygenation. Based on the patient's initial presentation, an estimation of total blood loss can be obtained and used as a guide for initial fluid replacement (Table 9.4).

The key to successful fluid resuscitation in trauma patients is to achieve a balance between organ perfusion and the risk of rebleeding or bleeding exacerbation. Persistent infusion of large volumes of intravenous fluids is not a substitute to definitive control of bleeding. Fluid overload in trauma patients can exacerbate the lethal triad of acidosis, hypothermia and coagulopathy. This can be avoided by accepting a lower-than-normal blood pressure and adopting a balanced approach to fluid administration; this is termed 'controlled resuscitation'. The aim is to manage blood loss, achieving a balance, rather than simply replacing volume losses, as bleeding in the neck is obvious, unlike the occult bleeding in the abdomen and pelvis. The key to this is reducing, or preferably stopping, the bleeding until definitive management can be achieved.

The incidence of vascular injuries in neck trauma varies in the literature from 25% to 70% of the patients attending the emergency department with a penetrating neck wound. The majority of these involve the venous vessels, followed by carotid artery and vertebral artery injuries. Following initial fluid resuscitation, further management of bleeding is guided by patient's haemodynamic status and site of injury.

THE CRITICALLY UNSTABLE PATIENT

The haemodynamically compromised patient with active bleeding or other hard signs (Table 9.2) of vascular injury will require urgent wound exploration and vascular repair following initial fluid resuscitation, as discussed. The site of active bleeding should be compressed while necessary arrangements are made for a safe transfer to theatre. At this point, involvement of other specialities may be considered: neurosurgery or interventional radiology for trauma in neck zone III and cardiothoracic or interventional radiology for neck zone I.

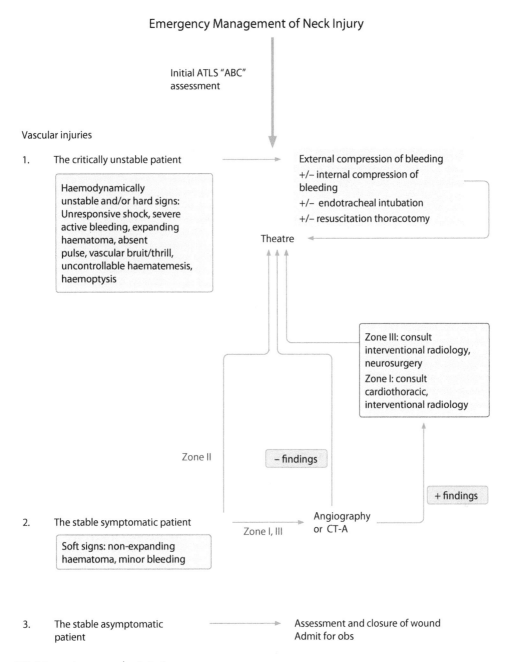

Figure 9.3 Managing vascular injuries.

Table 9.4 Estimated blood loss based on patient's initial presentation

	Class I	Class II	Class III	Class IV
Blood loss (mL)	Up to 750	750–1500	1500–2000	>2000
Blood loss (% blood volume)	Up to 15%	15–30%	30–40%	>40%
Pulse rate (bpm)	<100	100–120	120–140	>140
Systolic blood pressure	Normal	Normal	Decreased	Decreased
Pulse pressure (mm Hg)	Normal or increased	Decreased	Decreased	Decreased
Respiratory rate	14–20	20–30	30–40	>35
Urine output (mL/hr)	>30	20–30	5–15	Negligible
CNS/mental status	Slightly anxious	Mildly anxious	Anxious, confused	Confused, lethargic
Initial fluid replacement	Crystalloid	Crystalloid	Crystalloid and blood	Crystalloid and blood

Simple external compression will suffice in temporarily controlling the bleeding in most cases. When retro-clavicular bleeding is present or a bleeding source is located near the skull base, external compression may not control the bleeding. Intra-wound digital compression with a gloved index finger should be attempted. Insertion and inflation of a Foley balloon catheter into the wound, followed by external compression or closure of the superficial elements of the wound with sutures, has been reported to control bleeding in difficult scenarios. If the bleeding persists following balloon inflation, the catheter should be deflated and repositioned. Insertion of a second catheter can also be attempted. A Kelly's clamp can be used to keep the catheter under tension. Packing can be removed in theatre in a controlled manner, followed by surgical repair of the defect once the situation is stabilised.

If these measures fail to control the bleeding prior to transfer to theatre, urgent endotracheal intubation should be considered to apply further internal pressure on the site of haemorrhage. When the patient is in extremis and transfer to theatre is not an option, blind clamping of a suspected bleeding site can be attempted, even though this is known to be associated with increased risk of further vascular and nerve damage. Resuscitation

thoracotomy and clamping of bleeding vessels under direct vision is the last resort treatment when the patient reaches the emergency department with an imminent cardiac arrest.

In a patient with suspected air embolism, they must be placed in the Trendelenburg position and satisfactory venous volume ensured. This will have a secondary effect of increasing bleeding in the head and neck and should be followed up with local pressure and, once venous blood volume is replaced, the position should be corrected to normal to reduce further venous bleeding.

THE STABLE PATIENT WITH SOFT SIGNS OF VASCULAR INJURY

Imaging of the neck can identify clinically significant vascular injuries. Four-vessel catheter angiography is the gold standard investigation for recognition of vascular injuries in stable but symptomatic patients with soft signs of internal organ damage (Table 9.2). The advantage of this imaging modality, in addition to its high level of sensitivity and specificity, is that endovascular repair can be performed at the same sitting. Nevertheless, the unavailability of catheter angiography in many centres and the risk of cerebrovascular complications associated with the intervention have led to an increasing role for alternative non-interventional first-line investigations.

Computed tomography angiography (CT-A)

This is faster to perform, is not associated with complications and has high sensitivity and specificity. CT-A can identify extravasation injuries, presence of pseudoaneurysms, vessel dissection or occlusion, and anteriovenous fistula formation (Table 9.5). The proximity of the injury to big vessels will help identify its source and guide surgical or endovascular management. Vascular occlusion is the most common type of vessel injury in penetrating neck trauma, followed by pseudoaneurysm

formation, whereas vascular dissection is a rare finding.

Ultrasound scan of the neck (USS neck)

USS has also been proposed as an imaging modality in the emergency setting and is frequently available in emergency departments. Nevertheless, its value is controversial, as it is heavily operator dependent.

Magnetic resonance imaging (MRI)

MRI is not recommended as an emergency imaging modality for neck trauma. It is a time-consuming

Table 9.5 Vascular injury types and management options

Type of injury	Radiological findings	Management
Extravasation	• Pooling of contrast outside but in close proximity to a vessel • Lack of vascular enhancement in the damaged vessel	Conservative management
Pseudoaneurysm	• Disruption of damaged vessel wall (complete/partial) • Widening of parent vessel with outpouching of contrast	Surgical ligation Endovascular embolisation Bypass surgery Conservative management
Dissection (+/− intramural haematomas)	• Widening of vessel contour with narrowed central lumen • Intraluminal filling defects	Endarterectomy Surgical ligation Bypass surgery and grafting Anticoagulants Conservative management
Occlusion (partial/complete)	Lack of vascular enhancement	Surgical or endovascular revascularisation Conservative management
Arteriovenous fistula	Equal contrast enhancement in artery and vessel	Endovascular repair with conventional angiography Embolisation Surgical repair

investigation that can significantly delay treatment. Direct observation of the patient for signs of clinical deterioration or emergent management is not possible while the patient is under the magnetic field, and urgent intervention, if needed, is challenging.

THE STABLE ASYMPTOMATIC PATIENT

The haemodynamically stable and asymptomatic patient may be admitted to the hospital for a period of observation. In the presence of penetrating neck trauma, the depth of the wound can be evaluated in the emergency department, followed by primary wound closure if there are no signs of damage to important structures.

DEFINITIVE MANAGEMENT OF VASCULAR INJURIES

Depending on the zone of injury, different surgical approach can be utilised. An anterior sternocleidomastoid incision will suffice in most occasions to provide access to the injured vessel. A zone I injury may require a median sternotomy incision extending to the sternocleidomastoid region. An additional supraclavicular incision may be used. In zone II injuries when both sides of the neck are affected, or where there is evidence of a transcervical injury, the addition of a transverse cervical incision will give an improved surgical field access. Zone III injuries are often very challenging to be accessed surgically. Dislocation of the mandible with or without resection might be required for optimal surgical approach.

Arterial vascular injuries can be repaired either surgically or with the use of interventional radiology. Surgical approaches include vessel ligation or recanalisation. Repair of an injury to the common carotid or internal carotid artery with revascularisation of the vessel, as opposed to ligation, is associated with better outcomes. When revascularisation is not possible, arterial ligation can be attempted, but this is mainly indicated for patients with a pre-operative Glasgow Coma Scale of less than 8, as they are expected to have unfavourable outcomes irrespective of the surgical repair used.

Surgical repair should preferably be performed with the assistance of vascular surgeons.

In the event of a major bleeding originating from a venous injury, ligation of the bleeding vessel can be performed, and it is not linked with adverse outcomes. Nevertheless, in the presence of bilateral internal jugular injuries, preservation of one of the two vessels with revascularisation is important in avoiding complications of intracranial venous hypertension and cerebral oedema. Venous injuries close to the skull base may require packing to control the bleeding.

If local expertise is not available at the presenting hospital, then temporary control of the injuries, as discussed earlier, and the patient's stabilisation in the intensive care unit must be initiated, followed by definitive repair of the injuries when the appropriate personnel and resources are in place. This may necessitate hospital transfer.

MANAGEMENT OF DIGESTIVE TRACT INJURIES

Injuries to the pharynx and oesophagus are rare entities but have possible life-threatening complications. The incidence of pharyngo-oesophageal injuries varies in available studies – between 1% and 6.5%. Blunt pharyngo-oesophageal injuries are a very uncommon entity. Early identification of these injuries is crucial to avoid complications including mediastinitis, sepsis and abscess formation. High index of suspicion is required, as an oesophageal injury carries a mortality rate of up to 20%. Acute onset of haematemesis; dysphagia or odynophagia following a neck injury, as well as the presence of surgical emphysema or visible mucosal tear on performing flexible nasal endoscopy, are the main symptoms and signs suggestive of a pharyngo-oesophageal injury.

Investigations include anteroposterior (AP) and lateral neck and chest x-ray to look for evidence of soft tissue surgical emphysema or presence of air in the pre-vertebral plane. Presence of positive signs on plain radiography mandates the need for more detailed scans to further delineate the area of injury. CT findings suggestive of an injury to the oesophagus are: focal oesophageal wall defect or thickening; gas or fluid collection in close proximity to the oesophagus; and fluid collection in the mediastinum or evidence of inflammatory changes. Further evaluation of the injury should be carried out by performing a water-soluble contrast swallow. This can give valuable information about the size and extent of the leak. Endoscopic evaluation of the oesophagus by performing a rigid pharyngoscopy and oesophagoscopy can also identify the defect. The surgical diagnostic option is of significant value in intubated and sedated patients or those who are not co-operative enough to undergo a swallow assessment.

The mainstay of treatment of pharyngo-oesophageal injuries includes: keeping the patient nil by mouth; initiating treatment with broad spectrum intravenous antibiotics; and placement of a nasogastric tube for nutrition or, alternatively, initiation of total parenteral nutrition through a peripherally inserted central venous line. The decision for early surgical exploration and repair of the defect varies depending on local experience and expertise.

Small confined leaks are likely to heal by adopting a conservative management protocol. Large leaks with involvement of the mediastinum will need early surgical intervention with an aim to drain the collection, leaving the defect to heal with the measures already mentioned. Attempts to repair the pharyngo-oesophageal wall tears with primary tissue closure are reported to have a low success rate. Moreover, they do not reduce the hospitalisation days or improve overall outcomes.

If primary surgical management is to be adopted, it should be within the first 24 hours of injury, as subsequent to that, tissue coagulation at the injured area makes primary repair difficult. In presence of other injuries requiring surgical intervention, pharyngeal injuries should be repaired at that time.

MANAGEMENT OF NERVOUS SYSTEM INJURIES

Nerve injuries can be open or closed and are further classified using the Seddon stratification system. According to this, nerve damage can be a result of neuropraxia, axonotmesis or neurotmesis.

Clinical evaluation must include:

- Assessment of the Glasgow Coma Scale score
- Cranial nerve examination
- Spinal cord assessment, looking for localising signs
- Brachial plexus injuries
- Phrenic and sympathetic chain assessment (Horner syndrome)

SPINAL CORD INJURIES

Neurogenic and osseous injuries to the cervical cord and spine can be associated with neck trauma. Presence of acute focal neurological deficit in the conscious patient must alert the clinician to the presence of a spinal cord injury. In the unconscious patient, neurogenic injuries should be excluded radiologically when the mechanism of injury implies possible trauma to the spinal cord. MRI is the investigation of choice in the otherwise stable patient unless there is the presence of metallic objects in the victim's body that contraindicates this modality. In such cases a CT scan can be performed. Breach of the dura should be considered when there is presence of gas, bone fragments or foreign bodies in the cervical spinal canal. Unstable fractures of the survival spine should also be considered and excluded. Urgent neurosurgical assessment is needed for further evaluation and management of these injuries.

BRACHIAL PLEXUS INJURIES

The majority of brachial nerve injuries are managed expectantly with delayed exploration. Nevertheless, certain situations require urgent surgical intervention. Open and significantly contaminated wounds should be explored and debrided and any nerve damage repaired. In the presence of vascular injuries requiring surgical intervention, nerve injuries should also be repaired at the same sitting. Brachial plexus localised lesions following a stab wound injury or other sharp laceration must be explored due to the high incidence of nerve transection. In these cases, there is no role for expectant management. If nerve sheath integrity is seen during wound exploration, it is advised to leave it intact, followed by frequent clinical evaluation and neurophysiological assessments.

Cranial nerve injuries and Horner's syndrome are rare findings in neck trauma. Acute and complete paresis of lower cranial nerves should alert the clinician for the presence of nerve transection if consistent with the mechanism of injury and region of the wound. Urgent surgical exploration and repair of damaged nerve must be attempted. No specific treatment of post-traumatic Horner's syndrome has been described.

A SPECIAL CASE: DOG BITE NECK INJURIES

Humans are often victims of animal attacks, with the commonest injury being a dog bite. The characteristics of a dog bite neck injury are often attributed only to the penetrating nature of the injury. Nevertheless, the blunt component of this special case of trauma should not be forgotten. The blunt force of this trauma may be its most serious component, causing crushing damage to major vessels, airway structures and nerves.

The assessment and management of the neck trauma will follow the same pattern as previously discussed, but additional steps should be followed to ensure adequate management of this type of injury. Careful examination of the wound is required to assess whether there are signs of infection. If the wound appears infected, blood cultures must be obtained for both aerobic and anaerobic bacteria. Microbiology samples must be obtained from the superficial and deepest part of the wound prior to thorough decontamination of the wound. Suspected infection should be treated empirically with antibiotic cover. The tetanus status of the patient should be checked and prophylactic tetanus toxoid injection administered if required.

If this is a fresh wound, encourage it to bleed unless it is already actively bleeding. The injured area must be explored and carefully cleaned and foreign bodies (e.g., teeth) removed, followed by primary closure of the wound after decontamination and debridement is completed. The peculiar dual blood supply of the head and neck skin enables this to be closed, protecting the deeper structures and reducing the ultimate cosmetic impact of the injury.

The stable and asymptomatic patient can be discharged following a period of observation after wound care is completed and a course of oral antibiotics is prescribed.

CONCLUSION

Neck trauma is a relatively uncommon presentation in emergency departments. It can be a source of anxiety for the managing physician due to the complex anatomy involved and the numerous important structures at risk of damage. Successful management is based on the adaptation of a stepwise approach to manage this condition. If no local expertise is available, stabilisation of the patient and transfer to a trauma unit for definitive management is required.

KEY LEARNING POINTS

- The management of neck trauma is complex due to the variety of structures that can be injured.
- The zones of the neck guide the clinician to the potential structures injured.
- Resuscitation should be performed according to ATLS principles.
- In imminent airway compromise, the definite risk of inaction is greater than the potential risk to the larynx or trachea of performing an emergency cricothyroidotomy or tracheostomy.
- Controlled fluid resuscitation aims to balance organ perfusion and the risk of rebleeding by accepting a lower than normal blood pressure and avoiding fluid overload.

- The haemodynamically compromised patient with active bleeding requires surgical intervention rather than further investigation.
- Not all subplatysmal penetrating injuries require exploration.
- Injuries from animal bites require through exploration.

FURTHER READING

Burgess CA, Dale OT, Almeyda R, Corbrridge RJ. An evidence based review of the assessment and management of penetrating neck trauma. *Clin Otol*. 2012; 37: 44–52.

Demetriades D, Salim A, Brown C, Martin M, Rhee P. Neck injuries. *Curr Probl Surg*. 2007; 44(1): 13–85.

National Association of Emergency Medical Technicians. 2010. Chapter 4, Kinematics of Trauma. In: *Prehospital Trauma Life Support*. 8th edition. Burlington, MA: Jones and Bartlett, pp. 43–85.

National Institute for Health and Care Excellence. 2015. *Bites – human and animal. Scenario: managing a cat or dog bite* [online]. Available at: cks.nice.org.uk/bites-human-and-animal #!scenario:2. (Accessed 18 December 2016.)

Rathlev NK, Medzon R, Bracken, ME. Evaluation and management of neck trauma. *Emergency Med Clin North Am*. 2007; 25(3): 679–694.

Saito N, Hito R, Burke P, Sakai O. Imaging of penetrating injuries of the head and neck: current practice at a level I trauma center in the United States. *Keio J Med*. 2014; 63(2): 23–33.

Sperry JL, Moore EE, Coimbra R, Croce M, Davis JW, Karmy-Jones R, McIntyre RC Jr., Moore FA, Malhotra A, Shatz DV, Biffl WL. Western Trauma Association critical decisions in trauma: penetrating neck trauma. *J Trauma Acute Care Surg*. 2013; 75(6): 936–940.

10

Acute airway assessment and management

ADONYE BANIGO AND KIM W AH-SEE

INTRODUCTION

The airway, or the airway tract, is part of the respiratory system. It runs from the nose and mouth, where air is inspired, to the alveoli, where gaseous exchange takes place. The airway can be divided into the upper airway (the nasal and oral cavities, pharynx and larynx up to the level of the glottis) and the lower airway (the subglottis, trachea, bronchi and bronchioles housed in the lungs). In addition to their structural differences, the upper and lower airways also differ in their respiratory dynamics, as detailed in this chapter. The relatively unprotected nature of the upper airway and the extrathoracic trachea increases the risk of traumatic damage. The following sections concern the emergency management of pathology of the upper airway and part of the lower airway (subglottis and trachea).

Every organ and system in the body possesses the capacity to alter its physiology in response to stresses. This allows time for the stresses to be eliminated by the body's immune system and for a return back to the organ's normal physiology. This process happens not infrequently with the airway, producing minor symptomatology, and does not require significant external input to alter its course (e.g. upper respiratory tract infections). However, there are some stresses that trigger a sinister course of events. In these cases the airway has used its compensatory mechanisms, but these are either insufficient or not rapid enough to make up for the functional or structural overload caused by the disease process. The airway becomes an acute airway, which is one that is decompensating and life-threatening. It produces significant symptomatology and it requires emergency intervention to halt and reverse its progression.

This chapter will discuss the key principles of the acute adult airway patient, and how these patients should be assessed and managed.

PRINCIPLES

The acute airway exists as a continuum from early to late, with associated symptoms and signs at each stage (see Figure 10.1). This may not have been appreciated by the referring clinician but is very important because, whilst one patient with an acute airway may require treatment with high flow oxygen, nebulised adrenaline and steroids, another may require an emergency tracheostomy at the bedside. Both patients have been positioned at different points on the acute airway continuum, and patients require regular reassessments, as they will move along this scale in either direction depending on the success (or failure) of treatment given.

Patients with early signs and symptoms can be managed medically with appropriate drugs and admission and observation in an appropriate setting like ITU, HDU, theatre recovery or a well-staffed ENT ward. With these patients, consideration of surgical intervention can wait until the most senior head and neck surgeon arrives.

Patients with late signs and symptoms must also receive drug treatment, but they are more likely to require immediate surgical intervention, and in these cases there may be no time to wait for the most senior surgeon to arrive for that decision to be made.

SIGNS

The assessment of an acute airway patient involves taking a history and examining the patient with simultaneous management. This needs to be performed promptly and, given that these patients are often too unwell to give a history, identifying objective signs of an acute airway is pertinent. These signs are listed here with their definitions and descriptions:

Stridor – is defined as high-pitched, noisy breathing resulting from narrowing of the larynx and/or trachea. It is a hallmark sign of upper airway obstruction. Although stridor is often used synonymously to describe an inspiratory noise, stridor can be inspiratory (narrowing at or above the glottis level), expiratory (narrowing of the intrathoracic airway, commonly referred to as wheeze) or biphasic (narrowing of the trachea). Table 10.1 describes the differences between inspiratory and expiratory stridor in more detail.

Stertor – is defined as low-pitched, noisy breathing resulting from narrowing of the pharyngeal airway. Snoring is stertor during sleep.

Suprasternal retraction/flaring of nostrils/ intercostals recession – these are all signs of

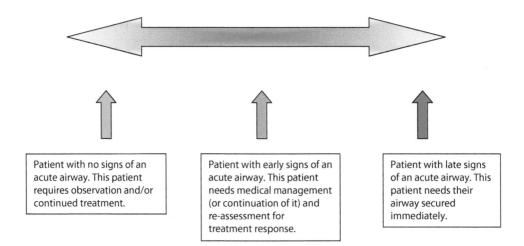

Patient with no signs of an acute airway. This patient requires observation and/or continued treatment.

Patient with early signs of an acute airway. This patient needs medical management (or continuation of it) and re-assessment for treatment response.

Patient with late signs of an acute airway. This patient needs their airway secured immediately.

Figure 10.1 Diagram acute airway continuum.

Table 10.1 Differences between intrathoracic airway and extrathoracic airway

Inspiratory stridor versus expiratory stridor

As mentioned on p. 98, narrowing of the extrathoracic airway causes an inspiratory stridor, while intrathoracic airway narrowing causes an expiratory stridor (wheeze). This difference occurs because of the influence of airway dynamics.

Extrathoracic airway	Intrathoracic airway
This is predominantly influenced by Bernoulli's principle.	This is predominantly influenced by intrapleural pressure changes.
The speed of air movement on inspiration leads to a decrease in pressure on the extrathoracic airway and a tendency to collapse. The opposite applies in expiration. Hence, the consequence of any reduction in airway diameter has a more adverse effect on inspiration.	On inspiration, the outward negative intrapleural force increases the diameter of the intrathoracic airway. The opposite applies in expiration. Hence, the consequence of any reduction in airway diameter has a more adverse effect on expiration.
In addition, pedunculated lesions of the supraglottis and glottis are drawn into the airway on inspiration.	

accessory muscle use as inspiratory effort increases to overcome the obstruction.

Restlessness/agitation – this can be due to hypoxia or anxiety; in an acute airway situation, the former must be ruled out.

Hoarseness – is defined as any change in voice quality. Although more commonly associated with glottis and supraglottic lesions, lesions of the oropharynx can also lead to voice changes classically described as a 'hot potato voice'.

STEPS

Assessment of an acute airway begins when the referring call is received. It must be rapid and thorough. There are two broad features of the acute airway that should be elucidated from the initial call and subsequent assessment: the severity of the acute airway and the cause of the acute airway:

1. **The severity of the acute airway**

Most of these signs can be ascertained using the Look, Listen and Feel approach:

Look – for cyanosis, agitation, obtunded, use of accessory muscles, respiratory rate

Listen – for abnormal breath sounds, hoarseness

Feel – for tracheal deviation, air escape from neck wounds, capillary refill time, heart rate

The severity of the acute airway will determine the priorities of management. For the patient with early signs, the priorities are to reach a diagnosis and instigate medical management. For the patient with late signs, the priority is to secure the airway.

2. **The cause of the acute airway**

There is often not enough time to collate a thorough history, as the patient may be too distressed. In some cases the history is obvious, e.g. a patient with a post tonsillectomy bleed, or a trauma patient. The features in Table 10.2 make the diagnosis more likely but are not exclusive to the diagnosis.

MANAGEMENT

The management of an acute airway can be divided into three broad categories: *pre-arrival* (this is from the time you receive the emergency call to when you arrive at the patient's bedside), *at the scene* (i.e. at the patient's bedside), and *post intervention* (decisions concerning management over the next few hours, including destination ward and other investigations required).

Table 10.2 Common causes of an acute airway

	Infective	Malignancy	Angioedema	Paradoxical vocal cord movement	Anaphylaxis
Age	<40	>40	<60	<30 female	Any age
Duration	Hours to days	Weeks to months	Minutes to hours	Days	Seconds to minutes
Associated features	Sore throat, fever	Smoker, drinker, self-neglect	ACE-inhibitor use, family history	Recent stress/ anxiety (exams, work)	Exposure to known allergen

PRE-ARRIVAL

A brief history is taken when the referral is received to ascertain the severity of the acute airway and potential cause. The referring team should be instructed to administer medical management listed below before your arrival and to contact the on-call anaesthetist. Due to the stressful situation, it is important to check that they have understood your instructions by asking them to repeat the instructions you have given. This is called Closed Loop Communication.

Oxygen via facemask (heliox if available, easier to breathe in due to reduced density)

Nebulised adrenaline 1 mL of 1:1000 with 4 mL saline

IV steroids (6.6 mg dexamethasone or hydrocortisone)

IV broad-spectrum antibiotics

Contact anaesthetist

Get the airway trolley, if available. If not, gather sizes of oropharyngeal and nasopharyngeal tubes, endotracheal tubes, cricothyroidotomy sets and tracheostomy tubes.

Flexible nasendoscope (you may need to take one with you or arrange for one to be delivered by the emergency team of the hospital)

AT THE SCENE

The patient is assessed for objective signs of an acute airway, listed in Table 10.3. Ensure the above

Table 10.3 Early and late signs of an acute airway

	Severity of the airway: signs	
	Early	Late
Talking	Able to talk in full sentences	Unable to talk in full sentences, unable to talk at all
Stridor	Soft	Harsh/loud, or quietening as the patient is tiring
Intercostal/subcostal recession, tracheal tug	Not present	Present
Colour of skin and mucous membranes	Pink, well perfused	Pale, blue, cyanosed
Respiratory rate	14–30	>30 or <14
Oxygen saturation	94% and above	<94%
Heart rate	100–120	>120 or <60
Blood pressure	Normal or high	Decreased
Level of consciousness	Obtundation (due to hypercarbia)	Agitation (due to hypoxia)
Capillary refill time	<2 seconds	>2 seconds

Table 10.4 Assessing an airway for risk of difficult intubation

L	Look externally	Look externally for features likely to predict difficulty, e.g. retrognathia, overbite, short neck, severe cervical arthritis, poor mouth opening
E	Evaluate the 3-3-2 rule	For ease of intubation, there should be proper alignment of the pharyngeal, laryngeal and oral axes: 3 finger breadths between the patient's incisors 3 finger breadths between the hyoid bone and chin 2 finger breadths between the thyroid notch and the floor of the mouth
M	Mallampati grading	Assess the degree of adequate visualisation of the oropharynx
O	Obstruction	Review the diagnosis and whether it carries the risk of obstructing the airway, e.g. epiglottitis, angioedema
N	Neck mobility	This can be limited due to severe cervical arthritis or immobilisation due to a neck collar

medical management listed has been administered and the anaesthetist is present or on their way.

Flexible nasendoscopy should be performed as soon as possible for non-traumatic cases to confirm the diagnosis and assess the severity. This is one of the most valuable tools in the ENT specialist's armamentarium. It will determine whether the patient needs a definitive airway and the likely success of intubation.

If an airway is deemed difficult, then the most senior anaesthetist should be called for assistance, if available, or preparations for a surgical airway should be made. Fibre-optic awake intubation is also an option. The mnemonic LEMON is used for the assessment for difficult intubation (Table 10.4).

Securing the airway versus definitive airway

The decision to secure an airway is made either because the airway continues to decompensate despite drug administration or the patient is tiring and there is concern that they may not be able to support their own airway for much longer. The aim of securing the airway is to use the least invasive adjunct but ensure it provides the most control of the airway. An airway is secure when the technique used lies distal to the level of the obstruction. Any adjunct can be used to secure the airway as long as it lies distal to the obstruction, examples are shown in Table 10.5. Securing the airway is often used synonymously with establishing the airway; hence, they are referring to the same process.

A definitive airway is described as a tube placed in the trachea with the cuff inflated, held in place with tape and connected to an oxygen-enriched assisted ventilator. Only cuffed endotracheal tubes and cuffed tracheostomies are definitive airways. Scenarios where a definitive airway is required are described in Table 10.6.

The surgical airway

FRONT OF NECK ACCESS – CRICOTHYROIDOTOMY/EMERGENCY TRACHEOSTOMY

The inability to establish a definitive airway via an oral or nasal route in a deteriorating patient is the indication for a surgical airway, i.e. cricothyroidotomy or tracheostomy. This can be due to distortion

Table 10.5 Options for securing the airway

Level of obstruction	Early	Late
Oral cavity/oropharyngeal	Oral airway (Guedel), nasopharyngeal airway, ET intubation	Cricothyroidotomy/emergency tracheostomy
Laryngeal	ET intubation +/− fibre-optic guidance	Cricothyroidotomy/emergency tracheostomy

Table 10.6 Indications for a definitive airway

Indication	Examples
Failure of other interventions	Desaturation, poor ventilation or apnoea with oropharyngeal, nasopharyngeal or laryngeal mask airway in situ
Protection of the airway	Bleeding into the airway, vomitus in the airway, inhalation injury, expanding neck haematoma, prolonged seizure activity

of the glottis due to tumour, oedema or complex laryngeal fracture, or an inability to view the glottis due to severe bleeding or vomitus.

There is often confusion as to whether to perform a cricothyroidotomy or emergency tracheostomy at the bedside for a patient with late signs of an acute airway who is about to completely obstruct. Cricothyroidotomy refers to opening of the cricothyroid membrane using a needle (referred to as needle cricothyroidotomy as pictured in Figure 10.2) or a scalpel (also known as surgical cricothyroidotomy).

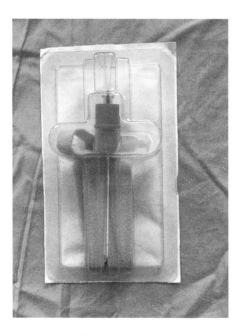

Figure 10.2 Needle cricothyroidotomy cannula.

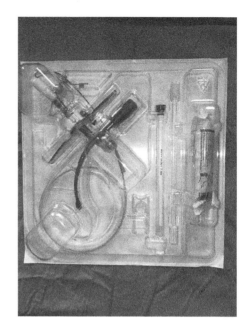

Figure 10.3 Seldinger-technique (also known as percutaneous tracheostomy) set.

The former opening can then be established using a cannula, whilst the latter is made with a tracheostomy tube. In an out-of-hospital setting, any appropriate hollow tube with firm walls would suffice. Cricothyroidotomy is theoretically a quick and simple temporising measure. However, cricothyroidotomy sets (particularly with the Seldinger technique) can often be an unfamiliar tool, which is highly disadvantageous in an emergency situation. In such cases, the intervening specialist should use a non-Seldinger technique cricothyroidotomy or perform a surgical tracheostomy, if they are more comfortable with the latter. Seldinger-technique tracheostomy sets as shown in Figure 10.3 (also known as percutaneous tracheostomy) are also available, but these are not appropriate for an emergency setting given the procedure length and the need for hyperextension of the neck, which is risky in a trauma situation. Percutaneous tracheostomies are more appropriate for a controlled setting, e.g. intubated ITU patient requiring a tracheostomy.

NEEDLE CRICOTHYROIDOTOMY STEPS

Place the cannula through the cricothyroid membrane into the trachea below the level of obstruction.

A jet insufflator can be connected to the cannula and used to deliver oxygen.

If a jet insufflator is not available, connect the cannula to high flow oxygen (15 L/min) with a Y-connector or by cutting a hole on the side of the tubing.

Intermittent insufflation is performed by placing your thumb over the Y-connector or side hole for 1 second on and 4 seconds off.

A patient can be adequately oxygenated for 30 to 45 minutes using this technique.

SURGICAL CRISCOTHYROIDOTOMY STEPS

Make a skin incision through the cricothyroid membrane.

Dilate the incision using a curved haemostat or tracheal dilator.

Insert a small cuffed tracheostomy tube through the opening (an endotracheal tube can also be used).

EMERGENCY TRACHEOSTOMY STEPS

A tracheostomy refers to the opening of the trachea.

The steps are the same as for a surgical cricothyroidotomy, except this incision is made on the trachea at the level of the second and third rings.

In an emergency situation this is best performed via a vertical incision with a number 11 blade from the skin into the trachea. This vertical incision avoids damage to the anterior jugular veins and problematic bleeding.

When the tracheostomy is formalised in theatre, a cartilage splitting technique should be used, which avoids removal of cartilage rings. Removal of cartilage rings can predispose to future tracheal stenosis.

Following front of neck access in an emergency situation, further formal examination in a theatre environment, where bleeding can be controlled and the surgical site inspected, is essential. It would also be an appropriate time to examine the primary pathology and take any photographs or biopsies if appropriate. If a cricothyroidotomy was performed, this would need to be converted to a surgical tracheostomy. In the time between gaining front of neck access and arrival in theatre, any airway intervention performed at the bedside will need to be secured with tapes around the patient's neck, and the tube may need to be physically held during transfer, to prevent dislodgement.

Following insertion of the definitive airway, it must be confirmed to be in the right place before by auscultating equal breath sounds bilaterally it is completed with tapes tied around the patient's neck. Auscultation of gurgling or rumbling noises (borborygmi) suggests the tube is in the oesophagus, and it must be repositioned immediately. A carbon dioxide detector showing CO_2 in the exhaled air is the confirmation that the airway has been successfully intubated. When the tube has been tied in place, it must be checked for dislodgement whenever the patient is moved. A chest x-ray can be performed when the patient is stable; this would further confirm correct intubation and may pick up a pneumothorax, which is not uncommon in a difficult emergency intubation. A gum elastic bougie should be used for predicted difficult airways or if the initial attempt was unsuccessful. Figure 10.4 shows a range of trachestomy tubes by different manufacturers, some only appropriate for short term use whereas others can be used longer term.

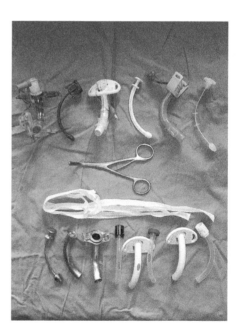

Figure 10.4 Selection of tracheostomy tubes in the top and bottom of the photograph with their inner cannulas and introducers. In the middle of the photograph lies a tracheal dilator forceps to aid insertion of a tracheostomy tube, and tapes to secure the tracheostomy tube.

POST INTERVENTION

Once the airway has been secured or the decision has been made that the airway can be managed conservatively, then the patient should be assessed fully, including assessment for other injuries and medical conditions.

Trauma patients must be treated with special consideration for other injuries, especially cervical spine injury, and the neck positioning during assessment and management is crucial; immobilisation may be required.

There should be a discussion about the need for further imaging (x-rays, CT scanning, etc.) and the most appropriate destination ward for the patient.

Trauma setting

The assessment and management of the airway in a trauma patient takes priority over the management of all other conditions resulting from the trauma. Poor delivery of oxygenated blood to vital organs is the quickest killer of the trauma patient. The airway can be maintained by using manoeuvres (jaw thrust, chin lift) or adjuncts (oropharyngeal, nasopharyngeal, or laryngeal mask airway), or it can be secured using a definitive airway.

Patients with maxillofacial trauma, neck trauma and laryngeal trauma are at high risk for developing an acute airway. This can be due to disruption of the larynx or trachea, or obstruction of the airway due to haemorrhage, increased secretions or foreign bodies (including dislodged teeth). Patients with altered levels of consciousness (especially in head injuries) who are obtunded and/or have thoracic injuries can still warrant a definitive airway to deliver adequate ventilation and prevent aspiration. The development of an acute airway in a trauma patient can be sudden and complete, progressive and recurrent and/or insidious and partial. It is important that the assessment and management involves maintenance of cervical spine protection until the possibility of spinal cord injury has been excluded by clinical assessment and appropriate radiographic studies. Patients who are wearing a helmet will need it to be removed using a two-person technique in which one provides inline immobilisation whilst the other removes the helmet.

Patients with altered levels of consciousness are at risk of hypopharyngeal obstruction due to backward displacement of the tongue. This can be corrected using a chin lift or jaw thrust manoeuvre and maintained with an oropharyngeal or

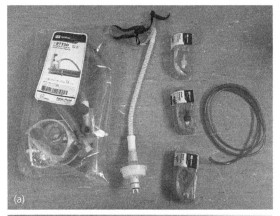

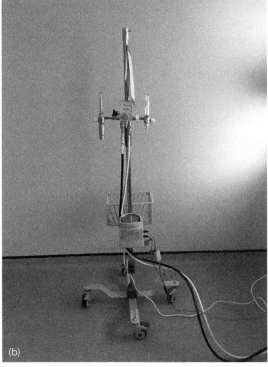

Figure 10.5 Optiflow kit. In (a) going from left to right lies the breathing circuit, a nasal cannula with the headstrap, different sized nasal cannulae and some spare tubing. (b) Shows the integrated heated humidification oxygenation system that the breathing circuit is connected to.

nasopharyngeal airway bearing in mind that nasopharyngeal airways are contraindicated in suspected skull base fractures. A laryngeal mask airway can also be used, but a plan must be made to insert a definitive airway.

The Transnasal Humidified Rapid-Insufflation Ventilatory Exchange (THRIVE), also known as Optiflow, is recognised to have a role in providing oxygenation during difficult airway management; its components are photographed in Figures 10.5a and b. It allows a smooth process of securing the airway by providing adequate saturation and avoids the repeated cycles of successive laryngoscopy, resultant hypoxaemia and responsive re-oxygenation. It can be used to oxygenate apnoeic patients for short airway procedures and can be useful in airway foreign body extraction.

KEY LEARNING POINTS

- Acute airway compromise is an ENT emergency.
- Urgent assessment is required as part of an ATLS process.
- Stridor can help indicate the level of obstruction.
- Initial medical management may provide temporary relief.
- A front of neck airway will be required if clinical signs worsen or the patient tires.
- "THRIVE" is a useful adjunct to managing the acute airway.

FURTHER READING

American College of Surgeons. *Advanced Trauma Life Support for Doctors*, 8th Edition, 2008. Published by American College of Surgeons.

Gleeson MJ, Clarke RC. *Scott-Brown's Otorhinolaryngology, Head and Neck Surgery*, 7th Edition, 2008. Published by CRC Press.

Lalwani AK. *Current Diagnosis and Treatment Otolaryngology – Head and Neck Surgery*, 3rd Edition, 2011. Published by McGraw-Hill Education.

Patel A, Nouraei SAR. The Transnasal Humidified Rapid-Insufflation Ventilatory Exchange (THRIVE): a physiological method of increasing apnoea time in patients with difficult airways. *Anaesthesia* 2015 March;70(3):323–329.

11

Food bolus/foreign body obstruction of the upper aerodigestive tract

KIM TO AND RICHARD ADAMSON

FOOD BOLUS/FOREIGN BODY OBSTRUCTION

INTRODUCTION

Food bolus/foreign body obstruction is not uncommon, with an estimated annual incidence of 13 episodes per 100,000 (Longstreth, Longstreth, & Yao, 2001). In adults, the most common cause of obstruction is food bolus impaction, which increases in incidence with age. This has been related to the use of dentures, which can impair oral sensation and mastication. In younger adults, eosinophilic oesophagitis is increasingly prevalent, with studies suggesting 33–54% of cases are caused by the condition (Truskaite & Dlugosz, 2016). Other causes include Schatzki's ring, peptic stricture, oesophageal diverticulum, post-surgical stricture, achalasia, hiatus hernia and oesophageal carcinoma (Triadafilopoulos, Roorda, & Akiyama, 2013). True foreign body obstructions are less common, but can occur in psychiatric and mentally impaired patients, in prisoners, in those with alcohol intoxication and in the elderly (Ikenberry et al., 2011).

Fortunately, 80–90% of food bolus/foreign bodies will pass spontaneously, and removal is only required in 10–20% of patients (Birk et al., 2016). Patients with sharp or corrosive foreign bodies need urgent removal due to the recognised complication of oesophageal perforation, which can lead to mediastinitis, sepsis and multi-organ failure. The reported mortality rate for mediastinitis is between 30 and 49% (Ridder et al., 2010). It is recommended that patients should be treated within 24 hours, as foreign bodies impacted for longer are at 14.1 times higher risk of major complications (Loh, Tan, Smith, Yeoh, & Dong, 2000).

HISTORY

In most adults, there is a clear history of acute onset dysphagia with inability to swallow following ingestion of a food bolus/foreign body. This may not be the case in the elderly or mentally impaired, and a collateral history may be required. The aim is to take a thorough history eliciting the following key points.

1. **Onset and duration** – ensures timely management of the patient.
2. **Nature of food bolus/foreign body**
   - *Food bolus* – Enquire about the type of food bolus and whether it contained any bone. A meat bolus can be managed initially with medical therapy. An impacted food bolus containing bone, shells from seafood or sharp fruit pits will require urgent removal (Ibrahim, Chauhan, & Nikkar-Esfahani, 2016; Park, Lim, Song, & Lee, 2016).
   - *Foreign body* – Enquire about the nature and size of the object. Large objects are unlikely to pass spontaneously and sharp objects will require urgent removal.
   - In elderly patients, it is worth asking about dentures; have a high index of suspicion if they cannot be found at home.
3. **Location in the throat** – If it is at the level of the thyroid cartilage, it may well be in the upper oesophagus. Below this level, it is difficult to determine where it is in the oesophagus. It is well known that the area of discomfort often does not correlate to the level of impaction, particularly in distal obstructions (Ikenberry et al., 2011; Wilcox, Alexander, & Clark, 1995).
4. **Ability to eat and drink** – A patient who is managing to eat and drink with no symptoms is unlikely to have a foreign body. However, beware of those who may have partial obstruction and may still be able to tolerate fluids and soft diet.
5. **Previous episodes** – This may reveal the underlying cause and previous area of impaction. If the patient is known to gastroenterology, refer to the on-call team. If the patient has presented for the first time, they will need further investigation as an outpatient.

6. **Symptoms suggestive of perforation** – Neck pain, sore throat, odynophagia, haematemesis, retrosternal pain, back pain, temperature and dyspnoea.
7. **Past medical history, allergies and drug history** – This information is useful to determine any contraindications to medical treatment.

EXAMINATION

We would recommend an ABC approach. The aim is to assess if the airway is compromised; to determine if the food bolus/foreign body is in the upper or lower oesophagus; the urgency of removal; and if there are any complications.

A – Airway

- Is the patient's airway stable or unstable?
- Signs suggestive of an unstable airway include: dysphonia, inability to talk in sentences, drooling, choking, stridor, spitting out saliva constantly and inability to protect own airway.
- Encourage the patient to spit out saliva, or use a Yankauer sucker.
- Look in the oral cavity – is there a foreign body?
- If you have concerns that the airway is unstable and/or there is a foreign body obstructing the upper airway, get help from your senior ENT surgeon immediately and contact the on-call anaesthetic team.

B – Breathing

- Take respiratory rate and oxygen saturation.
- Auscultate the chest – is there evidence of a wheeze or reduced breath sounds to suggest inhalation of the foreign body?
- Give the patient oxygen as necessary.

C – Circulation

- Take heart rate, blood pressure and temperature.
- Get intravenous access and take bloods, including FBC, U&E, CRP, coagulation screen and blood cultures (if pyrexial).
- Consider starting the patient on intravenous fluids and antibiotics as necessary.

Try to assess the location of the foreign body:

- Oral cavity – Fish bones can embed themselves in the tonsil – remove them with Magill's forceps.
- Perform fibre-optic nasolaryngoscopy at this stage and carefully look for the following:
  - A foreign body in the laryngopharynx
  - Common places for foreign bodies include the vallecular, tongue base and piriform fossa
  - Pooling of saliva suggestive of complete oesophageal obstruction
- Palpation of the tonsils and tongue base is also helpful to identify any foreign bodies such as fish bones.
- Palpate the neck for any signs of surgical emphysema secondary to perforation.
- Water test – Ask the patient to swallow a small mouthful of water and time how long it takes for the water to be regurgitated. A rough guide is that immediate regurgitation would suggest a high oesophageal obstruction, while delayed regurgitation after 10 seconds or more would suggest a lower obstruction. Lower oeosphageal obstructions should be referred to gastroenterology for endoscopy (oesophagogastroduodenoscopy).

INVESTIGATION

- Lateral soft tissue neck x-ray (Figure 11.1)
  This is a quick investigation with a low radiation dose and can be helpful in up to 51.6% of cases of foreign body obstruction (Karnwal, Ho, Hall, & Molony, 2008). It should be used in conjunction with the history and examination findings. If you are not confident with the interpretation of the x-ray, enlist the help of a radiologist. Look for signs of:
  - A radiopaque foreign body. A common mistake is to confuse calcification of the laryngeal cartilage as bone.
  - Widening of the pre-vertebral soft tissue (normal maximum width is up to 7 mm C1-4 and up to 22 mm C5-7), tenting of the oesophagus with gas shadow in the upper oesophagus and loss of cervical lordosis (Tysome & Kanegaonkar, 2012).
  - Air in the subcutaneous tissues suggestive of perforation.

- CT scan
  This is not routinely used in the investigation of acute foreign body obstruction. However, a CT scan of the neck and chest is indicated if oesophageal perforation is suspected (Birk et al., 2016). This can help to determine the location of the impacted foreign body and help to plan the surgical approach for removal. In the non-acute setting, a CT scan may be helpful in patients who represent with persistent symptoms and if you have a high index of suspicion. We would recommend discussing with a radiologist/senior ENT surgeon in these situations.

Contrast swallow is not recommended due to the theoretical risk of aspiration, and coating of the contrast medium can obstruct endoscopic examination (Khayyat, 2013). On the other hand, it is useful in the investigation of patients with recurrent food bolus obstruction in the outpatient setting.

MANAGEMENT

1. Medical
   The majority of food boluses will pass spontaneously, and given the risks associated with surgery, it is reasonable to observe the patient initially provided they are stable (Tsikoudas, Kochillas, Kelleher, & Mills, 2005). During this period, most clinicians in the UK would administer antispasmodic drugs – see Table 11.1 (Khayyat, 2013). However, a recent systematic review did not find any evidence that hyoscine butylbromide, gas-forming agents, glucagon or benzodiazepines were any more effective than watchful waiting (Khayyat, 2013; Leopard, Fishpool, & Winter, 2011).

2. Surgical
   If the decision is made to remove the food bolus/foreign body urgently or conservative management has failed, proceed with either upper rigid oesophagoscopy or endoscopy. The literature suggests this should be done within 24 hours. The choice between the two will largely depend on the nature of the foreign body, the level of obstruction and availability of endoscopy locally.

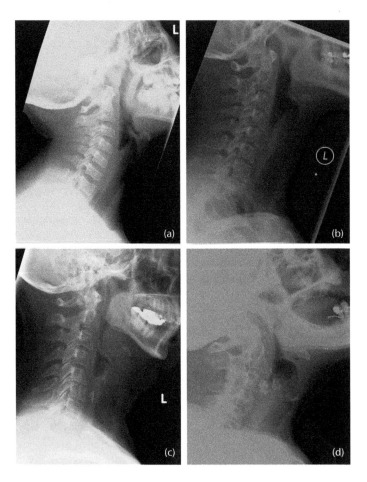

Figure 11.1 **(a)** Normal lateral soft tissue neck x-ray; **(b)** chicken bone; **(c)** mussel shell; **(d)** prune stone.

POST-TONSILLECTOMY HAEMORRHAGE

INTRODUCTION

Post-tonsillectomy haemorrhage (PTH) is the most common complication following tonsillectomy and can potentially be life-threatening. It can be classified as primary, which occurs within 24 hours of surgery, and secondary thereafter. Primary PTH is the result of inadequate haemostasis due to surgical technique, and most will occur within 12 hours of surgery (Chowdhury, Tewfik, & Schloss, 1988). Secondary PTH usually occurs on post-operative day 5–10 when the primary eschar sloughs away (Krishna & Lee, 2001; J Windfuhr & Seehafer, 2001). It has traditionally been suggested that

infection of the tonsil bed predisposes to secondary PTH, but evidence for this is lacking (Kumar, 1984; Stephens, Georgalas, Kyi, & Ghufoor, 2008). Moreover, secondary PTH can occur in patients treated with perioperative antibiotics and in those with negative throat swabs (Dhiwakar, Clement, Supriya, & McKerrow, 2012; Kumar, 1984).

The National Prospective Tonsillectomy Audit demonstrated the overall risk of PTH is 3.5% (0.6% primary, 3% secondary). The risk of returning to theatre for surgical arrest is 0.9%, with a higher risk associated with increasing age, male gender and the use of a 'hot' surgical technique (diathermy or coblation) (Brown et al., 2005). It is speculated that a 'hot' surgical technique can induce thermal damage, leading to local tissue necrosis and invasion by bacteria- and enzyme-containing saliva (JP Windfuhr, Schloendorff,

Table 11.1 Medical therapies in the management of food bolus obstruction

Medication	Dose	Contraindications	Side-effects
Hyoscine Butylbromide (Buscopan) (Joint Formulary Committee, 2016)	• 20 mg IV • Repeat after 30 minutes • 100 mg max per day	Pregnancy Myasthenia gravis Prostatic enlargement Urinary retention Bowel obstruction Pyloric stenosis Paralytic ileus Severe ulcerative colitis Significant bladder outflow obstruction Toxic megacolon Angle-closure glaucoma (caution) Cardiac disease (caution) (Medicines and Healthcare Products Regulatory Agency, 2017) Tachycardia	Constipation Dry mouth Urinary retention/ urgency Pupillary dilatation Photophobia Reduced bronchial secretions Transient bradycardia Skin dryness/flushing
Benzodiazepines (Joint Formulary Committee, 2016)	• Diazepam 10 mg IV • Repeat 10 mg after 4 hours if required	Compromised airway Respiratory depression Chronic psychosis CNS depression Obsessional and phobic states	Confusion (elderly) Amnesia Ataxia Drowsiness Lightheadedness Muscle weakness
Glucagon (Joint Formulary Committee; Bodkin, Weant, Baker Justice, Spencer, & Acquisto, 2016)	• 1 mg IV	Phaeochromocytoma Insulinoma	Nausea Vomiting Abdominal pain Hypotension Hypokalaemia
Effervescent agents (Karanjia & Rees, 1993)	• Fizzy drinks such as Coca-Cola	Unstable airway	Aspiration Perforation (rare)

Baburi, & Kremer, 2008b). Fortunately, the majority of PTH can be managed conservatively without the need for return to theatre or blood transfusion. However, it is important to note that a small herald bleed or repeated episodes of minor bleeding may precede a life-threatening PTH, and these patients should be admitted appropriately for observation. Mortality from PTH is reported with a varying incidence between 1 in 3000 to 28,700 (JP Windfuhr, Schloendorff, Baburi, & Kremer, 2008a).

REFERRALS

Most patients will present to the emergency department (ED) and will be in a resuscitation bay if they are actively bleeding. In the unlikely event that a general practitioner calls about a PTH presenting to the surgery, we would always recommend the patient to attend ED rather than the ENT ward in the first instance. They can be resuscitated and stabilised before being safely transferred to the most appropriate location.

HISTORY

A succinct and focused history is required to decide the most appropriate management in a timely manner. Take an AMPLE (Allergies, Medication, Past medical history, Last meal, Events leading) history, with the following key points:

1. **Date of operation** – Primary or secondary bleed?
2. **Onset, duration and frequency** – A patient who has active and ongoing bleeding is likely to need to go to theatre.
3. **Estimated blood loss, including any haematemesis/haemoptysis** – This may give you an idea of the severity of the PTH and any active bleeding you cannot see.
4. **Increasing pain, poor oral intake, fever and haliotosis** – Symptoms suggestive of an infective cause.
5. **Any personal/familial history of coagulopathy or liver disease**

EXAMINATION

Always take a systematic ABC approach so as not to miss any important steps in a stressful situation. The main concerns are airway and circulation. Figure 11.2 shows the equipment required when attending to a PTH.

A – Airway

- Sit the patient upright and encourage them to spit out any blood.
- Look in the mouth and identify any bleeding point/clot – this will be useful if the patient needs to go to theatre (Figure 11.3).
- Use suction (Yankauer) gently inside the mouth if bleeding is profuse.
- Consider calling for help and intubating the patient if aspiration and airway are at risk.

B – Breathing

- Take respiratory rate and oxygen saturation.
- Examination of chest – has the patient aspirated?
- If oxygen is needed, use oxygen delivered by nasal prongs unless the patient is in extremis and requires a non-rebreathable mask.

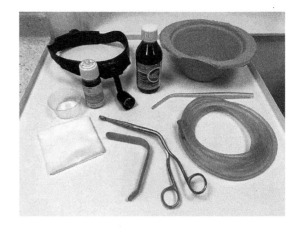

Figure 11.2 Equipment for post-tonsillectomy haemorrhage.

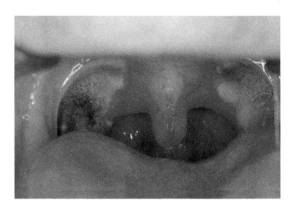

Figure 11.3 Appearance post-tonsillectomy. Note the clot on the right tonsil bed.

C – Circulation

- Take heart rate, blood pressure, capillary refill time and temperature – is the patient in hypovolaemic shock?
- Get IV access with two large-bore cannulas.
- Remember to send off bloods, including:
  - Full blood count
  - Urea and electrolyte
  - Coagulation screen
  - Group and save
  - Blood cultures, if pyrexial
  - Cross-match 2 units if the patient is haemodynamically unstable or the patient is returning to theatre.

- Resuscitate with intravenous fluids:
  - Consider activation of the major haemorrhage protocol if necessary.
  - Consider the use of O-negative blood if cross-matched blood is not yet available.
- Is the patient excessively swallowing to suggest they are actively bleeding or are they vomiting out fresh blood – active signs of bleeding?
- Attempt to arrest the bleed with medical measures (see below).

Keep the patient nil by mouth. If the patient has stopped bleeding and is haemodynamically stable, they can be admitted and transferred to the ENT ward. If a patient has active, ongoing or life-threatening haemorrhage, the patient is likely to be transferred directly to the emergency theatre. Remember to contact and alert your senior ENT surgeon.

MANAGEMENT

1. Medical
   1.1. 3% Hydrogen peroxide gargles
      - Check instructions on the back of the bottle, as brands may vary.
      - Dilute 1 part solution to 2 parts water and encourage the patient to gargle for 2–3 minutes. Repeat up to 3 times a day (Electronic Medicines Compendium, 2015).

        Hydrogen peroxide is best known for its bactericidal properties and is commonly used in the acute management of PTH. Its role in haemostasis was thought to be vasoconstriction; however, it has since been shown to be an endothelium-dependent smooth muscle relaxant (Shimokawa & Matoba, 2004). There is some evidence to suggest it may have prothrombotic properties and may reduce thrombus growth, but clinical evidence for its effectiveness in PTH is lacking (Hope & Lo, 2007). In a 10-year retrospective review of secondary PTH, Pai et al. (Pai, Lo, Brown, & Toma, 2005) did not show any difference in the rate of surgical intervention, hospital stay or readmission for further haemorrhage between the hydrogen peroxide and control groups. However, the study was performed in a paediatric cohort and, in addition, all patients received intravenous antibiotics.

   1.2. Topical adrenaline
      - If the patient can tolerate it, soak gauze in 1:1000 adrenaline and apply it against the bleeding point using Magills forceps for 5–10 minutes

        Adrenaline acts on α-adrenergic receptors to cause vasoconstriction. It is generally used as a temporising measure in severe bleeds while waiting to take the patient to theatre.

   1.3. Tranexamic acid

      If bleeding persists despite the measures already mentioned:

      1.3.1. Intravenous tranexamic acid (Sandoz, 2015)
         - Consider giving a STAT dose of 0.5–1 g tranexamic acid via slow intravenous injection.
         - The onset of action is immediate, with a half-life of 3 hours. It is renally excreted.
         - Contraindications: Active or past history of thromboembolic disease, severe renal impairment, history of convulsions and fibrinolytic conditions following consumptive coagulopathy (Sandoz, 2015).

      1.3.2. Topical tranexamic acid
         - Soak gauze in an ampoule of 500 mg/5 mL of tranexamic acid and apply it to the bleeding point with Magills forceps for 5–10 minutes.
         - There is evidence that topical tranexamic acid reduces bleeding and blood transfusion in surgical patients, but the risk of thromboembolism is uncertain (Ker, Beecher, & Roberts, 2013).

Tranexamic acid is a synthetic antifibrinolytic agent that reversibly inhibits lysine-binding sites on plasminogen. This inhibits its activation to plasmin on the surface of fibrin, thereby stabilising the fibrin clot (Dunn & Goa, 1999). Tranexamic acid reduces mortality and blood loss in major trauma patients, and it is widely used in elective surgery to reduce peri-operative blood loss (Mahdy & Webster, 2004; McCaul & Kredo, 2016; Perel, Ker, Morales Uribe, & Roberts, 2013). In a recent Cochrane review, Perel et al. (Perel et al., 2013) found that tranexamic acid can reduce the probability of having a blood transfusion by 30% in patients undergoing urgent and emergency surgery, although larger studies are required to assess mortality and thromboembolic adverse events.

1.4. Antibiotics
- There is no clear evidence to support the empirical use of antibiotics in secondary PTH (Ahsan, Rashid, Eng, Bennett, & Ah-See, 2007).
- If there is clinical evidence of infection, start the patient on intravenous antibiotics.
- Common organisms include *Staphylococcus aureus, Haemophilus influenzae, Streptococcus* (Lancefield groups A, B, C & G), mixed anaerobes and coliforms. Studies have shown frequent presence of bacteria that are resistant to amoxicillin, suggesting co-amoxiclav to be a more appropriate antibiotic (Stephens, Georgalas, Kyi, & Ghufoor, 2008).

2. Surgery
The indications for theatre and surgical arrest of PTH include:
- Active haemorrhage
- Persistent haemorrhage despite conservative measures
- Cardiovascular compromise

If the decision is made to take the patient back to theatre, you need to contact:
1. Your senior ENT surgeon, if you have not already done so
2. Emergency theatre coordinator
3. On-call anaesthetist

Explain to the patient the need to return to theatre and take consent as follows:
Operation: Examination under anaesthetic plus arrest of post-tonsillectomy haemorrhage
Risks: Pain, infection, further bleeding, blood transfusion
Surgical technique:
- Use a Yankauer sucker to remove any blood clots in the oral cavity.
- Attempt to identify the bleeding point.
- Direct pressure with adrenaline soaked swab may be helpful if bleeding is profuse.
- We would recommend using electrocautery as the tissues are generally quite sloughy and friable, making it difficult to ligate any bleeding points (except in primary bleeds).
- If this fails, some surgeons suggest suturing the tonsil pillars together and packing the tonsil bed with a haemostatic agent such as Surgicel® (Randall & Hoffer, 1998). However, there have been case reports where the packing has displaced, causing choking and aspiration (Handler, Miller, Richmond, & Baranak, 1986; Jacques, Nash, Kenway, & Vlastarakos, 2013). We therefore would not routinely recommend this.
- If bleeding still persists, your options are:
  - Pack the oral cavity and keep the patient intubated for 24 hours
  - Embolisation
  - External carotid artery ligation
- Remember to use a nasogastric tube to suction out any blood in the stomach at the end of the procedure to prevent aspiration on extubation.

RECOVERY

In our practice, patients will generally stay for 24 hours observation before being discharged home, as long as their pain is under control and they are managing oral intake. There is no evidence on the optimal duration of hospital stay, probably because it is impossible to predict if and when a patient may bleed again. The reported risk of repeated episodes of PTH come from large retrospective case series and is between 9.9 and 11.7% (Attner, Haraldsson, Hemlin, & Hessen Soderman, 2009; JP Windfuhr, Verspohl, Chen, Dahm, & Werner, 2015). They can occur anytime between post-operative day 1–15, and the longest reported time following tonsillectomy is post-operative day 58 (JP Windfuhr et al., 2008b). It is important to remember that patients presenting with repeated episodes of PTH should be taken seriously, as this can be a typical course of life-threatening PTH. It is also prudent to investigate if the patient has an underlying coagulation disorder in repeated episodes of PTH.

KEY LEARNING POINTS

- Around 80–90% of food bolus/foreign bodies will pass spontaneously within 24 hours.
- Sharp or corrosive foreign bodies must be removed urgently to prevent complications.
- The water test is a useful tool to assess the level of obstruction.
- Most post-tonsillectomy bleeds can be managed conservatively with hydrogen peroxide gargles.
- There is lack of evidence to support the use of empirical antibiotics in secondary post-tonsillectomy bleeds.

REFERENCES

Ahsan, F., Rashid, H., Eng, C., Bennett, D. M., & Ah-See, K. W. (2007). Is secondary haemorrhage after tonsillectomy in adults an infective condition? Objective measures of infection in a prospective cohort. *Clin Otolaryngol*, 32(1), 24–27.

Attner, P., Haraldsson, P. O., Hemlin, C., & Hessen Soderman, A. C. (2009). A 4-year consecutive study of post-tonsillectomy haemorrhage.

ORL J Otorhinolaryngol Relat Spec, 71(5), 273–278. doi: 210.1159/000245160. Epub 000242009 Oct 000245110.

Birk, M., Bauerfeind, P., Deprez, P. H., Hafner, M., Hartmann, D., Hassan, C., . . . Meining, A. (2016). Removal of foreign bodies in the upper gastrointestinal tract in adults: European Society of Gastrointestinal Endoscopy (ESGE) Clinical Guideline. *Endoscopy*, 48(5), 489–496. doi: 410.1055/s-0042-100456. Epub 102016 Feb 100410.

Bodkin, R. P., Weant, K. A., Baker Justice, S., Spencer, M. T., & Acquisto, N. M. (2016). Effectiveness of glucagon in relieving esophageal foreign body impaction: a multicenter study. *Am J Emerg Med*, 34(6), 1049–1052. doi: 1010.1016/j.ajem.2016.1003.1016. Epub 2016 Mar 1049.

Brown, P., Ryan, R., Yung, M. et al. (2005) National prospective tonsillectomy audit – final report. London: Royal College of Surgeons of England. Retrieved from www.rcseng.ac.uk/-/media/files/rcs/library-and-publications/non-journal-publications/national-prospective-tonsillectomy-audit-final-report-2005.pdf

Chowdhury, K., Tewfik, T. L., & Schloss, M. D. (1988). Post-tonsillectomy and adenoidectomy hemorrhage. *J Otolaryngol*, 17(1), 46–49.

Dhiwakar, M., Clement, W. A., Supriya, M., & McKerrow, W. (2012). Antibiotics to reduce post-tonsillectomy morbidity. *Cochrane Database Syst Rev*, 12:CD005607.(doi), 10.1002/14651858.CD14005607.pub14651854.

Dunn, C. J., & Goa, K. L. (1999). Tranexamic acid: a review of its use in surgery and other indications. *Drugs*, 57(6), 1005–1032.

Electronic Medicines Compendium. (2015). Hydrogen Peroxide Solution 3% BP 10 Vols. Retrieved from www.medicines.org.uk/emc/medicine/25449

Handler, S. D., Miller, L., Richmond, K. H., & Baranak, C. C. (1986). Post-tonsillectomy hemorrhage: incidence, prevention and management. *Laryngoscope*, 96(11), 1243–1247.

Hope, A., & Lo, S. (2007). Hydrogen peroxide mouthwash in post-tonsillectomy haemorrhage. *Clin Otolaryngol*, 32(3), 218–219.

Ibrahim, N., Chauhan, I., & Nikkar-Esfahani, A. (2016). 'A problematic plum pit in the piping': a case of traumatic oesophageal perforation. *BMJ Case Rep, 2016.* (pii), bcr2015213807. doi: 2015213810.2015211136 /bcr-2015212015-2015213807.

Ikenberry, S. O., Jue, T. L., Anderson, M. A., Appalaneni, V., Banerjee, S., Ben-Menachem, T., . . . Dominitz, J. A. (2011). Management of ingested foreign bodies and food impactions. *Gastrointest Endosc, 73*(6), 1085–1091. doi: 1010.1016/j.gie.2010.1011.1010.

Jacques, T., Nash, R., Kenway, B., & Vlastarakos, P. (2013). Pitfalls of operative management of secondary post-tonsillectomy haemorrhage – a case report. *B-ENT, 9*(4), 335–337.

Joint Formulary Committee. (2016). *British National Formulary.* 72 ed. London: BMJ Group and Pharmaceutical Press.

Karanjia, N. D., & Rees, M. (1993). The use of Coca-Cola in the management of bolus obstruction in benign oesophageal stricture. *Ann R Coll Surg Engl, 75*(2), 94–95.

Karnwal, A., Ho, E. C., Hall, A., & Molony, N. (2008). Lateral soft tissue neck X-rays: are they useful in management of upper aero-digestive tract foreign bodies? *J Laryngol Otol, 122*(8), 845–847. Epub 2007 Aug 2015.

Ker, K., Beecher, D., & Roberts, I. (2013). Topical application of tranexamic acid for the reduction of bleeding. *Cochrane Database Syst Rev*(7), CD010562. doi: 010510.011002/14651858. CD14010562.pub14651852.

Khayyat, Y. M. (2013). Pharmacological management of esophageal food bolus impaction. *Emerg Med Int, 2013:924015.* (doi), 10.1155/2013/924015. Epub 922013 May 924013.

Krishna, P., & Lee, D. (2001). Post-tonsillectomy bleeding: a meta-analysis. *Laryngoscope, 111*(8), 1358–1361.

Kumar, R. (1984). Secondary haemorrhage following tonsillectomy/adenoidectomy. *J Laryngol Otol, 98*(10), 997–998.

Leopard, D., Fishpool, S., & Winter, S. (2011). The management of oesophageal soft food bolus obstruction: a systematic review. *Ann R Coll Surg Engl, 93*(6), 441–444. doi: 410.1308/003588411X003588090.

Loh, K. S., Tan, L. K., Smith, J. D., Yeoh, K. H., & Dong, F. (2000). Complications of foreign bodies in the esophagus. *Otolaryngol Head Neck Surg, 123*(5), 613–616.

Longstreth, G. F., Longstreth, K. J., & Yao, J. F. (2001). Esophageal food impaction: Epidemiology and therapy. A retrospective, observational study. *Gastrointest Endosc, 53*(2), 193–198.

Mahdy, A. M., & Webster, N. R. (2004). Perioperative systemic haemostatic agents. *Br J Anaesth, 93*(6), 842–858. Epub 2004 Jul 2026.

McCaul, M., & Kredo, T. (2016). Antifibrinolytic drugs for acute traumatic injury. *S Afr Med J, 106*(8), 777–778. doi: 710.7196/SAMJ.2016 .v7106i7198.11042.

Medicines and Healthcare Products Regulatory Agency. (2017). Hyoscine butylbromide (Buscopan) injection: risk of serious adverse effects in patients with underlying cardiac disease. Retrieved from www.gov.uk/drug -safety-update/hyoscine-butylbromide-busco pan-injection-risk-of-serious-adverse-effects -in-patients-with-underlying-cardiac-disease

Pai, I., Lo, S., Brown, S., & Toma, A. G. (2005). Does hydrogen peroxide mouthwash improve the outcome of secondary post-tonsillectomy bleed? A 10-year review. *Otolaryngol Head Neck Surg, 133*(2), 202–205.

Park, I. H., Lim, H. K., Song, S. W., & Lee, K. H. (2016). Perforation of esophagus and subsequent mediastinitis following mussel shell ingestion. *J Thorac Dis, 8*(8), E693–697. doi: 610.21037/jtd.22016.21007.21088.

Perel, P., Ker, K., Morales Uribe, C. H., & Roberts, I. (2013). Tranexamic acid for reducing mortality in emergency and urgent surgery. *Cochrane Database Syst Rev* (1), CD010245. doi: 010210.011002/14651858.CD14010245. pub14651852.

Randall, D. A., & Hoffer, M. E. (1998). Complications of tonsillectomy and adenoidectomy. *Otolaryngol Head Neck Surg, 118*(1), 61–68.

Ridder, G. J., Maier, W., Kinzer, S., Teszler, C. B., Boedeker, C. C., & Pfeiffer, J. (2010). Descending necrotizing mediastinitis: contemporary trends in etiology, diagnosis, management, and outcome. *Ann Surg, 251*(3),

528–534. doi: 510.1097/SLA.1090b1013e3181c
1091b1090d1091.

Sandoz Limited. (2015). Tranexamic Acid 500mg
Tablets. Retrieved from www.medicines.org
.uk/emc/medicine/24325

Shimokawa, H., & Matoba, T. (2004). Hydrogen
peroxide as an endothelium-derived hyperpo-
larizing factor. *Pharmacol Res, 49*(6), 543–549.

Stephens, J. C., Georgalas, C., Kyi, M., & Ghufoor,
K. (2008). Is bacterial colonisation of the tonsillar fossa a factor in post-tonsillectomy haemorrhage? *J Laryngol Otol, 122*(4), 383–387. Epub
2007 Apr 2020.

Triadafilopoulos, G., Roorda, A., & Akiyama,
J. (2013). Update on foreign bodies in the
esophagus: diagnosis and management. *Curr
Gastroenterol Rep, 15*(4), 317. doi: 310.1007
/s11894-11013-10317-11895.

Truskaite, K., & Dlugosz, A. (2016). Prevalence
of eosinophilic esophagitis and lymphocytic
esophagitis in adults with esophageal food
bolus impaction. *Gastroenterol Res Pract,
2016:9303858.* (doi), 10.1155/2016/9303858.
Epub 9302016 Jul 9303828.

Tsikoudas, A., Kochillas, X., Kelleher, R. J., & Mills,
R. (2005). The management of acute oesophageal obstruction from a food bolus. Can we be
more conservative? *Eur Arch Otorhinolaryngol,
262*(7), 528–530. Epub 2004 Dec 2009.

Tysome, J. R., & Kanegaonkar, R. (2012). *ENT: An
Introduction and Practical Guide.* London:
Hodder Arnold.

Wilcox, C. M., Alexander, L. N., & Clark, W. S.
(1995). Localization of an obstructing esophageal lesion. Is the patient accurate? *Dig Dis
Sci, 40*(10), 2192–2196.

Windfuhr, J., & Seehafer, M. (2001). Classification
of haemorrhage following tonsillectomy.
J Laryngol Otol, 115(6), 457–461.

Windfuhr, J. P., Schloendorff, G., Baburi, D.,
& Kremer, B. (2008a). Lethal outcome of
post-tonsillectomy hemorrhage. *Eur Arch
Otorhinolaryngol, 265*(12), 1527–1534. doi:
1510.1007/s00405-00008-00699-00404.
Epub 02008 May 00428.

Windfuhr, J. P., Schloendorff, G., Baburi, D., &
Kremer, B. (2008b). Life-threatening post-
tonsillectomy hemorrhage. *Laryngoscope,
118*(8), 1389–1394. doi: 1310.1097/MLG
.1380b1013e3181734f3181737e.

Windfuhr, J. P., Verspohl, B. C., Chen, Y. S.,
Dahm, J. D., & Werner, J. A. (2015). Post-
tonsillectomy hemorrhage – some facts will
never change. *Eur Arch Otorhinolaryngol,
272*(5), 1211–1218. doi: 1210.1007/s00405
-00014-03025-00403. Epub 02014 Apr
00416.

SECTION 3

Emergencies in Otology

12

Acute otitis externa

SIMON A MCKEAN

INTRODUCTION

Otitis externa can be acute or chronic, diffuse or localised, and can be caused by infection, allergy, irritation or inflammation. It includes all inflammatory conditions of the auricle, external ear canal and outer surface of the tympanic membrane. It is a common problem which constitutes one in six new patient referrals and 30 per cent of people seen in an ear, nose and throat (ENT) emergency clinic. There are very few good quality trials of treatment for acute otitis externa.

CLINICAL FEATURES

HISTORY

Acute diffuse otitis externa affects up to 10 per cent of the population at some time in their lives. It generally develops within 48 hours and can last up to 3 weeks. The common symptoms are itching or pain (which can be severe) with variable discharge and a feeling of blockage, with a conductive hearing loss noted due to occlusion of the external canal.

Any chemical or physical irritation (including syringing and cotton bud abuse) can predispose to infection. Any cause of immunosuppression, including diabetes, can be a predisposing factor for otitis externa. Swimming[1] may underlie otitis externa, or 'swimmers' ear'. Any history of skin complaints should be noted. Contact dermatitis, eczema and psoriasis can affect the skin of the external canal. If there is any bony tenderness over the mastoid, or the pinna is protruding, consider mastoiditis as a differential diagnosis.

EXAMINATION

Look for any surrounding cellulitis and/or lymphadenitis. It may be important to demarcate the edge of the cellulitis to monitor treatment. With regards to the external canal, look for tenderness, erythema, oedema or narrowing (Figure 12.1). Obstruction of ear canal may necessitate aural toilette, wick placement or even the use of systemic antimicrobial agents. Examine to ensure there is not currently any foreign body in the ear canal. Cotton buds, hearing aids, middle ear ventilation tubes and even excess ear wax can traumatise the external canal skin, increasing susceptibility to infection.

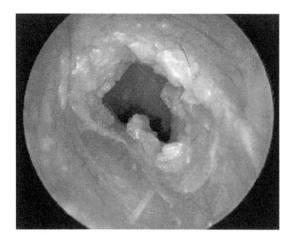

Figure 12.1 Otitis externa.

Look for discharge and note any smell, colour, blood staining, keratin or mucoid element. A green, offensive-smelling discharge may indicate infection with *Pseudomonas aeruginosa*. Fungal hyphae may sometimes be identified. The presence of a mucoid discharge suggests an open middle ear. The tympanic membrane must be fully examined before discharge from clinic, although this may not be possible on the first visit. Look for the presence of grommet, T tube or a tympanic membrane perforation and active middle ear. These may change the management, because of either the primary cause of the problem or its subsequent treatment (i.e. the use of potentially ototoxic medications). Cranial nerves (VII–XII) should be tested, since a palsy, although rare, may indicate deep extension of infection, such as skull base osteomyelitis.

DIFFERENTIAL DIAGNOSES

Other causes of otalgia, otorrhoea and inflammation of the external ear canal should be excluded. It is worth remembering that otalgia is commonly a referred pain from the teeth, tonsils, temporomandibular joint, larynx, neck or even sphenoid sinus. Cranial nerves V, IX and X transmit sensation from the middle and external ear.

Abscesses can develop (furunculosis) in the lateral third of the canal. This leads to severe pain, and the abscesses may rupture or need to be incised

and drained to give relief. (Figure 12.2). They are usually caused by *Staphylococcus aureus*.

Perichondritis in the younger population is often due to piercing of the pinna cartilage and can lead to widespread cellulitis (Figure 12.3). The combination of the crush injury to the cartilage and *Pseudomonas aeruginosa* is likely to be the cause. Relapsing perichondritis is the severe, episodic and progressive inflammation of the cartilage of the ear, nose and tracheobronchial tree, and has an autoimmune pathogenesis.

Myringitis means inflammation of the tympanic membrane. Primary myringitis can be due

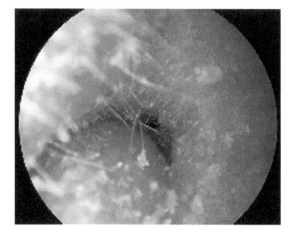

Figure 12.2 Furuncle.

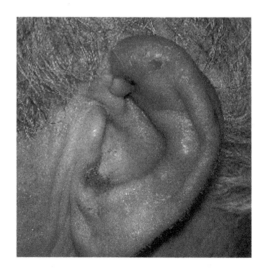

Figure 12.3 Perichondritis.

to trauma, infection or sudden pressure changes. Granular myringitis (Figure 12.4), due to infection, is seen as bubbles filled with blood on the surface of the tympanic membrane that can burst; however, the tympanic membrane itself is not perforated. Secondary myringitis occurs as a result of adjacent inflammation of the middle ear or the external canal. Bullous myringitis (Figure 12.5) is sometimes seen after there has been loss of the epidermal layer of the tympanic membrane.

Herpes zoster oticus consists of severe neuralgic otalgia with cutaneous vesicles and an acute peripheral facial palsy. The vesicles are found on the meatal and pre-auricular skin (Figure 12.6), along the canal itself and sometimes on the soft palate.

Skull base osteomyelitis (misleadingly also termed 'malignant otitis externa') is a rare but dangerous extension of infection into the mastoid and temporal

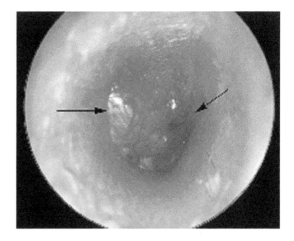

Figure 12.5 Myringitis – bullous.

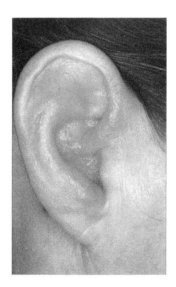

Figure 12.6 Zoster otitis.

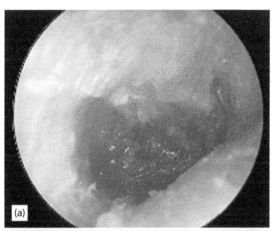

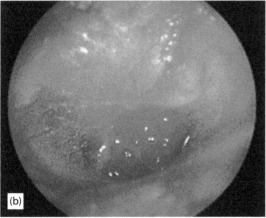

Figure 12.4 (a and b) Myringitis – granular.

bones. It is more common in immunocompromised patients, such as the elderly diabetic, and is often caused by Gram negative bacilli such as *Pseudomonas aeruginosa*. The patients often have severe deep otalgia and may develop cranial nerve palsies. Skull base osteomyelitis is diagnosed by high-definition computed tomography (CT) or magnetic resonance imaging (MRI) scans of the temporal bones. Isotope bone scans may also be useful. Treatment is with long courses of appropriate antibiotics, which may need to be given intravenously. Unfortunately, resistance of *Pseudomonas aeruginosa* to ciprofloxacin is now being reported, and this will have a significant

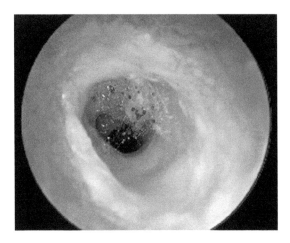

Figure 12.7 Otomycosis.

impact on the management of these patients. These patients also need nutrition, blood sugar control (if diabetic) and analgesia. (See Chapter 13.)

Benign necrotising otitis externa is also rare and is characterised by itching and pain with a variable discharge. Examination reveals focal bone exposure in the canal with minimal surrounding inflammation.

Keratosis obturans, which is of unknown aetiology, is characterized by a large amount of cerumen and keratin filling a ballooned external ear canal, which produces otalgia, otorrhoea and conductive hearing loss. It is usually bilateral and leads to erosion of the external canal.

Chronic otitis externa causes a continued sensation of itch with mild discomfort. It may be caused by repeated trauma, repeated exposure to infection (i.e. from an open middle ear), inadequate aural toilette, allergy, irritation or otomycosis.

Otomycosis (Figure 12.7) is most commonly caused by *Aspergillus* or *Candida* species. It is best treated by repeated careful microsuction and topical antifungals for no less than 2 weeks.

Neoplasms of the external canal skin are rare, but any non-healing ulcer should be biopsied.

TREATMENT

Aural toilette (especially to clear anterior recess)[2] may be treatment enough and is necessary for

diagnosis and visualisation of the tympanic membrane to exclude perforation.

Instillation of 3 per cent hydrogen peroxide (H_2O_2) can be useful to help clear the external canal but is recommended only if the tympanic membrane is intact. Previously, it was commonly used in the cleaning of open wounds. It helps with both the mechanical, physical clearance of debris and also has oxidising, antimicrobial effects. Although it is not ototoxic if used for brief periods in the middle ear, it does form a significant volume of gas. This could cause problems in the confines of the middle ear.

Analgesia is important. Pain symptoms are often overlooked but must be addressed and managed by appropriate analgesia, which may necessitate admission to hospital.

Topical antibacterial medications should be used for the initial treatment of diffuse, uncomplicated acute otitis externa. A systematic review concluded that topical antimicrobial therapy is highly effective for acute otitis externa, with clinical cure rates of 65–80 per cent within 10 days.[3] Remember that neomycin does not cover *Pseudomonas aeruginosa*, which is a common pathogen in otitis externa. It is also clear that aminoglycosides have measurable vestibulotoxic and ototoxic effects. Fluroquinolones (e.g. ciprofloxacin or ofloxacin) do not pose these threats and will treat both *Pseudomonas aeruginosa* and *Staphylococcus aureus*. Metronidazole gel can be useful if there is an otitis externa where anaerobes have been cultured.

In difficult cases a broad therapeutic approach may need to be taken. Tri-AdCortyl ointment contains steroid, neomycin and gramicidin and also an antifungal medication. After thorough microsuction, this ointment or similar combinations can be instilled into the ear canal and left until the next appointment. There is no clear therapeutic 'best option' for topical antibiotics in otitis externa.

Topical steroid drops alone may be useful for patients that have inflammation secondary solely to allergy or sensitisation rather than infection.

Topical antifungal drops such as clotrimazole solution should be combined with regular aural toilette.

Patients should be shown how to effectively insert ear drops. If possible, an assistant should administer the drops while the patient is lying on their side. The patient should remain in this position for 5 minutes. The anti-tragus can be gently massaged to encourage drops deeper into the canal. Topical acetic acid 2 per cent spray is often used as first line treatment in a primary care setting, as it has both antifungal and antibacterial action. It can be bought without prescription in the UK.

Patients are often advised to keep the ear dry. Cotton wool with petroleum jelly may be effective in keeping the ear dry while showering.

Patients should be advised not to scratch the ear or use cotton buds.[4] Any trauma to the skin can reduce its protective ability, therefore allowing initiation or extension of infection.

An external ear canal wick, such as the Pope otowick (Xomed), expands into the canal, improving delivery of topical medicines. Glycerine and ichthamol impregnated ribbon gauze has a hygroscopic effect to reduce canal oedema and good antibacterial effect against *Staphylococcus aureus* and *Streptococcus pyogenes*, but not *Pseudomonas aeruginosa*. 'Glyc and Ic' ribbon is a cheap option that may be useful for those with allergies to pharmaceutical carriers in drops or those who cannot manage to use drops effectively. Topical aluminium acetate drops are as effective as antibiotic drops but are expensive, difficult to obtain and need to be freshly prepared. They can be useful in diffuse, chronic disease.

Systemic antibiotics are unnecessary unless there is extension outside the ear canal, immunosuppression or local factors that hinder the delivery of topical preparations.

INVESTIGATIONS

Ear swabs are not routinely taken at a first appointment, but for treatment failures or chronic cases[5] they might be helpful. The most commonly identified pathogens in a UK series were *Pseudomonas aeruginosa*, followed by *Staphylococcus aureus*, anaerobes, *Streptococcus* species, *Candida* species and *Aspergillus* species. Blood glucose testing may reveal previously undiagnosed diabetes mellitus. Potential allergens and irritants include neomycin, benzalkonium chloride, propylene glycol and hearing aid mould materials. Up to one-third of patients may develop[6] sensitivity to either the carriers

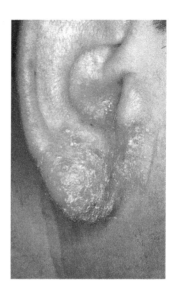

Figure 12.8 Contact dermatitis.

(i.e. propylene glycol) or the antibiotics themselves (i.e. neomycin). Nickel jewellery can cause sensitivity reactions. Also, household chemicals such as hairsprays or perfumes can be irritant (Figure 12.8). In chronic or recurrent disease, involvement of dermatologists may be beneficial, to perform contact allergy testing and to advise on further topical treatments.

KEY LEARNING POINTS

- Preventative measures should include avoiding both mechanical trauma and water ingress.
- Aural toilet is a cornerstone of treatment.
- Topical antibiotics are of benefit.
- Choice of topical antibiotic drop shows little difference in resolution of symptoms, except in the case of microbial resistance, and with the increased recognition of *Pseudomonas aeruginosa* infection, the topical use of quinolones is likely to be important.
- Remember potential allergens and the possibility of fungal infection in those ears that have already had prolonged treatment.

- Patients may have significant pain that needs to be managed.
- Effective delivery of medication is important; microsuction and the use of an ear wick can be beneficial.
- Intravenous antibiotics may be necessary.

REFERENCES

1. Springer GL, Shapiro ED. Fresh water swimming as a risk factor for otitis externa: a case control study. *Archives of Environmental Health*. 1985; 40(4): 202–6.
2. Sander R. Otitis externa: a practical guide to treatment and prevention. *American Family Physician*. 2001; 63(5): 927–36.
3. Rosenfeld RM, Singer M, Wasserman JM, Stinnett SS. Systematic review of topical antimicrobial therapy for acute otitis externa. *Otolaryngology – Head and Neck Surgery*. 2006; 134(4 Suppl): S24–48.
4. Yelland M. Otitis externa in general practice. *Medical Journal of Australia*. 1992; 156(5): 325–26.
5. Bluestone C, Casselbrandt M, Dohar J. *Targeted Therapies in Otitis Media and Otitis Externa*. Hamilton, Ontario: BC Decker, 2003.
6. Rasmussen PA. Otitis externa and allergic contact dermatitis. *Acta Otolaryngologica*. 1974; 77(5): 344–7.

13

Skull base osteomyelitis

STEPHEN JONES

INTRODUCTION

Osteomyelitis of the lateral skull base may be divided into two main conditions: necrotising (or malignant) otitis externa (NOE) and petrous apicitis (also known as Gradenigo's syndrome). NOE is much rarer than otitis externa, but should be considered in patients who have been diagnosed with otitis externa who fail to resolve, particularly those who fit the typical demographic group described in this chapter. Petrous apicitis is rarer still. Both conditions have the potential to cause significant disability or mortality and so it is important to consider the diagnosis and treat them appropriately as soon as possible.

NECROTISING OTITIS EXTERNA (NOE)

DEFINITION

NOE is infection of the external auditory meatus and neighbouring temporal bone, which may spread through the fissures of Santorini and osseocartilagenous junction to involve the rest of the temporal bone and jugular foramen. It most commonly affects older patients with diabetes or those who are immunocompromised in some way.

SYMPTOMS

The typical presentation is with ear discharge and severe otalgia, which is much worse than expected from clinical findings. If this picture is seen in the group of patients described earlier, or if appropriate treatment for otitis externa fails to resolve the infection, then the diagnosis should be considered.

SIGNS

Signs are oedematous, inflamed ear canal skin; discharge; and granulations arising from the ear canal (Figure 13.1). There may also be focal bone exposure in the ear canal. In the later stages, facial palsy, diplopia and lower cranial nerve palsies may be seen.

BACTERIOLOGY

NOE is most commonly caused by *Pseudomonas aeruginosa*. It may also be caused by other bacteria, including *Staphylococcus aureus*, *E. coli*, *Proteus mirabilis* and fungal species.

INVESTIGATIONS

Swabs should be taken from the ear canal to identify the causative organism. Various imaging modalities have a role to play in NOE. Some are useful in initial diagnosis and others for monitoring progress of treatment.

Computed tomography

CT will show bony erosion and thickening of the skin of the external ear canal (Figure 13.2). Often the ear canal and temporomandibular joint are involved initially, but all parts of the temporal bone may be affected. These changes would not be found in simple otitis externa. Erosion may extend

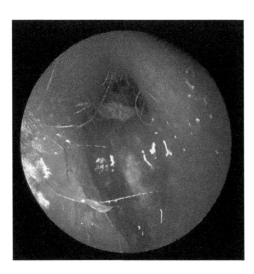

Figure 13.1 Endoscopic clinical photograph of typical granulations seen in the floor of the external auditory canal in NOE. http://eac.hawkelibrary .com/new/main.php?g2_itemId=353

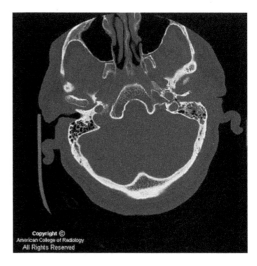

Figure 13.2 Axial CT scan of the temporal bones on bony windows demonstrating irregularity of the surface of the mastoid. http://neuroradiologyon thenet.blogspot.co.uk/2007/04/malignant-otitis -externa.html

inferiorly to involve the stylomastoid foramen or medially into the middle ear.

Magnetic resonance imaging

MRI may be useful for demonstration of the degree of soft tissue involvement. It is not generally used in NOE as commonly as other imaging modalities.

Technetium 99m scintigraphy

Technetium may be used in the diagnosis of NOE. Increased uptake will be seen in bone involved in the condition. These areas will remain apparent on scanning in the longer term, after infection has been successfully treated, and this investigation is not, therefore, useful in the monitoring of treatment.

Gallium 67 scintigraphy

Gallium scanning may be used for monitoring of treatment, as improvement correlates with resolution of the condition. It is less useful in initial diagnosis, as it is less specific than other imaging modalities. A baseline Gallium scan may be carried out for comparison with later studies to demonstrate successful treatment (Figure 13.3).

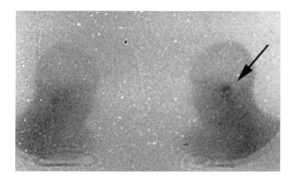

Figure 13.3 Gallium citrate Ga 67 scintigraphy in a 74-year-old male patient with diabetes mellitus and left-sided NOE. The left temporal bone shows enhanced uptake of ^{67}Ga (arrow). Taken from Handzel O, Halperin D. Necrotizing (malignant) external otitis. *American Family Physician*. 2003 68(2): 309–312.

DIFFERENTIAL DIAGNOSIS

The condition shares symptoms and signs with otitis externa, cholesteatoma and squamous cell carcinoma of the external auditory meatus. Some of these conditions may be excluded by examination or scanning, but biopsy may be required to ensure squamous cell carcinoma is excluded.

MANAGEMENT

CONSERVATIVE

As pain is a major feature in this condition, it is important that analgesia is given. Opiates are often needed and patients may need to remain in hospital to achieve good pain control.

Most commonly, systemic and topical ciprofloxacin is used due to the most likely bacteriology. If swabs suggest an alternative, antibacterial or antifungal may be required. Prolonged courses of treatment are required due to bone involvement. Generally, at least 6 weeks treatment is required. As the bioavailability of oral ciprofloxacin is good, it is not necessary to use intravenous antibiotics in patients who require it, meaning that they do not need to remain in hospital for prolonged periods for intravenous antibiotics. In diabetic patients it is essential that good diabetic control is achieved.

SURGICAL

Where conservative management is not successful, debridement of affected bone and grafting of exposed areas with soft tissue may be necessary. Biopsy may also be required to exclude squamous cell carcinoma in cases which fail to respond to conservative management or where there is doubt about the diagnosis.

HYPERBARIC OXYGEN

Hyperbaric oxygen therapy may have benefit in addition to antimicrobials, but evidence for this is limited.

COMPLICATIONS

The complications of NOE include some of the conditions described as presenting signs, such as facial palsy and lower cranial nerve palsies, which may go on to cause aspiration pneumonia and where untreated or diagnosed late may lead to death.

PETROUS APICITIS/ GRADENIGO'S SYNDROME

DEFINITION

Petrous apicitis is usually seen as a complication of acute otitis media (AOM) or mastoiditis, where the apex of the petrous temporal bone becomes involved by the infection. It is rare in comparison to many of the other complications of AOM.

SYMPTOMS AND SIGNS

Patients generally have the typical features of the preceding condition with otorrhoea, systemic upset and possibly swelling behind the affected ear, but will also have diplopia, due to lateral rectus palsy on the same side, and trigeminal nerve involvement causing periorbital pain on the affected side. It is seen more commonly in children than in adults.

BACTERIOLOGY

As would be expected in a complication of AOM, the bacteriological cause is often similar. This includes *Streptococcus pneumoniae*, *Streptococcus pyogenes*, *Haemophilus influenzae*, *Staphylococcus aureus* and *Psuedomonas* species. Specimens may be obtained from ear discharge or aspiration from the middle ear by myringotomy.

INVESTIGATIONS

Computed tomography

CT scanning in petrous apicitis (Figure 13.4) will demonstrate lysis of bone at the apex of the petrous temporal bone and opacification of air cells in

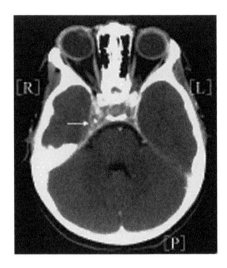

Figure 13.4 Axial CT scan image. Arrow indicates thrombosis of the right cavernous sinus. Taken from Successful prolonged conservative treatment of Gradenigo's syndrome in a 4-year-old girl: A case report and literature review. *International Journal of Pediatric Otorhinolaryngology* 2011 Extra, 6(2): 100–103.

the area, if present. If contrast is used, peripheral enhancement will also be seen. CT may also demonstrate any other infective complications, such as intracranial abscesses.

Magnetic resonance imaging

Similar to NOE, MRI will demonstrate soft tissue involvement in infection, such as meningeal inflammation surrounding the petrous apex (Figure 13.5).

Radioisotope Scanning

In petrous apicitis the apex of the temporal will demonstrate high uptake. This imaging modality is less commonly used compared to CT and MRI.

DIFFERENTIAL DIAGNOSIS

Patients with petrous apicitis will have a history of otalgia or ear discharge prior to the onset of squint. Other intracranial complications of infection spreading from the middle ear or

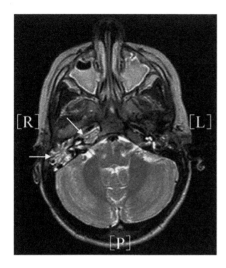

Figure 13.5 Axial T2 weighted MRI image. Hypersignal of the right mastoid and petrous apex indicated by the arrows. Taken from *Successful prolonged conservative treatment of Gradenigo's syndrome in a 4-year-old girl: A case report and literature review. International Journal of Pediatric Otorhinolaryngology* 2011 Extra, 6(2): 100–103.

mastoid may possibly cause lateral rectus palsy, although a solitary palsy without other complications would be rare in any other related cause. Imaging should differentiate between these differential diagnoses.

MANAGEMENT

Due to bony involvement, it is necessary to treat with an appropriate systemic antibiotic in the long term (generally 6 weeks). Topical antibiotics may also be used to treat ear discharge while present. Surgical drainage is often required, particularly if the condition occurs as a complication of acute mastoiditis. In most cases, the procedure of petrous apicectomy requires a translabyrinthine approach to the apex, which will cause complete loss of hearing and vestibular function on the affected side. It is sometimes possible to obtain drainage of the petrous apex via the mastoid without hearing loss if the temporal bone is well pneumatised. An extradural middle fossa approach to the petrous apex is also possible and

may allow access to the region without injury to the cochlea and vestibule, and preservation of the hearing and balance.

COMPLICATIONS

Complications are meningitis, intracranial abscess, involvement of lower cranial nerves, pre-vertebral or parapharyngeal abscess and carotid sympathetic sheath involvement. The condition may be fatal.

KEY LEARNING POINTS

- Osteomyelitis of the lateral skull base is a rare condition which is important due to the potentially serious consequences of failure to recognise and treat it.
- Both main conditions require early diagnosis and aggressive treatment to avoid permanent neurological deficits and mortality.

FURTHER READING

Acharya A, Reid A. Acute otitis media. In: Hussain SM, editor. *Logan Turner's Diseases of the Nose, Throat and Ear: Head and Neck Surgery.* Boca Raton, Florida, USA: CRC Press; 2016. pp. 403–409.

Gruber M, Roitman A, Doweck I, Uri N, Shaked-Mishan P, Kolop-Feldman A, Cohen-Kerem R. Clinical utility of a polymerase chain reaction assay in culture-negative necrotizing otitis externa. *Otology & Neurotology* 2015 36(4): 733–736.

Isaacson B, Mirabal C, Kutz JW, Lee KH, Roland PS. Pediatric otogenic intracranial abscesses. *Otolaryngology – Head and Neck Surgery* 2010 142: 434–437.

McKean SA, Hussain SM. Otitis externa. In: Hussain SM, editor. *Logan Turner's Diseases of the Nose, Throat and Ear: Head and Neck Surgery.* Boca Raton, Florida, USA: CRC Press; 2016. pp. 507–511.

Morrison G. Acute otitis media and mastoiditis. In: Hussain SM, editor. *Logan Turner's Diseases of the Nose, Throat and Ear: Head and Neck Surgery.* Boca Raton, Florida, USA: CRC Press; 2016. pp. 595–607.

Phillips JS, Jones SEM. Hyperbaric oxygen as an adjuvant treatment for malignant otitis externa. *Cochrane Database Systematic Reviews* 2005(2): CD004617.

Spielmann PM, Hussain SM. Diseases of the external ear. In: Hussain SM, editor. *Logan Turner's Diseases of the Nose, Throat and Ear: Head and Neck Surgery.* Boca Raton, Florida, USA: CRC Press; 2016. pp. 395–401.

Sudarshan SM. ENT head and neck radiology. In: Hussain SM, editor. *Logan Turner's Diseases of the Nose, Throat and Ear: Head and Neck Surgery.* Boca Raton, Florida, USA: CRC Press; 2016. pp. 659–690.

14

Acute otitis media

ALEX BENNETT

ANATOMY OF THE MIDDLE EAR CLEFT

The middle ear cleft encompasses the tympanic cavity, the Eustachian tube medially and the mastoid air cell system posteriorly. The roof of the tympanic cavity is the tegmen tympani: a thin plate of bone separating the middle ear cleft from the middle fossa of the cranium. It is continuous posteriorly with the tegmen mastoideum, which separates the middle cranial fossa from the mastoid air cell system. The petrosquamous suture line runs through the roof of the tympanic cavity. This suture only closes in adulthood, thereby providing a route for infection to access the extradural space in children. Veins draining the tympanic cavity into the superior petrosal sinus also run through this suture line and can provide a further pathway of access for infection. The posterior wall of the tympanic cavity is the aditus ad antrum – a large, irregular opening from the epitympanum anteriorly into the mastoid antrum posteriorly. The mastoid antrum communicates posteriorly with the mastoid air cell system; the outer wall of the mastoid air cell system is easily palpable behind the pinna, just below the skin. MacEwen's triangle is a direct lateral relation to the mastoid antrum.

EPIDEMIOLOGY AND PATHOLOGY

'Acute otitis media' (AOM) describes a viral or bacterial infection of the middle ear and mastoid air cell system which results in mucosal inflammation, is associated with a middle ear effusion and results in a variable collection of symptoms and signs. It is one of the most common illnesses in childhood, with a peak incidence between 6 and 18 months. 70% of children have had an episode by 2 years old and 90% by 6 years old. Episodes usually occur in autumn and winter when the causative viruses and bacteria are more prevalent.

Cases can be divided into four subgroups:

1. Sporadic – infrequent, isolated events commonly associated with upper respiratory tract infection
2. Resistant – persistence of middle ear infection beyond a short course (3–5 days) of antibiotic treatment
3. Persistent – persistence or recurrence of symptoms or signs of AOM within 6 days of completing a course of antibiotics
4. Recurrent – ≥3 episodes in 6 months, ≥ 4–6 episodes in 12 months

Recurrent AOM occurs in 20% of patients with AOM and has been reported in 5% of children under 2 years of age, with 25% of children who have their first episode of AOM before 9 months of age going on to develop recurrent acute otitis media.

The majority of episodes of AOM may be associated with viral infection. The typical respiratory tract viruses are respiratory syncytial virus (RSV), influenza A virus, parainfluenza viruses, adenoviruses and rhinovirus. Commonly identified bacterial pathogens include *Haemophilus Influenzae, Streptococcus* species, *Moraxella catarrhalis* and *Staphylococcus aureus*.

The route of access of pathogens to the middle ear cleft is variable. Direct access may be acquired from the nasopharynx via the Eustachian tube, although deposition in the middle ear cleft from the bloodstream may also be implicated. A third route of access is from the external auditory canal via a perforation or ventilation tube – this is most commonly associated with water exposure. Viral infection adversely affects Eustachian tube function through the release of inflammatory mediators, a reduction in the number of ciliated epithelial cells and an increase in mucus production. This contributes to the development of a negative middle ear pressure and consequently AOM. Viral infection also adversely affects host immunity, increasing susceptibility to bacterial infection; consequently, a viral upper respiratory tract infection may lead to a bacterial AOM. Bacterial adherence to nasopharyngeal epithelium may be increased by certain viruses – i.e. the development of biofilms which predispose to resistant, persistent and recurrent AOM.

RISK FACTORS FOR ACUTE OTITIS MEDIA

There is increasing evidence that genetic factors play a role in the risk of an individual patient developing AOM. Racial differences, in particular in relation to the shape, size and patency of the Eustachian tube, have been demonstrated with increased prevalence amongst American Indians, Eskimos and Australian Aboriginals. The influence of genetics on the immune mechanism also accounts for these variations, particularly immune deficiencies associated with low IgG2 subclasses. Atopy and maternal blood group A have also been associated with an increased risk of developing AOM.

Environmental factors are important, as it may be possible to influence these and thus reduce a patient's risk of developing AOM. Low socioeconomic status, particularly poor housing and overcrowding, is associated with an increased incidence of AOM. Day-care attendance, use of a pacifier and passive smoke exposure are all associated with an increased risk of AOM. Breastfeeding for 3 months confers protection against AOM.

Specific syndromes, particularly those associated with craniofacial anomalies or skull base abnormalities, are known to predispose to chronic otitis media, but whether this increases the risk of AOM is less clear. Patients with Down's syndrome and Turner's syndrome suffer more frequent episodes of AOM.

HISTORY AND EXAMINATION

Patients typically present with localizing ear symptoms including otalgia, hearing loss and possible otorrhoea. These usually follow an upper respiratory tract infection. There may also be symptoms suggestive of a more generalised systemic illness such as fever or irritability, and in children, the presence of poor feeding, vomiting, ear pulling and clumsiness. Diagnosis on the basis of history alone is difficult because the condition occurs most commonly in children who may not be able to give an appropriate history; some children may have no ear symptoms, and a large proportion may remain apyrexial throughout the episode.

Otoscopy can be particularly difficult in children; however, if a view of the tympanic membrane is achieved, this typically appears injected and bulging, indicating inflammation and fluid in the middle ear, which is under pressure (as in Figure 14.1). Mucopus in the middle ear gives the tympanic membrane a yellowish appearance. There may be evidence of mucopus in the middle ear if the tympanic membrane has spontaneously perforated, or if a ventilation tube is in situ.

Acute otitis media can be associated with intracranial, intratemporal and extratemporal complications. The incidence of such complications in adults in developed countries is estimated to be up to 2 per 100,000 population per year; the incidence of complications in children under 2 years old is 3 times higher. The incidence of intracranial complication developing in a patient admitted with otitis media is about 0.3%.

The most common complication in children, occurring in up to 10% of cases, is tympanic membrane perforation. This is commonly associated with a reduction in the degree of otalgia. Most heal spontaneously within 3 months, although a proportion of patients develop chronic perforations,

which may predispose to recurrent AOM, particularly in association with water exposure.

The most common complication in adults is acute mastoiditis; while it is a relatively common complication in adults, the incidence of AOM in adults is significantly lower than that in children, and acute mastoiditis is consequently predominantly a disease of childhood. There are four defined classes of mastoiditis:

1. Mucosal inflammation of the mastoid cavity which is visualised radiologically but not associated with the other signs that are typically associated with mastoiditis: this is not strictly a complication of AOM.
2. Acute mastoiditis with periosteitis: infection spreads through the cortex of the mastoid bone by emissary veins to involve the periosteum. The result is a full post-auricular crease, anterior deflection of the pinna and erythema, tenderness (typically over MacEwen's triangle, palpated through the conchal bowl) and mild swelling of the post-auricular region.
3. Acute mastoid osteitis: this is associated with breakdown of mastoid air cells and bone, and a sub-periosteal abscess may result. Development of zygomatic (Luc's) or cervical (Bezold's or Citelli's) abscesses may also occur.
4. Subacute ('masked') mastoiditis: this may occur in incompletely treated AOM after 10–14 days. Otalgia and systemic signs such as fever may persist, but there is an absence of the postauricular signs that are typically associated with mastoiditis. While seemingly benign, this stage must be considered and excluded, as it too can progress to serious complications.

Other complications, illustrated in Figure 14.2, include:

- Intracranial
  - Cerebritis
  - Extradural, subdural or intracranial abscess
  - Sigmoid sinus thrombosis
  - Otitic hydrocephalus
- Intratemporal
  - Labyrinthitis – due to round window permeability to bacterial toxins, resulting in vertigo and sensorineural hearing loss

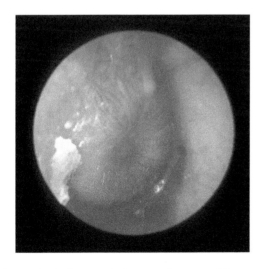

Figure 14.1 Otoscopic image of acute otitis media. Michael Hawke MD (Own work) [CC BY 4.0 (creativecommons.org/licenses/by/4.0)], via Wikimedia Commons.

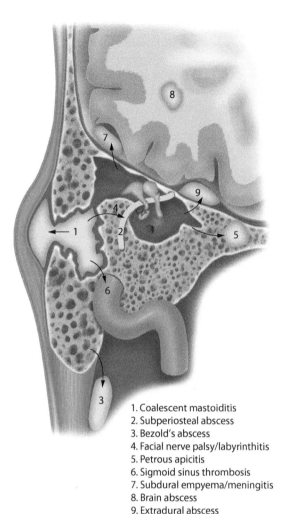

1. Coalescent mastoiditis
2. Subperiosteal abscess
3. Bezold's abscess
4. Facial nerve palsy/labyrinthitis
5. Petrous apicitis
6. Sigmoid sinus thrombosis
7. Subdural empyema/meningitis
8. Brain abscess
9. Extradural abscess

Figure 14.2 Complications of acute otitis media.

- Gradenigo's syndrome – Abducens nerve palsy, severe pain in the distribution of the trigeminal nerve, middle ear discharge/otorrhoea

INVESTIGATIONS

Tympanometry can be used to confirm the presence of fluid in the middle ear, but is not usually available for the assessment of patients presenting acutely.

A sample of pus is useful for microbiological culture, particularly in cases resistant to first line medical therapy or when complications of AOM have occurred. Microbiological culture often fails to demonstrate a specific bacterial growth, suggesting that in many cases middle ear inflammation persists beyond eradication of the primary organism. Nasopharyngeal swabbing for bacterial culture has a weak correlation with middle ear pathogens and is not recommended clinically.

In severe or complicated cases, blood tests, including full blood count, inflammatory markers (such as CRP) and blood cultures are indicated.

Where complications of acute otitis media are suspected to have occurred, a high resolution CT scan of the temporal bones (and neck, if required) with contrast is indicated, as it may demonstrate osteitis, abscess formation and intracranial complications. The timing of this investigation is guided by the clinical status of the patient. Imaging is also indicated in patients who fail to improve on antibiotic therapy.

ACUTE MANAGEMENT OF ACUTE OTITIS MEDIA

MEDICAL

The natural history of AOM is spontaneous resolution – otalgia settles in the majority of patients within 24 hours. Analgesia and antipyretic administration with paracetamol and NSAID may be all that is required.

A recent Cochrane review found antibiotics had no effect on pain between 3 and 7 or 11 and 14 days. Antibiotics also made no difference in the hearing loss at 4 weeks, rate of perforations or late AOM recurrence, while increasing the risk of antibiotic resistance. Antibiotics may, however, reduce the rate of mastoiditis. Antibiotics appeared to be of most benefit in children under 2 years of age with bilateral infection, with cochlear implants, Down's syndrome, cleft palate or immunodeficiency, or older children with a discharging ear. In others, an antibiotic prescription maybe delayed until symptoms persist beyond 4 days with no improvement.

The choice of antibiotic is governed by local microbiological protocol. A broad-spectrum antibiotic that covers the commonly encountered pathogens (e.g. amoxicillin or a macrolide such as clarithromycin) would be appropriate as a first line choice. Antibiotic resistance is increasing, however, necessitating the increased use of higher treatment doses or the use of antimicrobials capable of eradicating beta-lactamase producing bacteria.

SURGICAL

A myringotomy may be performed under local or general anaesthesia to reduce otalgia and provide a sample of pus for microbiological culture. This is particularly necessary in high-risk patients (e.g. immunocompromised), in those that have failed to respond to conventional treatment, in patients who are seriously unwell or where an intra-temporal or intra-cranial complication has occurred. A ventilation tube may be inserted to allow continued drainage and ventilation of the middle ear space. In adults, local anaesthesia can be achieved by the application of a topical anaesthetic such as 5% EMLA cream or 2% Xylocaine spray. In children and adults unable to tolerate a local anaesthetic, a general anaesthetic may be required. The presence of complications is also an indication for surgical drainage. Management of the complications of AOM may necessitate the involvement of other specialties (e.g. neurosurgery for intracranial complications, physicians/paediatricians for meningitis). Acute mastoiditis without abscess formation (class 2) is successfully treated in 75% of cases by high dose intravenous antibiotics and myringotomy (with or without ventilation tube insertion). Failure to improve or progression to class 3 necessitates drainage of the abscess. Drainage of the sub-periosteal abscess, myringotomy and ventilation tube insertion can usually be achieved; however, a cortical mastoidectomy can be challenging for the less experienced surgeon, as granulations make identification of landmarks difficult, and the facial nerve is relatively superficial in the young child. Where spontaneous rupture of the tympanic membrane has occurred, patients should be encouraged to keep their ears dry. The majority of such perforations will heal spontaneously within 3 months – appropriate follow-up is advisable to ascertain whether closure has occurred.

MANAGEMENT OF INTRA-TEMPORAL COMPLICATIONS

GRADENIGO'S SYNDROME (PETROUS APICITIS)

This rare complication may be due to medial spread of infection along the temporal bone or abscess formation at the petrous apex. Prolonged intravenous antibiotic therapy is required, and if a fluid collection is evident on CT scanning, transmastoid drainage should be undertaken to relieve pressure on the nervous structures. Traditionally, translabyrinthine approaches were undertaken, but function-preserving approaches avoiding the otic capsule are now preferred if technically possible. This topic is covered in more details in Chapter 13 (Skull Base Osteomyelitis).

LABYRINTHITIS

Intra-labyrinthine extension of infection can occur via the round window and will result in vertigo and sensorineural hearing loss. Appropriate intravenous antibiotic therapy, myringotomy and ventilation tube insertion are required. Vestibular sedatives followed by vestibular rehabilitation exercises will be required to address the vestibular loss. Hearing loss may be complete, so rehabilitation depends on the functional loss and status of the contralateral ear.

MANAGEMENT OF INTRACRANIAL COMPLICATIONS

This is covered in depth in Chapter 19 (Intracranial Emergencies Related to the Ear).

KEY LEARNING POINTS

- Otitis media is most commonly of viral aetiology and needs supportive treatment only.
- Antibiotics should be reserved for specific indications and are not required in otherwise healthy adults or children with a short duration of symptoms.
- Myringotomy +/− ventilation tube insertion is useful to relieve symptoms, culture the middle ear pus and manage certain complications of AOM.
- The most common complication of AOM is acute mastoiditis, which can be treated with intravenous antibiotics until abscess formation is suspected, when surgical drainage is required.

FURTHER READING

Kangsanarak J, Navacharoen N, Fooanant S, Ruckphaopunt K. Intracranial complications of suppurative otitis media: 13 years' experience. *Am J Otol.* 1995;16(1):104–9.

Leskinen K, Jero J. Acute complications of otitis media in adults. *Clinical Otolaryngology.* 2005;30:511–16.

National Institute for Health and Care Excellence. Clinical Knowledge Summaries: Otitis Media – acute. Retrieved from cks.nice.org.uk/otitis-media-acute. Last updated: July 2015.

Proctor B. The development of the middle ear spaces and their surgical significance. *Journal of Otolaryngology.* 1964;78:631–49.

Tawfik KO, Ishman SL, Altaye M, Meinzen-Derr J, Choo DI. Pediatric acute otitis media in the era of pneumococcal vaccination. *Otolaryngol Head Neck Surg.* 2017;156(5):938–45.

15

Acute vertigo

RAHUL KANEGAONKAR AND MAX WHITTAKER

INTRODUCTION

Dizziness and vertigo are common symptoms. Epidemiological studies have shown that vertigo and balance disorders affect 30 per cent of the general population before the age of 65 years, rising to 60 per cent at 85 years.[1] Annually, 5 out of every 1000 patients present to their general practitioner complaining of symptoms classified as vertigo, with another 10 per 1000 with symptoms of dizziness or giddiness. In the elderly population, a balance disorder may result in falls, a leading cause of death in this age group.

PERIPHERAL VESTIBULAR SYSTEM

Each peripheral vestibular system consists of five confluent fluid-filled chambers: three semicircular canals responsible for the detection of angular acceleration, and the utricle and saccule for linear acceleration (horizontal and vertical, respectively). The neuroepithelium of the sensory patches, the maculae, of the utricle and saccule consist of elaborately arranged hair cells that project into a fibrocalcareous plate, the otoconial membrane. As this membrane is denser than the surrounding endolymph, head movement results in hair cell deflection and depolarisation. The maculae of the semicircular canals are confined to a crest within the dilated segment of each canal, the ampulla. Hair cells project into a gelatinous mass, the cupula, which is deflected as a result of head rotation. The semicircular canals function in pairs, with the two lateral, and posterior and contralateral anterior canals working in tandem, resulting in an increased firing rate in one semicircular canal and reduced firing rate of its counterpart. This allows gaze stabilisation on head rotation and is the basis of the vestibular-ocular reflex. Pathology affecting any part of this complex system can result in vertigo.

ASSESSMENT OF THE ACUTELY DIZZY PATIENT

The history is the most important aspect in assessing an individual with acute vertigo. A description of the symptom should be elicited – vertigo being a sensation of motion, such as spinning, falling or lateral movement. Associated features are important to elicit and can point towards a diagnosis. Visual or sensory aura may suggest a migrainous phenomenon, hearing loss or tinnitus, or aural pressure may suggest Ménière's disease. Neurological symptoms such as dysphasia, dysarthria or loss of consciousness prompt a central neurological diagnosis and must be referred and investigated appropriately. Palpitations, chest pain or syncope suggest a cardiovascular cause and, again, should be referred and investigated appropriately. If the acute vertigo has been recurring in episodes, an important diagnostic factor is the

duration of events: Vertigo lasting for seconds to a minute would suggest benign paroxysmal positional vertigo (BPPV), a few hours would suggest Ménière's disease, and several hours to days would suggest an acute peripheral vestibular loss. Each diagnosis is considered in more detail in the following sections.

A thorough neurotological examination is required: spontaneous and evoked nystagmus must be identified, preferably using Frenzel lenses to remove visual fixation suppression. Nystagmus can be a challenging sign to assess without Frenzel lenses, but specific characteristics of this sign may be essential in differentiating between a peripheral and central aetiology (note Table 15.1). A cranial nerve examination, assessment of smooth pursuit and conjugate eye movements can all point towards a central cause if abnormal. A head impulse test can identify catch-up saccades and suggest the site of a peripheral lesion. A Dix–Hallpike test is important to identify BPPV; otoscopy is important to identify middle ear disease.

INVESTIGATIONS

A pure tone audiogram is required in every patient with vertigo. A magnetic resonance imaging (MRI) scan is required if a central cause is suspected, and a computed tomography (CT) scan is required if the vertigo is thought to be secondary to a middle ear pathology or due to a bony dehiscence of the otic capsule (e.g. superior semicircular canal dehiscence). Other investigations will be directed at specific diagnoses considered in the following sections.

Table 15.1 Differentiation between spontaneous nystagmus of peripheral and central origin

	Peripheral	Central
Nystagmus	Combined torsional and horizontal	Often pure vertical, horizontal or torsional
Fixation	Inhibited (i.e. reduced)	Usually little effect
Gaze	Unidirectional (follows Alexander's Law)	May be direction-changing
Mechanism	Asymmetry of peripheral vestibular tone	Imbalance in central oculomotor tone
Localisation	Peripheral vestibular apparatus or vestibular nerve	Central nervous system, usually brainstem or cerebellar

Source: Adapted from Baloh and Honrubia's Clinical Neurophysiology of the Vestibular System (2001).

BENIGN PAROXYSMAL POSITIONAL VERTIGO

HISTORY AND CLINICAL EXAMINATION

Benign paroxysmal positional vertigo (BPPV) is characterised by brief, intense bouts of rotatory vertigo associated with nausea and vomiting. With a lifetime prevalence of 2.4 per cent, this is the most common cause of vertigo.[2] The posterior canal is involved in the majority of cases (95 per cent), with the lateral canal affected in 5 per cent. The superior canal is rarely involved. Otoconial debris from the degenerating utricular macula is thought to be responsible. When the patient is prone, these calcium carbonate crystals settle within the most dependent part of the inner ear, most commonly the posterior

semicircular canal. Movement of this debris results in deflection of the cupula with over-excitation of the semicircular canal hair cells. Classically, patients experience severe rotatory vertigo on rolling over in bed. The symptom lasts seconds, but patients are left with marked unsteadiness for several hours thereafter. There is associated nausea and vomiting but, importantly, no hearing loss or tinnitus. Some may also experience diarrhoea. For most, this is an extremely frightening experience, with many patients fearing they are suffering a stroke. A tumbling or rolling vertigo may also be experienced when looking down or up suddenly ('top shelf syndrome'). As a result, patients are cautious when moving, in particular when rising or rolling over in bed when waking. A Dix–Hallpike test is used to confirm the diagnosis, with posterior canal BPPV producing – following a short latency – geotropic torsional nystagmus that completely settles (note Figure 15.1). Lateral canal

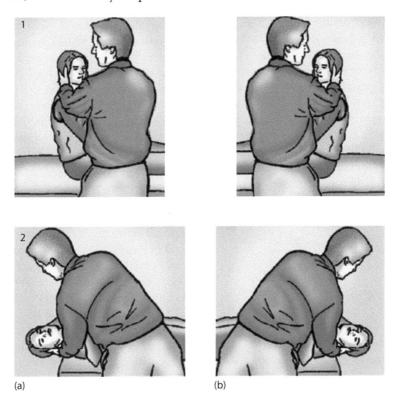

(a) (b)

Figure 15.1 **(a)** Dix-Hallpike positioning maneuver to the right. **(b)** Dix-Hallpike maneuver to the left. Observe for a latency of 2 to 6 seconds after positioning before the onset of nystagmus. Observe for nystagmus that is upbeating and torsional and duration of 10 to 30 seconds. The side with the downward ear is the attached side in benign paroxysmal positional vertigo of the posterior canal. (Reprinted with permission from Barrow Neurological Institute.)

BPPV produces a rapid, intense high-frequency nystagmus that equally abates completely. Persistent, vertical or direction-changing nystagmus should raise suspicion of central pathology and prompt an urgent MRI scan.

INVESTIGATIONS

A thorough neurotological examination is required to exclude concomitant pathology. A pure tone audiogram should be performed, but no additional investigations are required.

MANAGEMENT

Treatment involves returning the otoconial debris into the utricle, where it is believed to be reabsorbed. Manoeuvres to address posterior canal BPPV include the Epley, Semont and Brandt-Daroff exercises. Each has its merits; the Semont and Brandt-Daroff particle positioning manoeuvres can be performed by patients at home. The Epley manoeuvre is immediately curative in more than 85 per cent of patients (note Figure 15.2), but recurrence is common within the first year. A barbeque roll may be used to treat lateral canal BPPV (note Figure 15.3). Rarely, surgical intervention may be required in those with recurrent or unresponsive particle repositioning manoeuvres. Procedures used include posterior canal plugging, gentamicin ablation and surgical labyrinthectomy.

ACUTE PERIPHERAL VESTIBULAR LOSS

HISTORY AND CLINICAL EXAMINATION

There are various terms used to describe an acute peripheral vestibular loss (APVL). These include *vestibular neuritis*, *vestibular neuronitis* and *labyrinthitis*. Although these terms are often used interchangeably, the term *labyrinthitis* should be specifically reserved for cases where there is simultaneous vestibular and sensorineural hearing loss. An abrupt peripheral vestibular loss results in profound, continuous and severe rotatory vertigo. Nausea and vomiting are common, and patients are frequently bed bound for several days after the initial insult. Any movement will result in worsening of symptoms. The cause of APVL remains obscure, although both viral and vascular causes have been suggested.[3] The superior vestibular nerve pathway is generally affected, with relative sparing of the inferior vestibular nerve pathway. Signs include horizontal ocular nystagmus with the slow component towards the affected ear and skew deviation of the eye towards the affected ear in the initial phase. Nystagmus may be present in all directions of gaze in the initial phase (3rd degree nystagmus) and patients are extremely unsteady. As central compensation occurs, patients are gradually able to mobilise, and the nystagmus progressively reduces before settling entirely.

INVESTIGATIONS

Full audiovestibular testing will demonstrate a unilateral canal paresis on caloric testing, whilst true labyrinthitis results in a concomitant sensorineural hearing loss on pure tone audiometry. Imaging with CT or MRI should be considered if the head impulse test is intact, if there is concomitant new onset occipital headache or acute deafness (to identify a cerebellar infarction), or if neurological examination is suggestive of central pathology.

MANAGEMENT

Initial severe symptoms may be adequately managed with a peripheral vestibular sedative such as prochlorperazine. However, its use should be limited to 7 days, as it may eventually hinder central compensatory pathways and delay or even prevent rehabilitation. Whilst some patients recover fully without intervention, many continue to complain of disequilibrium on rapid head movement. Some develop imbalance when presented with visually rich patterns or crowds, owing to an over-dependence on visual information (*visual vertigo*). Mainstay treatment consists of customised vestibular rehabilitation, which has replaced the generic exercises previously recommended (e.g. Cawthorne-Cooksey exercises). This intervention involves encouraging patients to undertake increasingly more difficult exercises to promote central compensation. Visual vertigo may be treated by simultaneously

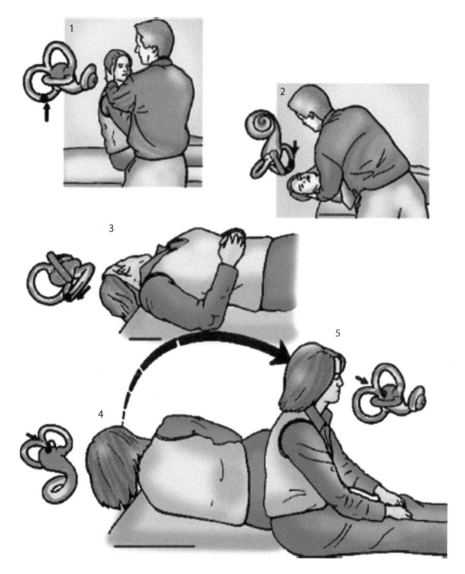

Figure 15.2 Canalith repositioning maneuver, also known as the "Epley maneuver." Step 1: Seat the patient on a table positioned so they may be taken back to the head hanging position with the neck in slight extension. Stabilize the head with your hands and move the head 45 degrees toward the side you will test. Move the head, neck and shoulders together to avoid neck strain or force hyperextension. Step 2: Observe for nystagmus and hold the position for ~10 seconds after it stops. Step 3: Keeping the head tilted back in slight hyperextension, turn the head ~90 degrees toward the opposite side and wait 20 seconds. Step 4: Roll the patient all the way on to his or her side and wait 10 to 15 seconds. Step 5: From the side-lying position, turn the head to face the ground and hold it there 10 to 15 seconds. Step 6: Keeping the head somewhat in the same position, have them sit up then straighten the head. Hold on to the patient for a moment because some patients feel a sudden but very brief tilt when sitting up. REPEAT: After waiting 30 seconds or so, repeat the whole maneuver. If there is not paroxysmal nystagmus or symptoms during Dix-Hallpike positioning (Steps 1, 2) then there is a high likelihood of success. (Reprinted with permission from Barrow Neurological Institute.)

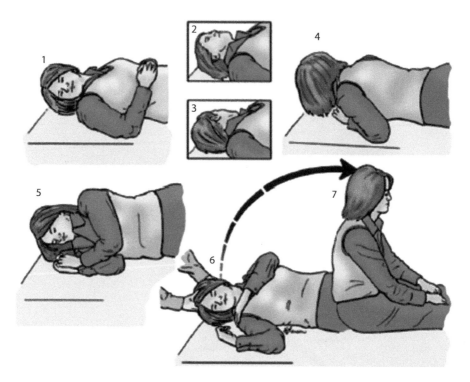

Figure 15.3 Lempert 360- (Barbeque) degree roll maneuver to treat horizontal canal BPPV. When the patient's head is positioned with the affected ear down, the head is then turned quickly 90 degrees toward the unaffected side (face up). A series of 90-degree turns toward the unaffected side is then undertaken there, the patients is turned to the face-up position and then brought up to the sitiing position. The successive head turns can be done in 15- to 20-second intervals even when the nystagmus continues. Waiting longer does no harm, but may lead to the patient developing nausea, and the shorter interval does not appear to detract from the effectiveness of the treatment. (Reprinted with permission from Barrow Neurological Institute.)

presenting subjects with a visually rich environment (e.g. projected moving dots on a screen). Any associated psychological complications should also be addressed. Complications of APVL include secondary BPPV (Lindsay Hemenway Syndrome) and poor/incomplete compensation.

MIGRAINE ASSOCIATED VERTIGO

HISTORY AND CLINICAL EXAMINATION

Migraine associated vertigo (also known as vestibular or vertiginous migraine) accounts for approximately one-third of patients presenting to a tertiary referral balance service. Although the aetiology of this condition remains obscure, symptoms are likely to be due either to a rapid change in blood flow within certain territories of the brain or to a spreading wave of hyper-excitability. Patients, with a female preponderance, classically present in their late 30s and 40s, and generally describe an initial 2- to 3-day spell of vertigo with marked disequilibrium that subsequently settles completely. Further spells are less intrusive, lasting 1 to 2 days. There is no associated hearing loss or tinnitus, but patients often report photophobia and phonophobia. As a result, most will rest in a dark, quiet room. There is an association with menstrual cycles in women, whilst in men symptoms are insidious. Most patients complain of a pervasive sense of disequilibrium. There is often a family or personal history of migraine. Clinical examination should be performed as previously described, but in this case is entirely unremarkable.

INVESTIGATIONS

Vestibular migraine is a diagnosis of exclusion, and full audiovestibular testing and MRI of the brain are required to exclude any central pathology.

MANAGEMENT

Initial treatment requires removal of classic dietary migraine triggers such as chocolate, cheese, caffeine, red wine, bananas, citrus fruits and processed meats. Should symptoms persist, serotonin 5HT agonists (triptans) may be used for acute spells and beta blockers, sodium valproate, topiramate and tricyclic antidepressants such as amitryptiline and pizotifen as prophylactic medication. Those who fail to settle may benefit from a neurology referral.

MÉNIÈRE'S DISEASE

HISTORY AND CLINICAL EXAMINATION

Ménière's disease is a relatively uncommon cause of vertigo, with an estimated incidence of 5 per 100,000 per year. Patients experience spontaneous, unpredictable bouts of severe rotatory vertigo. Episodes are often preceded by aural fullness in the affected ear and classically associated with hearing loss and roaring tinnitus. Although the exact aetiology is uncertain, post-mortem studies have demonstrated expansion of the scala media compartment of the inner ear. Symptoms are thought to arise owing to either rupture of Reissner's membrane and toxic overstimulation of the neuroepithelial elements of the inner ear, or an abnormality of longitudinal drainage of endolymph to the endolymphatic sac. Once a critical level is reached, endolymph drains into the utricle, stretching the cristae of the semicircular canals and resulting in profound vertigo.

INVESTIGATIONS

Fluctuating but progressive low-frequency sensorineural hearing loss is characteristic of this condition, although all frequencies are eventually affected. As such, serial pure tone audiograms are a useful adjunct in diagnosis, as well as patient monitoring. Caloric testing will reveal a peripheral vestibular deficit as the disease process progresses. Electrocochleography has been used to demonstrate an increase in the ratio between the amplitudes of the summating and action potentials suggestive of Ménière's disease. An MRI of the internal auditory meati is required to exclude central pathology (e.g. a vestibular schwannoma).

MANAGEMENT

Management is influenced by the level of hearing and vestibular function in both the affected and non-symptomatic ear. Destructive treatments should be undertaken with caution, as Ménière's disease may affect both inner ears in approximately 50 per cent of patients.

Medical

Medical treatment in the form of lifestyle changes (e.g. adopting a low-salt diet; avoiding alcohol, caffeine and stress) and medication are effective in controlling vertigo in approximately 85 per cent of patients. Pharmacological agents include betahistine, which, although it has no clinically proven benefit, is thought to prevent symptoms by vasodilatation in the inner ear with very few side-effects. Thiazide diuretics are thought to reduce the volume of the endolymph compartment, and antiemetic agents such as prochlorperazine are reserved for acute spells.

Surgery

If first-line treatments fail to control the attacks, surgery may be appropriate. If functional hearing exists in the affected ear, grommet insertion in isolation or combined with the Meniett device may be appropriate. The evidence base is poor for both these procedures. The device has been approved by the National Institute for Health and Care Excellence (NICE) for monitored usage. The use of steroid injection into the middle ear has been gaining momentum, but equally the evidence base is sparse. Endolymphatic sac decompression has been used in the management of Ménière's disease for many years. This is achieved via a cortical mastoidectomy, exposure of the posterior fossa dura and incision of the sac and/or insertion of a silastic tube. This has been a controversial procedure but has proponents, and indeed patients, who find it helpful.

Ablative treatments should be reserved for those cases failing to respond to conservative measures. Gentamicin ablation has gained popularity in some centres. By instilling gentamycin through the tympanic membrane into the middle ear, it avoids temporal bone dissection and aims to selectively eliminate vestibular function on the affected side. Usually, a single treatment is sufficient, although a small percentage may require two or, rarely, three injections. If Gentamycin is used judiciously, hearing is preserved, though a small risk of hearing loss is well recognised. Surgical labyrinthectomy (removal of all vestibular neuro-epithelium) or vestibular nerve section are reserved for those with intractable vertigo.

Customized vestibular physiotherapy

The vestibular hypofunction associated with Ménière's disease results in episodic dysequilibrium. Periods of decompensation may be misinterpreted as further attacks and should be distinguished by taking a careful history. As with acute peripheral vestibular loss, vestibular rehabilitation is also beneficial.

VESTIBULAR SCHWANNOMA

HISTORY AND CLINICAL EXAMINATION

Vestibular schwannomas are benign tumours originating from either vestibular nerve, most commonly the superior. With an estimated incidence of 1 in 100,000, they are a rare cause of vertigo and dizziness.

Full cranial nerve examination is essential, and may reveal facial weakness due to compression of the facial nerve if there is rapid growth or swelling, such as haemorrhage into a tumour or expansion of a cystic component. In the case of large tumours, trigeminal nerve function can also be affected, with reduced sensation and absent corneal reflexes.

INVESTIGATIONS

An asymmetric sensorineural hearing loss on pure tone audiometry should raise the suspicion of an underlying vestibular schwannoma. An MRI of the internal acoustic meati with gadolinium contrast is the gold standard investigation.

MANAGEMENT

Vertigo is managed by vestibular sedatives and vestibular rehabilitation exercises. These are also of benefit in those with static lesions or in the postoperative period following surgical excision. The majority of patients are initially managed conservatively, with serial imaging to assess the rate of growth of the tumour. Surgical intervention or stereotactic radiotherapy are reserved for tumours that continue to enlarge.

PERILYMPH FISTULA

HISTORY AND CLINICAL EXAMINATION

Perilymph fistulae are rare. They represent an abnormal communication between the perilymph of the inner ear and spaces surrounding the otic capsule. Acquired fistulae most commonly arise as a result of barotrauma, penetrating or blunt head trauma, or rapid changes in intracranial pressure. An iatrogenic fistula may occur following ear surgery for chronic ear disease or stapedectomy. Presentation is variable, with most patients describing fluctuating audiovestibular symptoms, including vertigo. Nystagmus may be evident on pneumatic otoscopy in 25 per cent of patients.

INVESTIGATIONS

Pure tone audiometry is mandatory and may demonstrate a fluctuating sensorineural hearing loss. Imaging is of limited value, although a pneumolabyrinth may be seen.

MANAGEMENT

In the acute setting, conservative measures such as bed rest and head elevation are appropriate. Surgical exploration or injection of either autologous blood or fibrin glue into the middle ear is reserved for those with persistent symptoms.[4,5]

KEY LEARNING POINTS

- Acute vertigo is a common presenting complaint.
- Assessment of the vertiginous patient requires a thorough history and neurotological examination.
- Patients with benign paroxysmal positional vertigo may be treated with particle repositioning manoeuvres.

REFERENCES

1. Shepard NT, Telian SA, 1996. Balance disorder patient. Basic anatomy and physiology review. Singular Publishing Group, Inc, pp. 1–16.
2. Fife TD. Benign paroxysmal positional vertigo. *Seminars in Neurology* 2009; 29(5):500–508.
3. De Ciccio M, Fattori B, Carpi A, Casani A, Ghilardi P, Sagripanti A. Vestibular disorders in primary thrombocytosis. *Journal of Otolaryngology* 1999;28(6):318–324.
4. Shinohara T, Gyo K, Murakami S, Yanagihara N. [Blood patch therapy of the perilymphatic fistulas – an experimental study]. *Nihon Jibiinkoka Gakkai Kaiho* 1996; 99:1104–1109.
5. Garg R, Djalilian HR. Intratympanic injection of autologous blood for traumatic perilymphatic fistulas. *Otolaryngology – Head and Neck Surgery* 2009;141:294–295.

16

Ear trauma

JOHN CROWTHER AND FAISAL JAVED

TRAUMA TO PINNA

PINNA LACERATION

Sharp trauma can result in a laceration of the skin and/or cartilage of the pinna. Blunt trauma or a bite (animal or human) can produce an irregular laceration. As exposed cartilage poses a risk for necrosis or infection, the wound should be washed thoroughly and laceration closed using 5-0 or 6-0 nonabsorbable interrupted sutures; however, it may be necessary to trim exposed cartilage or use a local skin flap to provide soft tissue cover. Tetanus vaccination should also be updated. Broad-spectrum antibiotics are prescribed for contaminated or bite wounds.

PINNA HAEMATOMA

This can occur after a blunt injury with contact sports or assaults. As cartilage blood supply relies on the blood vessels in the overlying perichondrium, collection of blood between the auricular perichondrium and cartilage can deprive the cartilage of its blood supply, resulting in cartilage necrosis and a deformed ear ('cauliflower ear'). Untreated, there is also a risk of abscess formation.

Drainage of the haematoma either by aspiration or by incision, usually under local anaesthetic, forms the mainstay of treatment. Compression to prevent recurrence can be provided by moulded pressure bandages or splints of various materials applied on both surfaces of the pinna for at least 48 hours.

EXTERNAL AUDITORY CANAL (EAC) TRAUMA

Inserting cotton buds or hairpins in the ear canal can traumatise the EAC skin. Clinical features include pain, bleeding or infection. Any foreign object should be removed. Button batteries cause chemical burns and should be removed urgently. The EAC should be kept dry until the skin has healed. Aural toilet and topical antibiotic/steroid drops are recommended in the presence of infection.

TYMPANIC MEMBRANE PERFORATION

A defect in the tympanic membrane (TM) (Figure 16.1) can be produced by direct trauma from a foreign body or indirectly from a relative change in pressure between the external and middle ear, e.g. from a slap to the ear or a blast injury. Clinical features include otalgia, hearing loss and/or blood stained otorrhoea.

Pure tone audiometry (PTA) can show a conductive hearing loss (CHL). An air-bone gap of over 30 dB should raise the suspicion of ossicular damage. Conservative management is advocated for traumatic perforations, as the majority will heal spontaneously. Patients should be advised to keep the affected ear dry. If the TM perforation shows no sign of healing after 3 to 6 months, surgical repair can be considered.

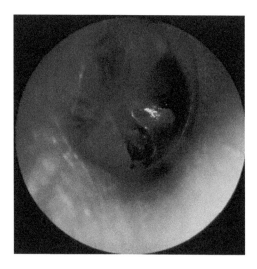

Figure 16.1 Right tympanic membrane showing an irregular inferior perforation secondary to a slap to the ear. Photo by Professor Brian O'Reilly.

TEMPORAL BONE FRACTURE

Falls, assaults and road traffic accidents may cause a temporal bone fracture. Fractures are classified as longitudinal or transverse, but most tend to be mixed. Longitudinal fractures comprise 80% of all temporal bone fractures and are frequently caused by a blow to the temporo-parietal region; the fracture line is parallel to the long axis of the petrous temporal bone. Transverse fractures comprise 20% of all temporal bone fractures. They are usually secondary to a blow to the frontal or occipital region; the fracture line runs at a right angle to the long axis of the petrous pyramid and may also run through the otic capsule. A temporal bone fracture should be suspected in the presence of Battle's sign (Figure 16.2a), peri-orbital ecchymosis (racoon sign), blood in the EAC, haemotympanum (Figure 16.2b), TM perforation, CSF otorrhoea and a lower motor neurone facial nerve palsy.

A computed tomography (CT) of the brain with high-resolution CT scan of the temporal bone should be obtained to confirm the diagnosis (Figure 16.3). The patient should be managed according to advanced trauma life support (ATLS) protocol, with concomitant intracranial and cervical spine injuries taking precedence over the temporal bone injury.

EXTERNAL AUDITORY CANAL INJURY

A laceration +/− step deformity of the bony canal may be visible on otoscopy. This is managed conservatively. Major haemorrhage should alert the clinician to possible damage of the jugular bulb or carotid artery. After resuscitation, urgent CT angiography is indicated to identify the source of bleeding with interventional radiology to control haemorrhage.

MIDDLE EAR INJURY

Haemotympanum

Bleeding behind an intact TM can result in haemotympanum. It is diagnosed by the characteristic appearance of a blue drum and is associated with

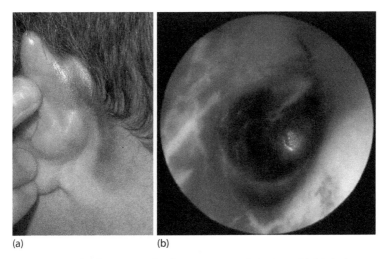

(a)   (b)

Figure 16.2 **(a)** Left post-auricular bruising, also known as Battle's sign. **(b)** Right haemotympanum and evidence of dried blood in the EAC. Photo **(b)** by Professor Brian O'Reilly.

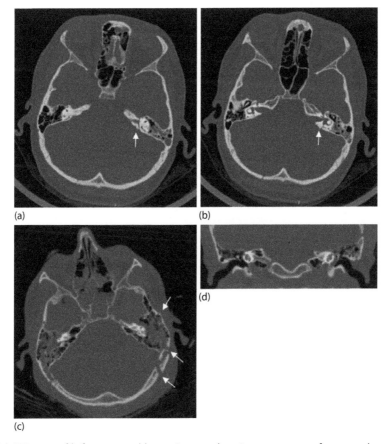

(a)   (b)

(c)   (d)

Figure 16.3 Axial CT scan of left temporal bone (arrow showing transverse fracture through the otic capsule at superior semicircular canal level) **(a)**, at lateral semicircular canal level **(b)**, comminuted fracture of left temporal bone (arrows showing multiple fracture lines) **(c)** and coronal CT scan, 1 year post-injury, showing the presence of CSF in the left middle ear **(d)**.

a CHL. Conservative management is advocated, as spontaneous resolution occurs in 73% of cases within 3 to 6 weeks.[1,2]

TM perforation

TM perforations can occur because of the fracture line involving the tympanic ring, implosion of the membrane secondary to blast trauma or penetration of the TM by particulate debris.[3] They are initially managed conservatively with water precautions, as the majority will heal spontaneously, but surgical repair can be considered if the perforation persists 3 to 6 months after the injury.

Ossicular chain injury

Incus dislocation (80%) is the most common ossicular chain abnormality, followed by stapes fracture.[1,2,4] Other injuries include fixation of ossicles in the attic, incudomalleolar separation, necrosis of incus long process and stapes footplate or malleus dislocation (Figure 16.4a).

A persistent CHL approximately 6 weeks to 3 months after the injury is suspicious of ossicular chain injury. The PTA will show a CHL with a large air-bone gap of up to 60 dB, with a Type A_d tympanogram in ossicular discontinuity (Figure 16.4b) and a Type A_s in ossicular fixation. High-resolution CT scans of the temporal bone may help in confirming ossicular damage. This can be managed conservatively with a hearing aid or surgically with tympanoplasty and ossicular reconstruction.

INNER EAR INJURY

Damage to the inner ear is more common with transverse fractures, as they are more likely to involve the otic capsule.

Sensorineural hearing loss

Sensorineural hearing loss (SNHL) is seen most commonly in fractures involving the otic capsule. Management is typically conservative with hearing aids; however, cochlear implantation may be required for patients with bilateral profound SNHL; this intervention may need to be performed soon after injury due to the risk of cochlear ossification.[5,6]

Vestibular disturbance

Vertigo following a temporal bone trauma can occur in up to 78% cases, with or without a temporal bone fracture.[7] Common causes include benign paroxysmal positional vertigo (BPPV), acute vestibular failure or perilymph fistula. BPPV is the most common cause of post-traumatic vertigo 61%),[8] occurring secondary to displaced otolith

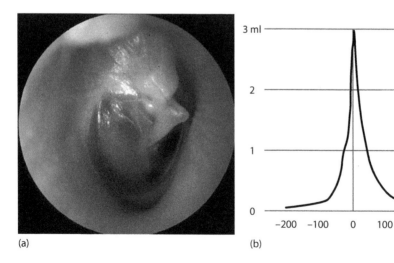

(a)   (b)

Figure 16.4 (a) Right tympanic membrane showing dislocation of the malleus head. (b) Right ear, Type A_d tympanogram. Photo (a) by Professor Brian O'Reilly.

particles in the posterior semicircular canal. A patient will have severe rotatory vertigo precipitated by head movements. A Dix–Hallpike test helps confirm the diagnosis and an Epley manoeuvre can be performed to reposition the displaced particles.

Perilymph fistula can occur due to the fracture line extending into the vestibular labyrinth or rupture of the oval or round window. Symptoms include fluctuating or progressive SNHL with or without vertigo or tinnitus.[9] Management is initially conservative with bed rest, head elevation and avoidance of straining; if symptoms do not resolve, then exploratory tympanotomy might need to be considered to identify and seal the site of perilymph leak. Patients with acute vestibular failure due to trauma benefit from vestibular rehabilitation to encourage central compensation.

An MRI should be considered in patients with persistent vertiginous symptoms, especially in the presence of associated sensorineural hearing loss to exclude any co-existing retrocochlear pathology.

CEREBROSPINAL FLUID OTORRHOEA

Cerebrospinal fluid (CSF) otorrhoea (or CSF rhinorrhoea in patients with an intact TM) can occur in approximately 33% patients.[10] A specimen of clear fluid can be sent to test for β_2-transferrin to confirm this.

Management is initially conservative with bed rest, head elevation and avoidance of straining, as the majority (81%) will resolve spontaneously in 5–7 days.[7] If the leak does not resolve within 1 week, then placement of a lumbar drain to reduce CSF pressure can be considered. Use of prophylactic antibiotics in the presence of CSF leak is unnecessary.[10] In the minority of cases where the leak persists despite conservative measures, surgical closure of the defect is recommended to prevent meningitis.

FACIAL NERVE INJURY

Facial nerve paralysis can occur in approximately 50% of transverse and 20% of longitudinal fractures.[7] It occurs most commonly in fractures involving the otic capsule. The two most important prognostic indicators of facial recovery following a temporal bone fracture include the time of onset (immediate or delayed) and the severity of the palsy (complete/total or incomplete/partial). This can be challenging to assess in patients with multiple injuries and especially in those who are sedated and ventilated. When possible, the facial nerve function should be assessed and documented using the House-Brackmann (HB) grading system. The decision to explore should be based on whether the facial palsy is complete and immediate, together with information from high-resolution CT imaging. Management options include nerve decompression, immediate anastomosis or cable nerve grafting using either the greater auricular or sural nerve.

Patients with partial or delayed facial palsy should be managed conservatively with a 1-week course of high dose prednisolone (1 mg/kg) if there is no contraindication (such as a traumatic brain injury). Approximately >90% patients will attain a HB Grade 1 or 2 facial nerve function with conservative management alone.[11] A management algorithm for management of post-traumatic facial nerve palsy is proposed in Figure 16.5.

IATROGENIC/SURGICAL TRAUMA

Trauma to ossicles, facial nerve and inner ear can occur during otologic surgery. Displacement or fracture of the stapes footplate from excessive manipulation of the ossicles may result in SNHL and balance disturbance. Removal of cholesteatoma from the lateral semicircular canal in the presence of a fistula may also cause SNHL and vertigo. Use of a facial nerve monitor may reduce the risk of facial nerve injury during surgery.

Sensorineural deafness is permanent, but balance disturbance should gradually improve with central compensation, aided by vestibular rehabilitation. Immediate facial nerve palsy after surgery may be secondary to local anaesthetic infiltration and hence should resolve when the anaesthetic wears off. If a facial palsy persists, any ear packs should be loosened or removed to relieve pressure on the nerve. A course of high dose oral steroids may be beneficial as in

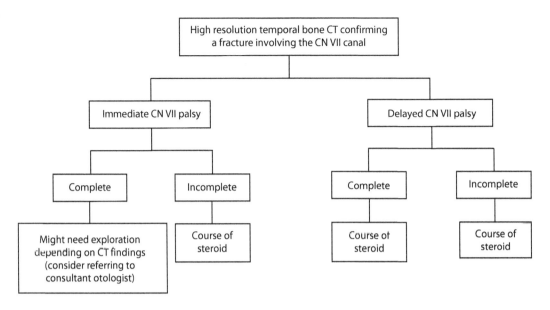

Figure 16.5 Algorithm for the management of post-traumatic facial nerve palsy.

idiopathic (Bell's) facial palsy. The operating surgeon should be notified and unless it is certain that the nerve is definitely intact, urgent re-exploration should be considered in those with persistent complete palsy.

BAROTRAUMA

Mechanical forces arising from pressure changes produce barotrauma. Middle ear barotrauma is the most frequent pressure-induced ear condition. Examples of large pressure changes include the rapid increase in external ear canal pressure from slap injuries typically sustained during assault, airplane descent, diving ascent or a blast injury. This can cause TM retraction, intra-tympanic membrane haemorrhage, middle ear effusion or, in severe cases, TM perforation. Symptoms include sensation of ear blockage with otalgia, which may be severe. Perilymph fistula can occasionally be caused by barotrauma and will lead to SNHL and balance disturbance. The fistula test may be positive in such cases.

Decompression sickness occurs when a reduction in ambient pressure (as occurs when divers are ascending from depth) causes the formation and release of bubbles of inert gases (typically nitrogen) within the tissues of the body. These expanding bubbles can damage the inner ear, causing hearing loss, tinnitus and balance disturbance.

Barotrauma can be prevented by taking measures to optimise Eustachian tube function, such as oral or topical nasal decongestants, prior to or during air travel. When diving, pressure in the ears must be regularly equalised prior to further descent. Decompression sickness can be prevented by divers complying with international guidelines on dive profiles and performing safety stops. Decompression sickness is managed with hyperbaric oxygen therapy.

ACOUSTIC TRAUMA (NOISE-INDUCED HEARING LOSS)

A temporary threshold shift can occur after exposure to loud sounds (>85 dB). This can recover within 24–48 hours. A permanent threshold shift occurs if there is constant or repeated exposure to loud sounds, e.g. working in a noisy factory, gunfire or loud music. This can cause irreversible

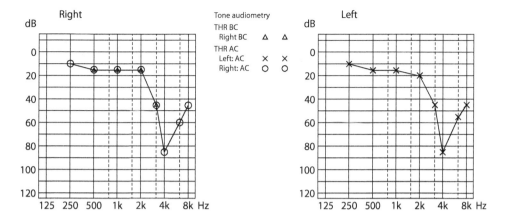

Figure 16.6 Symmetrical moderate to severe SNHL in the 4 KHz section from increased loud noise exposure.

SNHL. Extremely loud sounds >180 dB can produce an acute acoustic trauma.

Acoustic trauma causes maximal damage to the outer hair cells at the basal turn of the cochlea, where the high tones are tonotropically represented, producing a 3 to 6 KHz dip on a pure tone audiogram (Figure 16.6).

Ear defenders can prevent acoustic trauma: ear protection in the form of ear plugs or earmuffs is nowadays a legal requirement in industries with high background noise levels. Industries should also ensure employees are exposed to a maximum daily noise level of 85 dB(A) for less than 8 hours. In those with permanent SNHL, hearing aids should be considered.

KEY LEARNING POINTS

- Most traumatic tympanic membrane perforations will heal spontaneously within 3 months of the injury.
- A persistent conductive hearing loss with a healed tympanic membrane is suspicious of ossicular chain fracture/discontinuity or fixation.
- Most CSF otorrhea will heal spontaneously within a week of the injury and do not require prophylactic antibiotics.

REFERENCES

1. Nosan DK, Beneecke JE, Murr AH. Current perspective on temporal bone trauma. *Otolaryngology – Head and Neck Surgery* 1997;117:67–71.
2. Tos M. Course of and sequelae to 248 petrosal fractures. *Acta Otolaryngologica* 1971;85:1147–59.
3. Mills R, Nunez DA, Toynton SC. Ear Trauma. In: *Scott-Brown's Otorhinolaryngology, Head and Neck Surgery*. Volume 3. 7th edition. Published by Edward Arnold 2008;3496.
4. Lee D, Honrado C, Har-El G, Goldsmith A. Pediatric temporal bone fractures. *Laryngoscope* 1998;108:474–7.
5. Camilleri AE, Toner JG, Howarth KL, Hampton S, Ramsden RT. Cochlear implantation following temporal bone fracture. *The Journal of Laryngology and Otology* 1999;113:454–7.
6. Vermeire K, Brokx JP, Dhooge I et al. Cochlear implantation in post-traumatic bilateral temporal bone fracture. *ORL, Journal for Oto-Rhino-Laryngology and Its Related Specialties* 2012;74(1):52–6.
7. Brodie HA, Thompson TC. Management of complications from 820 temporal bone fractures. *American Journal of Otology* 1997;18:188–97.

8. Davies RA, Luxon LM. Dizziness following head injury: a neuro-otological study. *Journal of Neurology* 1995;242: 222–30.

9. Glasscock ME 3rd, Hart MJ, Rosdeutscher JD, Bhansali SA. Traumatic perilymphatic fistula: how long can symptoms persist? A follow-up report. *American Journal of Otology* 1992;13:333–8.

10. McGuirt WF Jr, Stool SE. Temporal bone fractures in children: a review with emphasis on long term sequelae. *Clinical Pediatrics* 1992;31:12–8.

11. Darrouzet V, Duclos JY, Liguoro D et al. Management of facial paralysis resulting from temporal bone fractures: our experience with 115 cases. Otolaryngology – *Head and Neck Surgery* 2001;125(1):77–84.

17

Emergency treatment of sudden hearing loss

CATHERINE RENNIE AND DAVID K SELVADURAI

Sudden sensorineural hearing loss (SSNHL) is an otological emergency. It often affects healthy individuals and is an alarming symptom that impacts on quality of life. The aetiology remains controversial, but early diagnosis and treatment can significantly improve hearing outcomes. The estimated annual incidence is 5–30 per 100,000 persons, and 99% of cases are unilateral. It is defined by a hearing loss of 30 dB or more, over at least three contiguous audiometric frequencies, that develops over 72 hours or less. This can be difficult to demonstrate clinically, as previous audiometry is rarely available. It is therefore accepted practice to compare the hearing level to that in the opposite ear.

Many possible causes for SSNHL have been identified; it may present as an isolated condition or be the presenting feature of a systemic disease process. If an underlying condition cannot be identified on history and physical examination, then SSNHL is said to be idiopathic in nature (termed idiopathic sudden sensorineural hearing loss, or ISSNHL). In the vast majority, 90–95%, a cause is never identified. Possible causes of SNHL are listed in Table 17.1. The most important diagnoses to exclude are vestibular schwannoma, stroke and malignancy.

A number of hypotheses have been proposed for the aetiology of ISSNHL. These include labyrinthine viral infection, vascular insult, intracochlear membrane rupture and autoimmune inner ear disease. There is, however, no conclusive evidence for any of these theories. The aetiology may be multifactorial: for example, a viral infection can cause nerve injury, vascular structure injury or injury to erythrocytes, leading to secondary microvascular insufficiency. Viruses can also cause inflammation resulting in vascular insufficiency. Autoimmune disease can lead to vasculitis through anti-endothelial cell antibodies.

In terms of severity, the hearing loss is divided almost equally into mild, moderate, severe and profound.

Table 17.1 Possible aetiology of sudden sensorineural hearing loss

Autoimmune	Circulatory	Infectious	Metabolic	Neoplastic	Neurologic	Toxic	Traumatic
Antiphospholipid syndrome	Alteration of microcirculation	Encephalitis	Hyperlipidaemia	Cerebellopontine angle tumours	Multiple sclerosis	Aminoglycoside antibiotics	Barotrauma
Autoimmune inner ear disease (AIED)	Vertebrobasilar insufficiency	Herpes virus	Thyrotoxicosis	Leukaemia	Migraine	Loop diuretics	Ear surgery
Cogan's syndrome	Sickle cell disease	HIV	Diabetes	Myeloma		NSAIDS	Inner ear decompression sickness
Granulomatosis with polyangitis	Cardiopulmonary bypass	Lyme disease				Salicylates	Noise exposure
Lupus erythrmatosus		Measles					Perilymph fistula
Polyarteritis nodosa		Mumps				Platinum based chemotherapy	Temporal bone fracture
Relapsing polychondritis		Meningococcal meningitis				General anaesthesia	
Rheumatoid arthritis		Rubella					
Sarcoid		Syphilis					
Sjogren's		Toxoplasmosis					
Ulcerative colitis							

CLINICAL ASSESSMENT

In assessing patients with SSNHL it is important to remember that between 32 and 65% recover spontaneously, and patients should therefore be counselled appropriately. The aim of clinical evaluation is to identify treatable causes of SSNHL.

Ten key areas to cover in the history are:

1. The onset. The shorter the history of hearing loss, the better the prognosis.
2. The baseline hearing level. SSNHL can be new or an incremental loss, and fluctuating hearing levels may point to Ménière's disease.
3. Unilateral or bilateral. A bilateral SHL could suggest ototoxicity or autoimmune disease.
4. The degree of hearing loss. A poorer prognosis is associated with an increasingly severe hearing loss.
5. Associated symptoms such as tinnitus, vertigo and aural fullness could represent a diagnosis of endolymphatic hydrops.
6. Vertigo is present in 30–40% of cases of SSNHL. It is a poor prognostic indicator.
7. Any history of trauma, diving, flying and intense noise exposure is relevant.
8. Past medical history. Any previous or concurrent viral infections. Systemic disease associated with sudden hearing loss should be explored, as SSNHL can rarely be the first presentation of a systemic disease.
9. Any previous ear surgery should be noted.
10. Ototoxicity should be excluded with a careful drug history.

Examination should include:

1. Otoscopy to exclude middle ear effusions, infections and cholesteatoma.
2. Tuning fork tests to distinguish a conductive hearing loss from a SNHL.
3. A fistula test to help identify a perilymph fistula.
4. A complete examination of the head and neck.
5. A thorough neurological examination of cranial nerves and cerebellar signs.

PERTINENT INVESTIGATIONS

1. Audiometry is required. A downward sloping audiogram is associated with a poorer outcome.
2. Vestibular schwannoma should be excluded with a gadolinium-enhanced MRI scan. This is also useful in evaluating multiple sclerosis and cerebrovascular accidents. Up to 20% of patients with vestibular schwannoma report a sudden drop in their hearing at some point in their history, although the incidence of vestibular schwannoma in patients who present with SHL is considerably lower. A surprisingly high prevalence of cerebellopontine angle tumours has been noted in SHL patients, ranging from 2.7% to 10.2% of patients who are evaluated with MRI. High-resolution CT of the temporal bones may be acceptable in cases where MRI is contraindicated.
3. Other investigations to rule out identifiable causes should be tailored to the patient's history. Laboratory tests, including FBC, ESR, urea and electrolytes, lipid profile, glucose, thyroid function tests, clotting screen, VDRL, serology for Lyme disease and autoantibodies (antinuclear antibodies, anticardiolipin antibodies, lupus anticoagulant, antineutrophil cytoplasmic antibodies), may be requested if clinically indicated. The American Academy guideline discourages routine laboratory testing.

PROGNOSIS

Four factors have been shown to affect recovery from ISSNHL:

1. Time elapsed since onset. Earlier presentation caries a better prognosis, as expected in a condition with a high spontaneous recovery rate.
2. Age over 60 carries a worse prognosis.
3. Vertigo is a poor prognostic indicator.
4. Audiogram. A profound hearing loss or a downward sloping audiogram have a poorer prognosis.

The rate of improvement in the first 2 weeks may predict long-term outcome. Long-term follow-up is recommended to identify conditions that are associated with this presentation. Some patients will benefit from ongoing audiological and psychological support for tinnitus and profound hearing loss.

TREATMENT

If a specific cause for a SSNHL is found, the patient should be managed accordingly. The high spontaneous recovery rate for ISSNHL and its low incidence make validation of treatment difficult. If it is idiopathic in nature, patients may be offered a course of oral corticosteroid. If systemic corticosteroids are contraindicated or there is no improvement with initial oral therapy, intratympanic corticosteroid (IT) as either primary or salvage therapy may be considered, and hyperbaric oxygen therapy (HBOT) may be useful within the first 3 months. A number of other treatments have been proposed, but evidence for their efficacy is lacking:

- Anti-inflammatory/immunosuppression: steroids, prostacyclin
- Antiviral agents: acyclovir, valcyclovir
- Vasodilators: 5% carbon dioxide with 95% oxygen (carbogen), papaverine, pentoxifylline
- Volume expanders/haemodilutors: hydroxyethyl starch, dextran
- Calcium antagonists: nifedipine
- Other agents and procedures: iron, vitamins, procaine, hyperbaric oxygen, ginkgo biloba, zinc, co-enzyme Q10.

CORTICOSTEROIDS

Steroid therapy is widely accepted as the standard treatment for SSNHL; however, the evidence is limited. Systematic reviews and meta-analyses revealed no evidence of benefit of steroids over placebo. Several authors have found that steroids had a significant effect on the recovery of hearing in patients with hearing loss between 40 and 90 dB, but the methodology of these studies has been criticised. A meta-analysis in 2010 of various medical treatments, including corticosteroids, showed a slight but not statistically significant improvement with medical therapy compared to placebo.

Although the evidence for corticosteroids is limited, treatment should be considered in view of the severity of the disability that may result from the condition. Spontaneous improvement in hearing is most common during the first 2 weeks; late recovery is rare. Early corticosteroid treatment is associated with the greatest hearing recovery, with reduced benefit after 4 to 6 weeks. 1 mg/kg/day (maximum dose of 60 mg day) of oral prednisolone as a single daily dose for 10 days is associated with the best treatment outcomes.

Systemic corticosteroids have a wide range of potential side effects across many organ systems. It is therefore important to assess the risks and benefits on a patient-by-patient basis. Systemic corticosteroids may not be an appropriate treatment for patients with insulin-dependent or poorly controlled diabetes, peptic ulcer disease and prior psychiatric reactions to corticosteroids. The severe side effects are rare during the short 10- to 14-day course of steroids recommended for SSNHL. Super-high-dose steroid therapy has been used in this condition but requires further study.

Intratympanic (IT) steroid therapy has been used as a treatment for SSNHL, particularly in refractory cases or those in which systemic steroids may be hazardous, but again, evidence is lacking. There have been large numbers of small studies, often with very small numbers; many are retrospective, without controls, and the steroid dosage, delivery method and frequency of injection has varied considerably, making it difficult to assess and compare outcomes. The main theoretical advantages of intratympanic treatment is the reduction in systemic corticosteroid side effects and better cochlear penetration. Intratympanic injection achieves higher inner ear steroid concentrations. IT steroids have been used as the primary treatment, in combination with other therapies and as salvage treatment. Although routinely used in clinical practice, IT steroids are associated with an inconsistent clinical response. This may be due to variability in diffusion across the round window membrane exacerbated by any inflammation or scar tissue in the round window niche, leading to unpredictable intracochlear bioavailability.

Adverse effects with IT steroids are infrequent. Pain, transient dizziness, infection, persistent tympanic membrane perforation and possible vasovagal episode during injection have all been reported.

Rauch conducted a large randomised controlled trial comparing oral versus IT steroid therapy for ISSNHL in 2011. This was conducted at 16 centres and recruited 250 patients. All patients were recruited within 14 days of onset of their SSNHL and followed up for 6 months. 121 patients received 60 mg/d of oral prednisone for 14 days with a 5-day taper and 129 patients received 4 doses over 14 days of 40 mg/mL of methylprednisolone injected into the middle ear. The results showed that for initial therapy of SSNHL, promptly administered and equivalently dosed oral and IT steroid appeared to be equally effective, with hearing improvement seen in more than 75% of treated patients. Since the results for the two groups were equivalent, decisions on the choice of treatment for an individual should be based upon the risk of potential side effects and cost. Side effects were reported in similar numbers in both groups, though the systemic group suffered more potentially serious issues such as raised blood sugar. The majority of side effects were self-limiting.

HYPERBARIC OXYGEN

Hyperbaric oxygen therapy (HBOT) delivers 100% oxygen to a patient at a pressure greater than 1 atmosphere to increase tissue oxygenation. This should enhance the physiological response to infection and ischaemia. HBOT has been used in the treatment of SHL since the 1960s. Numerous studies have investigated its use; however, very few are prospective randomised controlled trials. A Cochrane review included seven randomised controlled trials published between 1985 and 2004. Patients who presented early with ISSNHL showed statistically significant hearing improvement with HBO, but the clinical significance of this improvement is less clear.

A more recent prospective randomised control of HBOT for SSNHL compared HBOT + oral steroid with oral steroid alone. The results showed

no significant difference between the two groups. HBOT has also been used in combination with IT steroids, but no statistically significant difference was found between HBOT + IT steroid against HBOT + IV steroid.

Complications are fortunately rare but include damage to the middle ear, sinuses and lungs from pressure changes, temporary worsening of short-sightedness and oxygen poisoning. It is, however, a very expensive intervention that is not widely available. Therapy typically involves multiple 1- to 2-hour sessions over days to weeks.

SALVAGE

For patients who are refractory to systemic steroid therapy, salvage with IT steroid or HBOT have been investigated. There are now numerous case series, a number of RCTs and a meta-analysis looking at the use of IT steroids in this scenario. Despite methodological limitations, the majority do show improved hearing outcomes after IT steroid therapy, with improvement rates ranging from 8% to 100%. A meta-analysis showed a statistically significant greater improvement in hearing on pure-tone audiometry in patients who received salvage intratympanic steroids than in those who did not. The degree of clinical significance is questionable, as the improvement in audiological thresholds may not confer an improvement in usable hearing to the patient. HBOT has also been successfully used in the treatment of refractory SSNHL. In patients with permanent hearing loss, early discussion regarding rehabilitation options can reduce patient anxiety. Ideally, these discussions should take place when a hearing loss is first identified, as temporary aiding during treatment may be beneficial.

MEASURING OUTCOMES

The American Academy of Otolaryngology, Head & Neck Surgery (AAOHNS) have proposed recommendations for outcomes assessment which should be used in future reporting to allow a better understanding of this condition:

AAOHNS RECOMMENDATIONS FOR OUTCOMES ASSESSMENT

1. Unless a previous asymmetry of hearing was known or suspected, the unaffected ear should be used as the standard against which recovery should be compared;
2. A complete recovery requires return to within 10 dB HL of the unaffected ear and recovery of word recognition scores to within 5% to 10% of the unaffected ear;
3. Partial recovery should be defined in two ways based on whether or not the degree of initial hearing loss after the event of SSNHL rendered the ear nonserviceable (based on the AAO-HNSF definition); and
4. Anything less than a 10 dB HL improvement should be classified as no recovery.

Associated symptoms of tinnitus, sensation of fullness, vertigo or nausea following treatment should also be recorded.

CONCLUSION

SSNHL is an important condition that can have a significant impact on quality of life. Some patients respond spontaneously without intervention; however, certain interventions such as corticosteroid treatment may improve outcomes. Early steroid treatment is advocated, either systemic or intratympanic, and HBOT may be useful within the first 3 months. A definitive treatment paradigm requires further study and higher quality data collection.

KEY LEARNING POINTS

- There are many potential causes of sudden sensorineural hearing loss, but the diagnosis is elusive in up to 90%.
- An MRI scan to identify a vestibular schwannoma is required. Other investigations are tailored to the individual.
- Short-course, high-dose corticosteroid treatment is recommended despite a lack of high-quality evidence.

FURTHER READING

Labus J, Breil J, Stutzer H, Michel O. Meta-analysis for the effect of medical therapy vs. placebo on recovery of idiopathic sudden hearing loss. *Laryngoscope.* 2010; 120(9): 1863–71.

Mattox DE, Lyles CA. Idiopathic sudden sensorineural hearing loss. *Am J Otol.* 1989; 10(3): 242–7.

Rauch SD, Halpin CF, Antonelli PJ, Babu S, Carey JP, Gantz BJ et al. Oral vs intratympanic corticosteroid therapy for idiopathic sudden sensorineural hearing loss: a randomized trial. *JAMA.* 2011; 305(20): 2071–9.

Stachler RJ, Chandrasekhar SS, Archer SM, Rosenfeld RM, Schwartz SR, Barrs DM et al. Clinical practice guideline: sudden hearing Loss. *Otolaryngology – Head and Neck Surgery.* 2012; 146(3 suppl): S1–S35.

Wei BP, Mubiru S, O'Leary S. Steroids for idiopathic sudden sensorineural hearing loss. *Cochrane Database Syst Rev.* 2006; (1): CD003998.

18

Acute facial palsy

RICHARD M IRVING AND RAGHU NANDHAN SAMPATH KUMAR

INTRODUCTION

The face is the window to the mind and facial expression reflects the emotions and well-being of the individual. Hence, acute facial weakness is probably the most visible and distressing nerve palsy in the body. It manifests not only as a cosmetic deformity but also with functional problems of eyelid closure, oral continence and speech. The prevalence of acute facial palsy in the general population of the UK is about 1:5000, making it a comparatively common clinical entity. A systematic approach to the correct diagnosis for facial weakness and timely, appropriate management is vital in providing the best chance for its complete recovery.

APPLIED ANATOMY

The facial nerve is a mixed nerve containing motor, sensory and parasympathetic fibres; however, it is the motor component that predominates,
producing the greatest morbidity associated with conditions affecting the nerve. Each facial nerve has approximately 10,000 fibres, of which two-thirds are motor and the remaining one-third are sensory.

The facial nerve is the commonest cranial nerve to be involved in a functional deficit due to its long and tortuous course (Figure 18.1). It commences from the brainstem, running intracranially through the cerebellopontine angle and traverses a non-expandable bony canal within the petrous temporal bone, where it takes two acute bends (genus) through the middle ear cleft and exits through the stylomastoid foramen to traverse through the parotid gland to supply the hemifacial muscles.

The facial nerve comprises both upper and lower motor neurons. UMN weakness occurs due to lesions involving the motor cortex or internal capsule, while LMN weakness is due to affliction of the nerve in its intracranial, intratemporal or extracranial segments. Upper motor neuron palsy spares the forehead due to bilateral cortico-bulbar innervation, which results in weakness of the contralateral lower facial muscles only, while lower

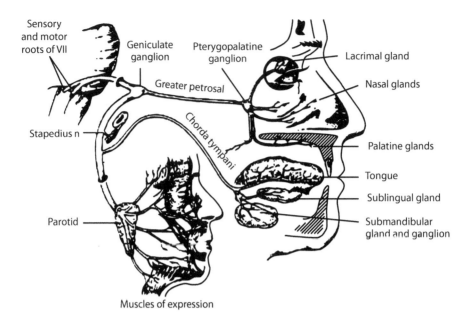

Sensory and motor roots of VII

Geniculate ganglion

Pterygopalatine ganglion

Greater petrosal

Lacrimal gland

Nasal glands

Chorda tympani

Stapedius n

Palatine glands

Tongue

Sublingual gland

Parotid

Submandibular gland and ganglion

Muscles of expression

Figure 18.1 Anatomical course and supply of the facial nerve.

motor neuron weakness involves the entire ipsilateral hemi-facial muscles.

The labyrinthine segment is the narrowest segment of the facial nerve canal and therefore susceptible to compression secondary to inflammation and to vascular insults, as it lacks epineurium and anastomosing arterial cascades. Idiopathic (Bell's) palsy is most commonly due to oedema at this segment. In such cases loss of tears and saliva may be features presenting along with facial palsy. Bell's palsy patients may also perceive pain around the stylomastoid foramen site, as the nerve is inflamed at this exit point.

Variations in the anatomical course of the facial nerve may exist both in its intratemporal and extracranial segments. The fallopian canal in the middle ear cleft maybe dehiscent in up to 50% of cases, especially if congenital ear malformations coexist. Facial palsy occurs in about 6% of acute otitis media, where this segment is involved.

PATHOLOGY OF ACUTE FACIAL PALSY

Acute facial nerve paralysis can result from numerous causes, as listed in Table 18.1, the most common being idiopathic or Bell's palsy, trauma, infection and neoplasia. Cases of bilateral facial palsy should alert the clinician to underlying systemic or neurological pathology, such as syphilis, Lyme disease or Guillain–Barré syndrome.

ASSESSMENT OF FACIAL PARALYSIS

History is paramount in identifying the aetiology of facial weakness. A thorough history regarding onset, duration and progress of weakness, past and preceding otological history, presence of coexistent neurological symptoms and systemic illnesses would help the clinician to arrive at a diagnosis from the differentials quoted previously. It is vital to perform a comprehensive ENT and head and neck examination, including otoscopy, to identify obvious pathology leading onto the facial palsy. Examination is incomplete without testing all cranial nerves and assessment of hearing and balance functions.

Bell's palsy is a diagnosis of exclusion of other causes and should not be the provisional diagnosis for commencing treatment, without confirmation. Red flags that warn against the diagnosis of Bell's

Table 18.1 Differential diagnoses of acute facial nerve palsy

Idiopathic	Bell's palsy
Infection	Acute or chronic otitis media
	Cholesteatoma
	Malignant otitis externa
	Skull base osteomyelitis
	Lyme disease
	Syphilis
	Herpes simplex
	Varicella zoster
	Ramsay Hunt syndrome
Trauma	Temporal bone/skull base fracture
	Gunshot/penetrating injuries
	Forceps delivery
Tumour	Schwannoma
	Meningioma
	Haemangioma/glomus
	Parotid malignancy
Surgery/ Iatrogenic	Mastoid operations
	Stapedotomy
	Cochlear implant
	Lateral skull base surgery
Neurological	Lacunar/brainstem infarct
	Guillain–Barré syndrome
	Multiple sclerosis
Miscellaneous	Sarcoidosis
	Diabetic neuropathy
	Radiotherapy/ osteoradionecrosis
	Melkersson–Rosenthal syndrome

palsy are obvious otological symptoms and the presence of bilateral facial palsy, slurred speech, hemiparesis/paraesthesia of the face and limbs, cerebellar signs, multiple cranial neuropathy, previous history of facial weakness or history of loco-regional cancers.

Recurrent or bilateral palsy warrants an urgent high-resolution CT/MRI scan to look for tumours or neurological causes. All trauma cases require CT scan of brain + petrous temporal bone to assess the site of nerve injury. Immediate post-traumatic total facial palsy indicates obvious trauma to the nerve, while delayed onset facial weakness in the background of a recent head injury suggests oedema of the nerve, which is most likely in anatomical continuity. Urgent ENT referral is important in both scenarios, and audiograms are indicated in all temporal bone trauma. Blood tests should be targeted at screening for infective source like syphilis, Lyme disease, HIV, TB and EBV. If infection is ruled out, an auto-immune screen, connective tissue screen and CSF analysis may be indicated.

Facial palsy should always be graded at first and all subsequent consultations. Several facial grading systems exist in an attempt to objectively quantify facial motor function. Facial grading scales are used in measuring recovery, potential deterioration and comparison of facial nerve outcomes across therapeutic modalities. The House–Brackmann (HB) score (Table 18.2), first described in 1985, is the most popular and widely used clinical measure of the degree of facial motor weakness. It comprises six grades, from normal (HB I) to total paralysis (HB VI).

The use of topodiagnostic tests to assess function of a branch of the facial nerve to determine the site of the lesion is of historical significance only. Routinely, taste, salivary flow tests, Shirmer's test and stapedial reflex are not done, as they have no prognostic value and provide limited clinical correlation.

Although not indicated in the acute setting, it is essential for the clinician to understand objective electrophysiological tests that help evaluate the degree of facial nerve dysfunction/potential recovery and can guide ongoing management – in particular, timing of surgical decompression and facial reanimation procedures. Currently, the two most common neurophysiology tests used are electroneuronography (ENoG) and electromyography (EMG).

ENoG relies on a functional contralateral nerve and is mainly of value in acute onset complete facial nerve paralysis. The amplitude of nerve conduction velocity stimulated at the stylomastoid foramen and detected with a surface electrode at the nasolabial fold correlates with a poor prognosis if greater than 95% reduction in amplitude occurs on the affected side within 3 to 21 days. It takes up to 3 days for Wallerian degeneration to occur, and after three weeks, due to concurrent degeneration and regeneration, ENoG is of less value.

Table 18.2 House–Brackmann grading

Grade	Gross	Resting tone	Forehead	Eye closure	Mouth
I	Normal symmetrical function in all areas				
II	Slight weakness	Normal	Moderate-good function	Complete closure with minimal effort	Slight asymmetry
III	Obvious weakness	Normal	Slight-moderate function	Complete closure with full effort	Slight weakness
IV	Disfiguring	Normal	None	Incomplete closure	Asymmetric
V	Barely perceptible motion	Asymmetric	None	Incomplete closure	Slight movement
VI	Total paralysis (No movement, loss of tone, no synkinesis, contracture or spasm)				

EMG studies are useful in cases of delayed recovery and in cases of bilateral facial nerve palsy. EMG measures voluntary motor unit potentials (the patient is asked to make forceful contractions) using needle electrodes placed in the orbicularis oris and orbicularis oculi muscles. Fibrillation potentials suggest Wallerian degeneration and arise 2 to 3 weeks following injury, while polyphasic potentials indicate early signs of reinnervation, which can precede clinical signs of recovery by 3 months. Electrical silence is a poor prognostic indicator and argues against attempts at facial reanimation designed to use the native facial musculature.

Common causes of acute facial paralysis are briefly discussed in the following sections.

1. BELL'S PALSY (ACUTE IDIOPATHIC FACIAL PARALYSIS)

Described by Sir Charles Bell in 1821, this is an idiopathic unilateral peripheral facial nerve palsy with some evidence to support a viral aetiology. Annual incidence is 20 to 30 cases per 100,000 people per year, with an equal sex incidence and a peak incidence of 40 years, although it can occur in all age groups. Patients who have had a single episode of Bell's palsy have an 8% risk of recurrence. Although Bell's palsy is the commonest cause of unilateral facial paralysis, accounting for 60–70% of all cases, it is a diagnosis of exclusion. The majority (85%) of patients will show partial recovery within 3 weeks of onset and all patients get some recovery. Poor prognostic factors include complete facial palsy at onset, age over 60 years, severe pain, no recovery by 3 weeks and associated conditions, e.g. hypertension and diabetes.

Bell's palsy normally presents with sudden onset of unilateral lower motor nerve facial palsy over a course of 24–48 hours. It is frequently preceded by periauricular paresthesia or otalgia. A viral prodome may exist, and dysgeusia, hyeracusis and facial numbness may be present. Tearing may be reduced, but paradoxically the patient may complain of excess tears due to loss of lower lid control. Examination includes assessment of facial nerve function, remaining cranial nerves, otoscopy and palpation of the parotid. Specifically, the degree of eye closure and presence of Bell's phenomenon should be determined, to quantify corneal risk. A baseline pure tone audiogram should be obtained, especially if the patient complains of hearing loss, as this is not typical in Bell's palsy. Ocular care takes precedence in cases where there is incomplete eye closure, to prevent sight threatening complications. Regular topical lubricants throughout the day with thicker viscosity lubricant at night should be prescribed with taping of eye shut at night. Referral to ENT and ophthalmology should be considered in all cases of total facial paralysis.

Treatment algorithm for Bell's palsy

1. Eye care – Hypromellose eye drops during the day/Lacrilube ointment + eye tape at night if incomplete eye closure (above Gr-III palsy).
2. Antibiotics – (only if suspected otitis media/URTI) amoxicillin orally 15–20 mg/kg (maximum 500 mg) three times a day for 14 days.

   If penicillin allergy (<12 years old) – azithromycin 10 mg/kg (maximum 500 mg) once a day for 3 consecutive days, then repeated for 3 consecutive days in week 2. If penicillin allergy (>12 years old) – doxycycline 100 mg twice daily for 14 days.
3. Steroids – Prednisolone 1 mg/kg (60 mg maximum) for 5–7 days if patient presents within 72 hours of symptom onset. PPI needs to be added with oral steroids. Good evidence from well-constructed clinical trials supports the value of corticosteroids in Bell's palsy.
4. Antivirals – Cochrane review suggests 'no significant benefit' of antivirals compared with placebo in producing complete recovery from Bell's palsy. Literature also shows that antivirals are significantly less likely than corticosteroids to produce complete recovery.
5. Recommended urgent referrals:

ENT – if unsure of diagnosis. All adults with associated red flags of ENT/H&N pathology and all children with facial palsy need referral to ENT.

Ophthalmology – indicated if eye is not fully closing at night (above Gr-III).

Neurology – if focal or evolving neurological signs, UMN or bilateral facial weakness and multiple cranial nerve palsy.

Physiotherapy – if weakness is still present at 6 weeks post-treatment follow-up (nerve conduction study recommended).

Outcome at follow-up depends upon the factors of age, aetiology, degree of palsy at first presentation, duration of weakness, presence of medical comorbidities/systemic illnesses and compliance with treatment. Prognosis is expected to be good, with complete resolution of weakness within 4 weeks in the majority of patients with Bell's palsy. If no recovery is observed by 3 weeks, an alternative diagnosis must be considered, with appropriate investigations in a specialist clinic for further management. The options for facial reanimation are aimed at improving cosmesis and restoring function. This may include facial physiotherapy, botulinum toxin injections and surgical reanimation techniques.

2. INFECTION

Bacterial causes for acute facial nerve paralysis include acute or chronic otitis media and skull base osteomyelitis. Facial paralysis secondary to acute otitis media is rare and tends to be more common in young children. Middle ear cholesteatoma is associated with facial paralysis in under 1% of cases; however, when the disease is in the petrous apex, this increases to close to 50%. Most cases of facial paralysis secondary to acute otitis media resolve with conservative management in the form of systemic antibiotics. Surgical options of myringotomy with or without ventilation tube may be indicated when spontaneous perforation of the tympanic membrane does not occur. A mastoidectomy may be indicated for suppurative complications, lack of clinical improvement or worsening of the facial palsy. Rarely, surgical decompression of the facial nerve is necessary. The converse generally is true for chronic otitis media or cholesteatoma or the delayed onset of facial paralysis, as this is probably secondary to erosion of the facial nerve canal, and early surgical intervention is warranted in the form of a mastoidectomy. Recovery can occur even if treatment is delayed for several months in facial paralysis secondary to cholesteatoma; however, optimal outcomes are achieved with early intervention.

Lyme disease and Ramsey Hunt syndrome are uncommon infections causing acute facial palsy. Lyme disease is a multisystem illness caused by the spirocheate *Borrelia burgdorferi*. It is transmitted by tick bites and can give rise to both unilateral or bilateral facial nerve paralysis. Erythema migrans is evident in the early stages of the disease with associated joint pain, fever and later symptoms of fatigue and neck stiffness. Enquiring about recent travel or outdoor activities such as hiking or camping is important to establish the aetiology. The diagnosis is confirmed by serology, and treatment is with long-term antibiotics. Ramsey Hunt syndrome is caused by the varicella zoster virus and is characterised by vesicles in the external ear, soft palate or tongue. It may be misdiagnosed as Bell's palsy, as the classic vesicles may not appear or may be delayed. Varicella zoster virus polymerase chain reaction (PCR) may help to distinguish between Ramsay Hunt syndrome and Bell's palsy patients. If the diagnosis is suspected, prompt treatment with steroids and antivirals is recommended. Despite treatment, the prognosis is poor, with fewer than half of patients achieving complete recovery of facial function.

3. TRAUMA

Both blunt and penetrating mechanisms of injury may result in acute facial nerve paralysis. Causes of injury include motor vehicle accidents, assault, stab and gunshot injuries, and iatrogenic injury. Temporal bone fractures account for 18–22% of skull fractures in patients treated for head trauma. Common sequelae of temporal bone fractures include facial nerve injury, damage to the cochleo-vestibular apparatus with associated sensorineural hearing loss, conductive loss, balance disturbance, tinnitus, vertigo and cerebrospinal fluid leak.

Traditional classification systems of longitudinal, transverse and mixed temporal bone fractures are still used but poorly correlate to clinical complications (Figure 18.2). More recently, petrous or otic capsule sparing versus non-petrous or otic capsule violating classifications have been suggested to provide improved clinical correlation, aiding early recognition of potential complications and

(30–50%) compared to longitudinal (10–25%) temporal bone fractures and in otic capsule involving fractures; it is less common in children. Gunshot-related temporal bone injury results in extensive injury to adjacent structures, with a much higher incidence of facial nerve paralysis compared to closed head injury. As a result, these injuries are more likely to require surgical exploration than blunt temporal bone fractures.

Due to the nature of force required, the majority of patients with temporal bone fractures will have multiple injuries, including possible intracranial and cervical spine injury. Therefore, initial assessment follows advanced trauma life support protocols with multidisciplinary involvement. Once the patient is stabilised, a complete neuro-otological examination is required, including otoscopy for haemotympanum/perforated eardrum, evidence of postauricular ecchymosis (Battle's sign), CSF leak from the ear or nose and, in the conscious patient, assessment of facial nerve function, nystagmus and hearing loss (bedside tuning fork test and formal audiometric testing at the earliest opportunity). In the critically ill patient, rapid imaging with high-resolution CT is essential to evaluate the temporal bone but also the intracranial contents and potential cervical spine injury.

In acute facial palsy post ear surgery, iatrogenic injury of the tympanic segment of the facial nerve is the most common site of injury, due to the prevalence of facial canal dehiscence or exposure secondary to cholesteatoma. The vertical segment is more prone to trauma during posterior tympanotomy

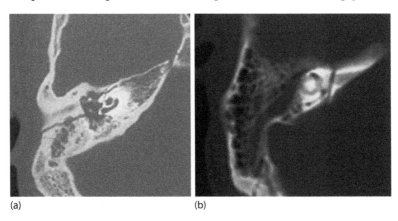

(a) (b)

Figure 18.2 (a) Longitudinal fracture of temporal bone; (b) Transverse fracture of temporal bone.

for cochlear implantation or combined approach tympanoplasty. The nerve can also be damaged in the cerebellopontine angle during skull base neurosurgery or in its extra-temporal segment while operating on the parotid gland.

In children the facial nerve approximates to that found in adults, except that it exits through the more superficially located stylomastoid foramen with ongoing development of the mastoid tip as a traction epiphysis from the time of birth. Hence, at birth there is a possibility of acute facial palsy due to forceps delivery, and there is also a higher risk of facial nerve injury in children due to surgery or trauma at this point of exit from the temporal bone.

In general, post-traumatic delayed onset or incomplete paresis almost always recovers, the majority within the first 3 months. Treatment involves high dose corticosteroids and eye care. The decision to explore a facial nerve following trauma is complex. Factors favouring exploration and indicating a severe injury to the nerve are a penetrating injury, immediate onset of paralysis, CT evidence of nerve canal disruption or bony spicule, loss of inner ear function, persistent CSF leak and 90% or greater degeneration on ENoG. Iatrogenic injury should be repaired at the time of surgery if noticed, or re-explored within days and the nerve repaired. Patients with persistent facial paralysis are observed for up to 9 months before considering reanimation and reinnervation techniques, to allow for natural recovery.

4. TUMOURS

Tumours account for less than 5% of patients with facial nerve paralysis. These may present with acute, but more commonly a recurrent or progressive, weakness. Schwannomas form the majority of intrinsic facial nerve tumours and can occur anywhere along the course of the facial nerve (Figure 18.3). Haemangiomas are extremely rare benign vascular tumours and tend to arise around the geniculate ganglion and internal auditory canal, reflective of the rich blood supply at these sites. Malignant involvement includes direct perineural spread via the facial nerve into the temporal bone by parotid mucoepidermoid and adenoid cystic carcinoma and squamous cell carcinoma.

Eliciting a past history of recurrent or progressive facial nerve paresis or absence of recovery after 3 months having been treated as Bell's palsy, and presence of facial spasms or twitching, are suggestive of a tumour. Hearing loss may be sensorineural with associated tinnitus or vertigo with tumours in the labyrinthine segment, or conductive with tumours in the horizontal segment. Examination should include assessment of facial nerve function, otoscopy, and palpation of parotid and neck. Thin-sectioned contrast-enhanced MRI in combination with high resolution CT of temporal bone is advised. All such patients need urgent referral to otologists for further management.

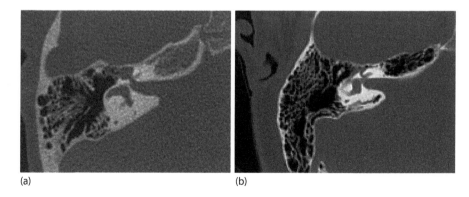

(a)   (b)

Figure 18.3 **(a)** Schwannoma of the right geniculate ganglion; **(b)** Normal geniculate ganglion for comparison.

Diagnostic clues in acute facial palsy:

- Vesicles – Ramsay Hunt syndrome
- Parotid lump – consider malignancy
- Children – acute otitis media/ cholesteatoma/mastoiditis
- Diabetic – skull base osteomyelitis
- Trauma – temporal bone fractures
- Surgery – iatrogenic injury
- UMN palsy/multiple cranial nerve palsy – neurological (stroke/infarct)
- Bilateral recurrent LMN palsy – Melkersson–Rosenthal syndrome

KEY LEARNING POINTS

- The facial nerve is the most common cranial nerve to be affected by disease.
- A good history and examination helps arrive at a diagnosis.
- Imaging is critical to diagnosis and exclusion of alternative pathology.
- Bell's palsy is a diagnosis of exclusion, and it recovers fully in most cases.
- Good evidence supports the use of steroids in treating Bell's palsy.
- Steroids + antivirals are indicated in Ramsay Hunt syndrome.
- Traumatic and iatrogenic facial palsy may need urgent surgery.
- Facial palsy of longer than 3 weeks warrants thorough re-evaluation.
- Early referral to an ENT specialist is critical to the outcome.

FURTHER READING

1. Sataloff RT, Selber JC. Phylogeny and embryology of the facial nerve and related structures. Part II: Embryology. *Ear Nose Throat J* 2003;82(10): 764–6, 769–72, 774.
2. May M, Klein SR. Differential diagnosis of facial nerve palsy. *Otolaryngol Clin North Am* 1991;24(3): 613–45.
3. House JW, Brackmann DE. Facial nerve grading system. *Otolaryngol Head Neck Surg* 1985;93: 146–7.
4. Gilden DH. Clinical practice. Bell's palsy. *N Engl J Med* 2004;351(13): 1323–31.
5. Axelsson S, Berg T, Jonsson L. Prednisolone in Bell's palsy related to treatment start and age. *Otol Neurotol* 2011;32: 141–6.
6. Siddiq MA, Hanu-Cenat LM, Irving RM. Facial palsy secondary to cholesteatoma: analysis of outcome following surgery. *J Laryngol Otol* 2007;121(2): 114–7.
7. Johnson F, Semaan MT, Megerian CA. Temporal bone fracture: evaluation and management in the modern era. *Otolaryngol Clin North Am* 2008;41: 597–618.
8. Moore PL, Selby G, Irving RM. Gunshot injuries to the temporal bone. *J Laryngol Otol* 2003;117(1): 71–4.
9. Doshi J, Irving R. Recurrent facial nerve palsy: the role of surgery. *J Laryngol Otol* 2010;124(10): 1202–4.
10. Alaani A, Hogg R, Saravanappa N, Irving RM. An analysis of the diagnostic delay in unilateral facial palsy. *J Laryngol Otol* 2005;119(3): 184–8.
11. Salib RJ, Tziambazis E, McDermott AL, Chavda SV, Irving RM. The crucial role of imaging in detection of facial nerve haemangiomas. *J Laryngol Otol* 2001;115(6): 510–3.
12. Josef Finsterer. Management of peripheral facial nerve palsy. *Eur Arch Otorhinolaryngol* 2008;265: 743–52.
13. Hohman MH, Hadlock TA. Etiology, diagnosis, and management of facial palsy: 2000 patients at a facial nerve center. *Laryngoscope* 2014;124: E283–93.

19

Intracranial emergencies related to the ear

PARAMITA BARUAH AND DUNCAN BOWYER

The proximity of the middle ear to the intracranial cavity allows potential spread of infection and development of intracranial complications. Routine antibiotic use has significantly reduced the frequency of complications of otitis media; however, intracranial spread of infection still occurs and has a high mortality in case series (Table 19.1).[1–4] Acute otitis media (AOM) and chronic otitis media (COM) may both lead to intracranial complications. Before antibiotics were widely available, approximately half of cases were associated with AOM; today the majority arise on a background of COM.

EPIDEMIOLOGY

In the pre-antibiotic era, intracranial complications developed in 2–6% of acute otitis media patients, proving fatal in 75% of cases.[4] In 1995, Kangsanarak *et al* reviewed 24,321 patients with otitis media, revealing an intracranial complication rate of

0.36%.[1] Most of these complications occurred in patients in their second decade. Paediatric patients form an important cohort that present with intracranial complications related to acute otitis media. In a nationwide study in the USA, 61,783 paediatric admissions over 12 months with otitis media were analysed, of which 181 (0.3%) also had meningitis, 48 (0.1%) had venous sinus thrombosis and 37 (0.1%) had an intracranial abscess.[5]

PATHOPHYSIOLOGY

Middle ear infection can spread outside of the temporal bone by three mechanisms: bony erosion, thrombophlebitis or direct spread. Bony erosion results from an osteitic process that often develops under an area of granulation. Thrombophlebitis of the mastoid emissary veins that drain to the sigmoid sinus is a route of access to the intracranial cavity. Finally, direct spread of infection occurs through preformed pathways, such as those resulting from

Table 19.1 Mortality from intracranial complications secondary to otitis media

	Gower et al (deaths/cases)	Singh and Maharaj (deaths/cases)	Osma et al (deaths/cases)	Kangsanarak et al (deaths/cases)
Meningitis	9/76 (12%)	1/22 (5%)	12/41 (29%)	4/43 (9%)
Brain abscess	1/6 (17%)	12/93 (13%)	2/10 (20%)	9/29 (31%)
Subdural/epidural abscess	0/3	2/36 (6%)	0/14	3/35 (9%)
Cerebritis/encephalitis	–	–	1/1 (100%)	0/16
Sinus thrombosis	0/5	0/36	0/1	4/16 (25%)
Otitic hydrocephalus	0/5	–	–	0/7

previous tympanomastoid surgery, temporal bone fractures or via anatomical points of weakness.

The risk of developing intracranial complications from otitis media varies with the underlying ear disease. In a series of 87 patients presenting with otogenic intracranial pathology, AOM was the underlying aetiology in only 5.[1] Of the 82 patients with COM and intracranial complications, 80% had squamous epithelial disease (cholesteatoma) and 20% mucosal disease. Singh and Maharaj[3] also found that intracranial complications were more commonly associated with cholesteatoma (59%).

DIAGNOSIS

Signs and symptoms of intracranial sepsis are often subtle, and a high degree of clinical suspicion is required. A history of headache, nausea and vomiting, or altered alertness are suggestive. It is essential to perform a complete neurological examination in addition to otologic examination. If intracranial sepsis is suspected, a contrast-enhanced CT of the temporal bones and brain should be urgently organised. Pus from ear discharge or following myringotomy, and blood cultures, should be sent for antimicrobial sensitivities to direct therapy.

MENINGITIS

Otogenic meningitis is the most common intracranial complication of otitis media[1,2] and often coexists with other complications, both intracranial

and extracranial. The early stages of the illness can be non-specific, with generalised headache and fever or irritability in a child. This progresses to neck stiffness, photophobia and vomiting. Further decline results in lethargy, seizures and coma.

Initial patient management involves stabilisation and rehydration. CT imaging allows exclusion of coexisting intracranial pathology and obstruction of CSF drainage, which precludes lumbar puncture. MRI is increasingly replacing CT as a diagnostic test due to its high sensitivity in detecting subtle intracranial findings and meningeal enhancement, which is diagnostic for the condition (Figure 19.1).

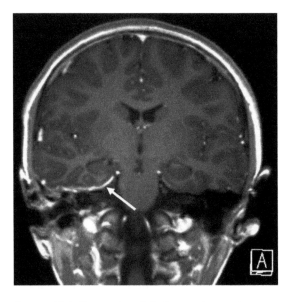

Figure 19.1 Coronal gadolinium-enhanced T1-weighted MRI of a 3-year-old child with otogenic meningitis, demonstrating dural enhancement (arrow).

Lumbar puncture allows CSF sampling for microbiological analysis.

Broad-spectrum antibiotics are commenced promptly and modified as bacterial sensitivities become available. Early use of corticosteroids is associated with less hearing damage and neurological sequelae, as well as a trend towards lower mortality.[6] Definitive surgical management of the underlying ear disease is performed once the patient has been stabilised. This may involve myringotomy and ventilation tube insertion (AOM), cortical mastoidectomy (mastoiditis) or tympanomastoidectomy (cholesteatoma). Serial audiograms are recommended, as hearing loss can occur as a late complication.

BRAIN ABSCESS

Brain abscesses associated with middle ear disease are more common in developing countries.[1-3] In a series of 122 consecutive patients diagnosed with brain abscess, otitis media was the third most common underlying source.[7] Otogenic brain abscesses are slightly more common in the temporal lobe than in the cerebellum (Figure 19.2).[8,9] Their natural history typically occurs over 2–3 weeks. In the initial inoculation phase there is localised encephalitis and oedema followed by a quiescent phase during which the inflammatory response attempts to contain and encapsulate the infective focus that eventually develops into a space-occupying lesion. Initial symptoms are typically mild and progress to high fever, headache, and nausea and/or vomiting, followed by changes in level of consciousness and focal neurologic deficits as a result of mass effect. A lesion in the temporal lobe may lead to an ipsilateral headache, aphasia and possibly a visual field defect. Lesions in the cerebellum may cause ataxia, dysmetria and nystagmus.

Initial management of an otogenic brain abscess involves stabilisation and broad-spectrum antibiotics. Positive cultures usually reveal polymicrobial infection including anaerobes. Neurosurgical drainage of the abscess is combined with surgical management of the middle ear and mastoid disease if the patient is sufficiently stable. Otologic surgery may be delayed by 4–6 weeks in some cases.[10]

SUBDURAL EMPYEMA

A subdural empyema is a collection of pus that develops between the dura and arachnoid layers.

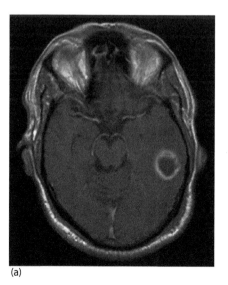
(a)

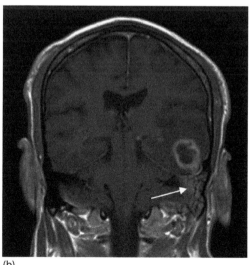
(b)

Figure 19.2 Axial (a) and coronal (b) contrast-enhanced T1 MRI demonstrating an otogenic temporal lobe abscess. Note fluid-containing mastoid air cells (arrow).

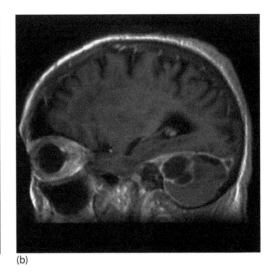

(a)   (b)

Figure 19.3 Axial **(a)** and sagittal **(b)** contrast-enhanced T1 MRI demonstrating a subdural abscess within the posterior fossa with coexisting sigmoid sinus thrombosis.

It is a rare complication of otitis media and can develop by direct extension or thrombophlebitis. Infection spreads readily once it enters the subdural layer because the anatomical barriers are limited. The clinical picture deteriorates rapidly, in keeping with an expanding intracranial mass. The patient is toxic and progresses quickly from severe headache, fever, vomiting and malaise to falling consciousness level and focal neurological signs. Confirmation of the diagnosis is made with neuroimaging (Figure 19.3). Treatment is emergency neurosurgical drainage and intravenous antibiotics (initially driven by local empirical policy and subsequently by culture sensitivities). Management of the underlying ear disease is addressed only once the patient has been stabilized. The condition has a high mortality rate (13% with subdural empyema compared to 0% with epidural abscess in a series of 31 children), and residual neurological deficits are common.[11]

EXTRADURAL ABSCESS

An extradural (epidural) abscess is a collection of pus between the dura and the adjacent temporal bone. It occurs when infection spreads directly through defects in the middle or posterior fossa bony plates or, alternatively, via bone erosion by granulation tissue or cholesteatoma. They are often asymptomatic and can be discovered coincidently on imaging or during mastoid surgery. Alternatively, they present with otalgia, headache and low-grade pyrexia. Extradural abscesses frequently coexist with other intracranial complications, particularly sigmoid sinus thrombophlebitis. Surgical management involves the removal of granulation tissue and drainage of pus through a mastoidectomy with postoperative intravenous antibiotics. Antimicrobial therapy is usually continued for several weeks, with repeat imaging as directed by the clinical scenario.

SIGMOID SINUS THROMBOSIS

Thrombosis of the sigmoid (lateral) sinus occurs through direct spread of infection or from retrograde thrombophlebitis of the veins that drain the middle ear cleft. Initial intimal inflammation of the vessel wall leads to mural thrombus formation. As this becomes infected, the resulting attraction of fibrin, blood cells and platelets causes enlargement of the thrombus and eventually venous occlusion. The thrombus may then propagate into the internal jugular vein (IJV) or, retrograde, towards the cavernous sinus. Dislodgement of the clot at the leading edge of the thrombus produces septic emboli, characterised by spiking fever and metastatic abscess formation.

The classical clinical description of sigmoid sinus thrombosis is a 'picket-fence' spiking temperature coinciding with septic embolisation. However, it is no longer a reliable sign, due to widespread use of antibiotics.[12] Patients often complain of otalgia and neck pain. Propagation of the clot into the IJV may be palpated as a cord-like structure in the neck. The presence of severe headache, vomiting or depressed conscious level should alert the clinician to the possibility of additional intracranial pathology. MRI with magnetic resonance venography (MRV) has high sensitivity in detecting sigmoid sinus thrombosis, but a CT scan is often more accessible in the acute setting and a filling defect may be seen in the affected sinus (Figure 19.4). In around one-third of cases, CT contrast accumulates in the collateral veins surrounding the non-enhancing thrombus, known as the 'empty delta sign'. Sigmoid sinus thrombosis is estimated to occur in 3–12% of cases of acute mastoiditis with complete clinical recovery in 76–84% of cases.[13] The condition is managed with intravenous antibiotics, with or without surgical debridement. The extent of any surgical intervention remains controversial; accepted practice includes routine opening of the sigmoid sinus and removal of the infected clot, aspiration of the sinus and opening only if pus is evacuated, or simple cortical mastoidectomy to remove surrounding infected material. The role of anticoagulation is also unclear. A review of otogenic sigmoid sinus thrombosis has suggested that complications of embolisation and sepsis are lower in this cohort than in non-otogenic thrombosis and that anticoagulation is only used in selected cases.[14] Other authors have described the use of anticoagulation for 3–6 months after surgical management of sigmoid sinus thrombosis. Follow-up imaging reveals partial or full canalisation of the sinus in up to 87% of cases.[15]

OTITIC HYDROCEPHALUS

Otitic hydrocephalus is a rare complication of otitis media and is often associated with sigmoid sinus thrombosis.[16] This is postulated as a key factor in the development of raised intracranial pressure, possibly by preventing CSF reabsorption into the cranial venous sinuses. Approximately 25–33% of patients with sigmoid sinus thrombosis will have otitic hydrocephalus.[17,18] Patients complain of a diffuse headache in the early stages, progressing to lethargy, blurred vision (from retinal vein occlusion) and diplopia (abducens nerve palsy). MRI scanning demonstrates normal ventricular volume, but a raised intracranial pressure is discovered on lumbar puncture. Management is

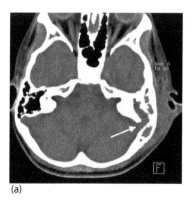
(a)
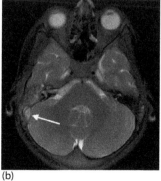
(b)
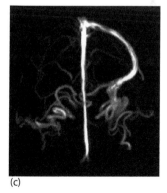
(c)

Figure 19.4 (a) Axial CT demonstrating a breach in the sigmoid sinus plate and probable sinus thrombosis (arrow). Thrombosis was confirmed intraoperatively. (b) Axial T2 MRI provides superior diagnostic imaging in suspected sigmoid sinus thrombosis. (c) Magnetic resonance venography (MRV) identifies absent venous flow in the right sigmoid and transverse sinuses due to thrombosis.

high-dose intravenous corticosteroids, diuretics and hyperosmolar agents such as mannitol, and lumboperitoneal shunts to normalise intracranial pressure. Surgical correction of the underlying ear disease is performed only once the patient has become neurologically stable.

KEY LEARNING POINTS

- The proximity of the middle ear to the middle and posterior cranial fossa allows potential spread of infection and development of intracranial complications.
- Routine use of antibiotics has made otogenic intracranial sepsis less common, but when they do occur, they still carry a significant risk of long-term morbidity/mortality.
- Intracranial complications of otitis media often coexist with other complications, both intracranial and extracranial.
- Signs and symptoms are often subtle, and a high degree of clinical suspicion is required.
- A history of headache, nausea and vomiting, or altered alertness are suggestive of intracranial spread of infection.
- Cross-sectional imaging is essential in the diagnosis and directing management of intracranial sepsis.

REFERENCES

1. Kangsanarak, J., Navacharoen, N., Fooanant, S. et al. Intracranial complications of suppurative otitis media: 13 years' experience. Am J Otol 1995; 16:104–109.

2. Osma, U., Cureoglu, S. & Hosoglu, S. The complications of chronic otitis media: report of 93 cases. J Laryngol Otol 2000; 114:97–100.

3. Singh, B. & Maharaj, T. J. Radical mastoidectomy: its place in otitic intracranial complications. J Laryngol Otol 1993; 107:1113–1118.

4. Gower, D. & McGuirt, W. F. Intracranial complications of acute and chronic infectious ear disease: a problem still with us. Laryngoscope 1983; 93:1028–1033.

5. Lavin, J. M., Rusher, T. & Shah, R. K. Complications of pediatric otitis media. Otolaryngol Head Neck Surg 2016; 154:366–370.

6. Brouwer, M. C., McIntyre, P., de Gans, J. et al. Corticosteroids for acute bacterial meningitis. Cochrane Database Syst Rev 2010:CD004405.

7. Yen, P. T., Chan, S. T. & Huang, T. S. Brain abscess: with special reference to otolaryngologic sources of infection. Otolaryngol Head Neck Surg 1995; 113:15–22.

8. Isaacson, B., Mirabal, C., Kutz, J. W., Jr. et al. Pediatric otogenic intracranial abscesses. Otolaryngol Head Neck Surg 2010; 142:434–437.

9. Mathews, T. J. & Marus, G. Otogenic intradural complications: a review of 37 patients. J Laryngol Otol 1988; 102:121–124.

10. Sennaroglu, L. & Sozeri, B. Otogenic brain abscess: review of 41 cases. Otolaryngol Head Neck Surg 2000; 123:751–755.

11. Smith, H. P. & Hendrick, E. B. Subdural empyema and epidural abscess in children. J Neurosurg 1983; 58:392–397.

12. Manolidis, S. & Kutz, J. W., Jr. Diagnosis and management of lateral sinus thrombosis. Otol Neurotol 2005; 26:1045–1051.

13. Wong, B. Y., Hickman, S., Richards, M. *et al.* Management of paediatric otogenic cerebral venous sinus thrombosis: a systematic review. *Clin Otolaryngol* 2015; 40:704–714.

14. Bradley, D. T., Hashisaki, G. T. & Mason, J. C. Otogenic sigmoid sinus thrombosis: what is the role of anticoagulation? *Laryngoscope* 2002; 112:1726–1729.

15. Ulanovski, D., Yacobovich, J., Kornreich, L. *et al.* Pediatric otogenic sigmoid sinus thrombosis: 12-year experience. *Int J Pediatr Otorhinolaryngol* 2014; 78:930–933.

16. Symonds, C. P. Otitic hydrocephalus. *Brain* 1931; 54:55–71.

17. Garcia, R. D., Baker, A. S., Cunningham, M. J. *et al.* Lateral sinus thrombosis associated with otitis media and mastoiditis in children. *Pediatr Infect Dis J* 1995; 14:617–623.

18. Syms, M. J., Tsai, P. D. & Holtel, M. R. Management of lateral sinus thrombosis. *Laryngoscope* 1999; 109:1616–1620.

SECTION 4

Emergencies in Paediatric ORL

20

Acute otitis media and its complications

SIMONE SCHAEFER AND IAIN BRUCE

INTRODUCTION

Acute otitis media (AOM) is one of the most common medical conditions of childhood and an important reason for seeking review in primary care. It is defined as the presence of inflammation in the middle ear, associated with an effusion and accompanied by the rapid onset of symptoms and signs of middle ear inflammation.[1,2] This should be distinguished from otitis media with effusion (OME, 'glue ear'), where the presence of effusion in the middle ear is not associated with these acute features. Although most children will suffer from AOM during childhood, a subgroup has recurrent AOM (rAOM), defined as having three or more episodes over the past 6 months or four or more episodes over the past year.[2] By the age of 3 years, approximately 50% to 85% of all children will have had at least one episode of AOM and 33% will have had two or more episodes.[3,4] The peak age-specific incidence lies between 6 and 15 months.[3]

Although the complication rate from AOM is low, there are a number of complications potentially associated with AOM, sometimes associated with high morbidity and rarely mortality (Table 20.1). Therefore, it is important to rapidly differentiate the child with complicated AOM from all the other children presenting with AOM.

PATHOPHYSIOLOGY

The identification of risk factors for developing a complication of acute otitis media is difficult due to the low incidence of complications, but there are a few recognised predisposing factors – firstly,

Table 20.1 Complications of acute otitis media

Intratemporal	Intracranial	Extracranial
Acute mastoiditis	Lateral sinus thrombosis	Bezold's abscess (along sternocleidomastoid muscle)
Facial nerve palsy	Extra- and subdural abscess	Citelli's abscess (posterior to the mastoid)
Subperiosteal abscess	Meningitis	Luc's abscess (along root of zygoma)
Bacterial labyrinthitis	Intracranial sepsis	Septic emboli
Apical petrositis (Gradenigo's syndrome)	Otitic hydrocephalus	

the bacterial virulence of the infecting agent, with the most commonly identified causal bacteria being *Streptococcus pneumoniae*, *Haemophilus influenzae* and *Moraxella catarrhalis*. However, *Streptococcus pyogenes*, *Pseudomonas aeruginosa* anaerobes and *Staphylococcus aureus* are often involved in AOM with complications. Secondly, the extent of pre-existing cell tracts and dehiscence in the temporal bone may present a pathway for pathogens, therefore providing an easy route for the spread of infection outside the middle ear cleft (Figure 20.1). Furthermore, inadequate host defences (e.g. immunodeficiency) predispose to the development of complications of AOM.

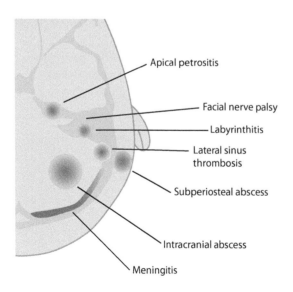

Figure 20.1 Spread of infection in complicated acute otitis media.

GENERAL SYMPTOMS AND SIGNS

Children with AOM will often present to their primary care physician complaining of otalgia or with symptoms suggestive of otalgia, such as 'pulling', 'tugging' or 'rubbing' the ear. However, in younger children, the presenting symptoms can be much less specific and include fever, irritability and poor feeding. A history of altered mental state or lethargy may suggest the development of an intracranial complication.

Typically, the findings on otoscopy are an erythematous and bulging tympanic membrane. Besides otoscopy, clinical evaluation should seek to identify extracranial, intratemporal and intracranial complications, as suggested by fluctuation of the soft tissues overlying the mastoid bone, a protruding ear, altered conscious level, cranial neuropathies and signs of meningism.

When a complication is diagnosed, a multidisciplinary treatment plan should be established involving the otolaryngologist, paediatrician, neurologist, neurosurgeon and microbiologist, depending on the case.

INTRATEMPORAL COMPLICATIONS

ACUTE MASTOIDITIS

Acute mastoiditis (AM) is the most common complication of AOM, with an incidence of about

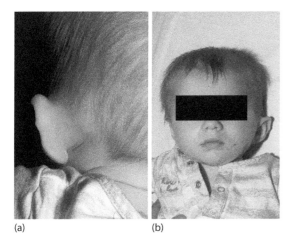

(a)   (b)

Figure 20.2 Clinical presentation of acute mastoiditis: postauricular swelling, skin erythema and loss of the postauricular sulcus **(a)** and protrusion of the auricle **(b)**.

1 to 2 per 10,000 children in the general population, and representing 2.4% of all children admitted with otitis media in a nationwide study in the US.[5,6] It is characterised by inflammation of the mastoid air-cell system, osteitis and possible extension into the surrounding structures.

The most frequently occurring signs are post-auricular swelling with loss of the post-auricular sulcus, skin erythema, tenderness and protrusion of the auricle (Figure 20.2). Furthermore, sagging of the wall of the posterosuperior ear canal can be seen on otoscopy, in addition to the previously described tympanic membrane abnormalities seen in AOM. Other accompanying findings might include facial nerve palsy and signs of intracranial extension.

A computed tomography (CT) scan with contrast is the most widely used imaging modality, due to its ability to show bony erosion, abscess formation, sinus thrombosis and intracranial sepsis (Figure 20.3). The timing of a CT scan is debatable.

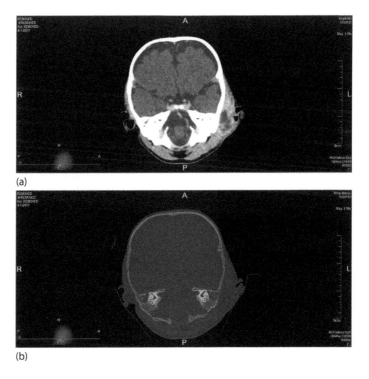

(a)

(b)

Figure 20.3 CT in acute mastoiditis (same patient as Figure 20.2) **(a)** CT with contrast showing a subperiosteal abscess. **(b)** CT without contrast showing decortification of the mastoid bone with postauricular swelling on the left side and opacification of both mastoids.

Some authors suggest performing a scan on every patient with AM to avoid missing any intracranial complications, whilst others consider that this might expose a significant number of patients to unnecessary irradiation.[7,8] A CT scan should be arranged if intracranial complications are suspected, when the response to conservative treatment with intravenous antibiotics is poor, when there is diagnostic doubt and pre-operatively prior to a cortical mastoidectomy. For intracranial complications, additional magnetic resonance imaging (MRI) can be useful to determine the extent of the disease.

In the absence of symptoms and signs of complications, intravenous broad spectrum antibiotics are the first-line treatment of AM. Some clinicians may consider a myringotomy or ventilation tube insertion at the initial stage of management, with both necessitating general anaesthesia (GA). When a subperiosteal abscess has formed, treatment will usually consist of a cortical mastoidectomy with drainage of the pus collection within the soft tissues (Figure 20.4). Incision and drainage (I&D) or needle aspiration of the abscess alone, have been shown to be effective in some studies. A cortical mastoidectomy should be performed for complications of AM and considered if the response to conservative management is poor (Figure 20.5). It should also be performed when there is a suggestion of cholesteatoma on the CT imaging, with underlying cholesteatoma in 7.5% of patients presenting with AM.

APICAL PETROSITIS

In apical petrositis the infection in the middle ear cleft has spread into the apical region of the petrous bone. Patients may present with a triad of retro-auricular pain, otorrhoea and abducens nerve palsy, also known as Gradenigo's syndrome. Imaging studies in the form of CT with contrast and/or MR scan are necessary to confirm the diagnosis (Figure 20.6).

More recently, a conservative approach for treating this condition is becoming more prevalent, with several authors showing full recovery with ventilation tube insertion and intravenous antibiotics alone.[9,10]

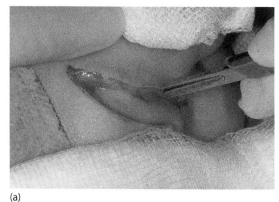
(a)

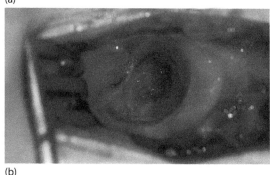
(b)

Figure 20.4 Cortical mastoidectomy in acute mastoiditis with subperiosteal abscess. (a) Incision and drainage of the subperiosteal abscess. (b) Subsequent cortical mastoidectomy (note the inflamed and highly vascular tissue).

FACIAL NERVE PALSY

The course of the facial nerve runs through the middle ear, making the nerve susceptible to inflammatory damage in AOM. Furthermore, 6–10% of the general population have a dehiscence of the facial nerve canal in the middle ear, as a variant of normal anatomy. The incidence of facial nerve palsy (FNP) in patients with AOM has been reported as 12.6–16.7%.

Myringotomy with, or without, ventilation tube insertion is common for FNP complicating AOM, combined with a cortical mastoidectomy when there is concurrent AM. Although a role for steroid treatment is established in idiopathic facial nerve palsy, no consensus exists regarding steroid use in FNP complicating AOM. However, if there are no patient-specific contraindications to steroid use,

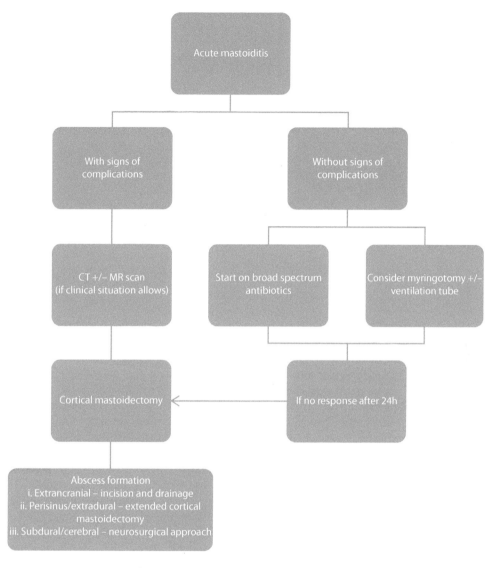

Figure 20.5 Treatment strategy for acute mastoiditis.

the same treatment strategy as for idiopathic FNP could be followed.[11]

LABYRINTHITIS

Although rare (1.8–2% of intratemporal complications), suppurative (bacterial) labyrinthitis can cause significant morbidity. It must be distinguished from serous labyrinthitis, where there is a non-purulent inflammation of the labyrinth. Via the internal auditory meatus (IAM), labyrinthitis can either cause meningitis or itself complicate meningitis.

The diagnosis of labyrinthitis is a clinical one, with presenting features including hearing loss, tinnitus, vertigo and nystagmus. Suppurative labyrinthitis should be suspected when symptoms are severe and/or progressive and is often associated with other complications. Imaging studies may be requested to exclude any intracranial pathology.

A serous labyrinthitis can often be treated conservatively with antibiotic therapy and systemic

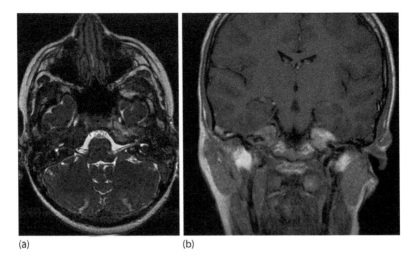

(a)   (b)

Figure 20.6 Left-sided apical petrositis evidenced by contrast enhancement on MR imaging – (a) axial and (b) coronal cuts.

corticosteroids. Suppurative labyrinthitis is likely to require more invasive treatment, depending on the extent of involvement of the temporal bone structures. Treatments include myringotomy and ventilation tube insertion in AOM and cortical mastoidectomy in AM. The recovery rates for inner ear function after suppurative labyrinthitis are poor, with most patients having a resultant profound hearing loss (71–100%).

INTRACRANIAL COMPLICATIONS

INTRACRANIAL SEPSIS

The spread of an otogenic infection to involve the intracranial structures can lead to various complications, including meningitis, intracranial abscess formation, subdural empyema and epidural abscess. Although antibiotic treatment, immunisations, increase in social welfare and wide access to healthcare have led to a significant decrease in the incidence and mortality of these complications, they continue to occur, with the emerging incidence of bacterial resistance to antibiotics being a complicating factor.

Symptoms of AOM and/or AM may be accompanied by neurological symptoms, including headache, nausea and vomiting, altered mental state (drowsiness), diplopia, seizures and extremity weakness.

A CT with contrast and MR scan are essential to confirm the diagnosis and the extent of intracranial involvement. Treatment of otogenic intracranial sepsis, in the absence of significant abscess formation, consists of a cortical mastoidectomy combined with long-term (at least 6 weeks) intravenous broad-spectrum antibiotic treatment. Multidisciplinary consultation with neurology and neurosurgery specialities should always be undertaken. However, if further intervention is deemed necessary, the intracranial abscess can be drained by aspiration through the mastoid cavity or via a craniotomy, depending on the localisation and extent of the abscess. More recently, conservative management with antibiotic treatment alone has also been utilised successfully, adding to the debate regarding the most appropriate treatment strategy.

LATERAL SINUS THROMBOSIS

Otogenic lateral sinus thrombosis (LST) comprises septic thrombus involving the sigmoid (and possibly transverse) sinus with partial or complete occlusion of blood flow. The thrombus may result from direct extension from osteitis or septic granulation tissue overlying the sinus wall, or indirect extension of the infection through emissary veins. The infection may spread to the other dural sinuses and the internal jugular vein, or even cause systemic septic emboli. LST complicates approximately 2–3% of cases of AM. Despite improvement in treatment options, LST can cause serious long-term neurological morbidities and rarely death (mortality rate of 5–10%).

Patients presenting with LST commonly have a recent history of AOM and ongoing symptoms of otalgia and headaches. Further neurological history might include photophobia and diplopia. On examination, signs of AOM or AM may have already resolved secondary to previous antibiotic treatment. The presence of fever, lethargy, papilloedema and an abducens nerve palsy should alert to this possible complication.

Imaging studies must be performed to confirm the suspected diagnosis of LST. On CT with contrast imaging, LST may be associated with the 'Delta sign', a flow void in the sinus with enhancement of the infectious surrounding tissues (Figure 20.7). More recently, MR venography (MRV) has been used to further delineate the extent of the flow restriction and to visualise the contralateral venous system (Figure 20.8).

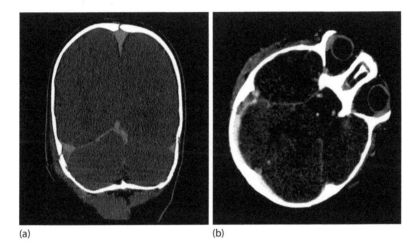

(a)   (b)

Figure 20.7 Lateral sinus thrombosis on CT scan. (a) Positive Delta sign of the right sigmoid sinus. (b) Lateral sigmoid sinus thrombosis extending into the transverse sinus.

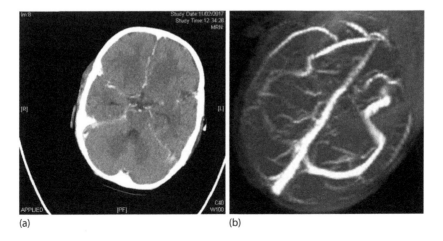

(a)   (b)

Figure 20.8 Lateral sinus thrombosis on MR venography. (a) Right sigmoid sinus thrombosis on contrast CT. (b) MR venography of the same patient showing occlusion of the right sigmoid and transverse sinus.

The treatment options for otogenic LST remain contentious and include combinations of intravenous antibiotics, anticoagulation and surgery. As with other intracranial complications of AOM, multidisciplinary care is mandatory. Currently, the most common surgical treatment is cortical mastoidectomy, potentially combined with ventilation tube insertion. No consensus exists regarding the role of needle aspiration of the sinus to confirm the diagnosis (superseded by MR venography), or surgical evacuation of the thrombus from the sinus. Likewise, the use of anticoagulants has not been standardised, with the decision to anticoagulate best taken by neurologists. Serial MR venography may be used to determine the extent of thrombus progression, or to monitor response to treatment. A systematic review including 190 children has found that anticoagulants were used in 59% of the cases without any major bleeding complications, and that for all children with a good clinical outcome, 56% received both surgery and anticoagulation. However, rates of complete recanalisation on follow-up imaging were similar for the 'anticoagulated' and the 'non-anticoagulated' group.[12]

OTOGENIC HYDROCEPHALUS

Otogenic hydrocephalus is characterised by the presence of increased intracranial pressure (ICP) and may accompany other intracranial complications, such as lateral sinus thrombosis (LST) or intracranial sepsis. Reported rates vary between 0.93% in AOM and 33% in LST. Symptoms include headache, nausea, vomiting and lethargy. Diagnosis and management of this complication is usually lead by neurologists and includes eye examination for papilloedema. As with other intracranial complications, surgical management is dictated by the location and severity of the ear infection.

BEZOLD'S ABSCESS

In 1881, Bezold described the formation of a neck abscess as a complication of mastoiditis. The

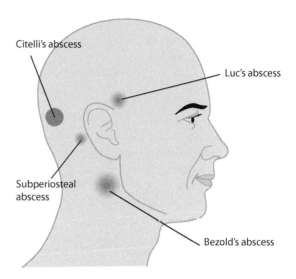

Figure 20.9 Extracranial complications of AOM.

abscess is caused by erosion of the mastoid tip along the digastric ridge with the spread of pus between the digastric and the sternocleidomastoid muscles (Figure 20.9). Subsequently, infection may spread inferiorly along the great vessels, the parapharyngeal or the retropharyngeal space.

Bezold's abscess has become a rare complication since the introduction of antibiotics and is especially rare in childhood, since its formation requires aeration of the mastoid tip, a finding uncommon in young children. The most common symptoms on presentation are otalgia, otorrhoea, neck swelling, neck pain, restricted movement of the neck and pyrexia. Because of the deep nature of the abscess, it is not always easily accessible to palpation.

Diagnosis is confirmed by a contrast-enhanced CT scan of the neck and temporal bones. A cortical mastoidectomy combined with incision and drainage of the abscess and broad spectrum antibiotics is the most commonly used treatment method.

LUC'S ABSCESS

Henri Luc first described the formation of a subperiosteal temporal abscess as a complication of AOM in 1913. A Luc's abscess extends over the zygomatic arch, with the route of spread of infection being via a breach in the anterior mastoid cortex directly communicating with the subperiosteal plane. The diagnosis should be suspected in a child with a fluctuant preauricular facial swelling with associated symptoms of malaise, pyrexia and a history suggestive of AOM. Depending on the findings, the need for a cortical mastoidectomy as well as incision and drainage of the abscess can be evaluated.[13]

CITELLI'S ABSCESS

Various descriptions of Citelli's abscess are given in the literature. Some authors describe it as being situated in the occipital region, posterior to the mastoid, in contrast to a subperiosteal post-auricular abscess that is situated over the mastoid. Pus travels either along the mastoid emissary vein or occipitotemporal suture, resulting in abscess formation and possible osteomyelitis of the calvarium. Other authors describe a Citelli's abscess as lying along the posterior belly of the digastric muscle. Diagnosis and management is the same as for a post-auricular abscess.

KEY LEARNING POINTS

- Acute otitis media is one of the most common conditions in childhood.
- Young children can present with atypical features such as fever, irritability and poor feeding.
- History taking and examination should focus on confirming the diagnosis and excluding intratemporal, intracranial and extracranial complications.
- Treatment of complications of acute otitis media is usually multimodal (antibiotic therapy combined with surgical intervention).
- Multidisciplinary involvement is essential in the management of intracranial complications.

REFERENCES

1. National Institute for Health and Care Excellence. (2015, July 1). *Otitis Media: Acute*. NICE Clinical Knowledge Summaries: cks.nice.org.uk/otitis-media-acute

2. Venekamp RP, Damoiseaux RA, Schilder AG. Acute otitis media in children. *BMJ Clin Evid* 2014; *9*(301): 1–21.

3. Venekamp RP, Sanders SL, Glasziou PP, Del Mar CB, Rovers MM. Antibiotics for acute otitis media in children. *Cochrane Database Syst Rev* 2015, Issue 6. Art. No.: CD000219. doi: 10.1002/14651858.CD000219.pub4.

4. Marchisio P, Bellussi L, Di Mauro G et al. Acute otitis media: from diagnosis to prevention. Summary of the Italian guideline. *Int J Pediatr Otorhinolaryngol* 2010; *74*(11): 1209–16.

5. Royal College of General Practitioners Research & Surveillance Centre. (2014/2015). Retrieved from Weekly Returns Service: www.rcgp.org.uk/clinical-and-research /our-programmes/research-and-surveillance -centre.aspx

6. Lavin JM, Rusher T, Shah RK. Complications of pediatric otitis media. *Otolaryngol Head Neck Surg* 2016; *154*(2): 366–70.

7. Luntz M, Bartal K, Brodsky A, Shihada R. Acute mastoiditis: the role of imaging for identifying intracranial complications. *Laryngoscope* 2012; *122*(12): 2813–17.

8. Tamir S, Schwartz Y, Peleg U, Perez R, Sichel JY. Acute mastoiditis in children: is computed tomography always necessary? *Ann Otol Rhinol Laryngol* 2009; *118*(8): 565–9.

9. Burston BJ, Pretorius PM, Ramsden JD. Gradenigo's syndrome: successful conservative treatment in adult and paediatric patients. *J Laryngol Otol* 2005; *4*(119): 325–9.

10. Janjua N, Bajalan M, Potter S et al. Multidisciplinary care of a paediatric patient with Gradenigo's syndrome. *BMJ Case Report* Published online 2016; 1–5. doi: 10.1136/bcr-2015-214337.

11. Cope D, Bova R. Steroids in otolaryngology. *Laryngoscope* 2008; *9*(118): 1556–60.

12. Wong BY, Hickman S, Richards M, Jassar P, Wilson T. (2015). Management of paediatric otogenic cerebral venous sinus thrombosis: a systematic review. *Clin Otolaryngol* 2015; *40*(6): 704–14.

13. Scrafton DK, Qureishi A, Nogueira C, Mortimore S. Luc's abscess as an unlucky complication of mastoiditis. *Ann R Coll Surg Engl* 2014; *96*: e28–e30.

FURTHER READING

Enoksson F, Groth A, Hultcrantz M et al. Subperiosteal abscesses in acute mastoiditis in 115 Swedish children. *Int J Pediatr Otorhinolaryngol* 2015; *79*(7): 1115–20.

Goldstein NA, Casselbrant ML, Bluestone CD, Kurs-Lasky M. Intratemporal complications of acute otitis media in infants and children. *Otolaryngol Head Neck Surg* 1998; *119*(5): 445–54.

Isaacson B, Mirabal C, Kutz JW Jr et al. Pediatric otogenic intracranial abscesses. *Otolaryngol Head Neck Surg* 2010; *3*(142): 434–7.

Maranhão AS, Godofredo VR, Penido Nde O. Suppurative labyrinthitis associated with otitis media: 26 years' experience. *Braz J Otorhinolaryngol* 2016; *82*(1): 82–7.

Mattos JL, Colman KL, Casselbrant ML, Chi DH. Intratemporal and intracranial complications of acute otitis media in a pediatric population. *Int J Pediatr Otorhinolaryngol* 2014; *12*(78): 2161–4.

Taylor MF, Berkowitz RG. Indications for mastoidectomy in acute mastoiditis in children. *Ann Otol Rhinol Laryngol* 2004; *113*(1): 69–72.

Wu JF, Jin Z, Yang JM et al. Extracranial and intracranial complications of otitis media: 22-year clinical experience and analysis. *Acta Otolaryngol* 2012; *132*(3): 261–5.

Zanoletti E, Cazzador D, Faccioli C et al. Intracranial venous sinus thrombosis as a complication of otitis media in children: critical review of diagnosis and management. *Int J Pediatr Otorhinolaryngol* 2015; *79*(12): 2398–403.

21

Acute sinusitis and its complications

NEIL BATEMAN

INTRODUCTION

Sinonasal infections are common in the paediatric population. Viral upper respiratory infections are commonplace, and a proportion of these will go on to cause a more prolonged episode of sinusitis. The majority of these infections do not go on to cause worrying complications. However, sinusitis in children can cause complications with potentially life-threatening or life-changing sequelae, and it is essential that any otolaryngologist caring for children has a good working knowledge of the potential complications, the clinical assessment of affected children, and their investigation and management.

PATHOPHYSIOLOGY

Acute sinusitis is defined as sinusitis, or an inflammation of the mucosal lining of the paranasal sinuses, which resolves within 12 weeks. Episodes lasting longer than this are termed chronic.

The majority of episodes of acute sinusitis are triggered by a viral upper respiratory tract infection (URTI). URTIs are exceptionally common in children and children will, on average, have six to eight per year. The overwhelming majority of these URTIs are viral in nature and self-limiting, requiring only symptomatic treatment. A small number may trigger an episode of acute sinusitis, and an even smaller proportion of these may go on to cause a complication.

Allergic rhinitis may contribute to mucosal oedema and contribute to the triggering of acute sinusitis, especially in older children.

MICROBIOLOGY

The most common bacteria implicated in acute sinusitis in children are *Streptococcus pneumoniae*, *Haemophilus influenzae* and *Moraxella catarrhalis*. Less commonly, *Staphylococcus aureus*, *Streptococcus pyogenes* and anaerobic bacteria are implicated.

ANATOMY

The ethmoid and maxillary sinuses are present at birth. The sphenoid and frontal sinuses undergo pneumatisation during childhood, and are present at the ages of 5 and 7–8 years, respectively, but are not completely developed until late adolescence.

COMPLICATIONS OF SINUSITIS

Complications of acute sinusitis may be classified as orbital, intracranial and osseous. Orbital complications occur with the greatest frequency in children, owing to the particularly thin paediatric lamina papyracea facilitating the spread of infection to the orbit.

ORBITAL

Orbital complications occur as a complication of infection of the ethmoid sinuses either by direct spread through a defect in the lamina papyracea or via communicating blood vessels. The schema for classification proposed by Chandler in 1970 has gained widest acceptance. The stages include:

1. Stage I – Pre-septal cellulitis
2. Stage II – Orbital cellulitis
3. Stage III – Subperiosteal abscess
4. Stage IV – Orbital abscess
5. Stage V – Cavernous sinus thrombosis

Pre-septal cellulitis refers to inflammation anterior to the orbital septum, which is a layer of connective tissue originating at the orbital margin and inserting into the trans plates of the eyelids. This structure acts as a barrier between the superficial soft tissues and the orbital contents. Clinically, cellulitis is confined to the eyelid. Pre-septal cellulitis has a different aetiology to orbital cellulitis and intra-orbital abscesses and commonly results from a primary skin infection, rather than sinus disease.

Post-septal cellulitis is a general inflammation of the orbital tissue without abscess formation. A subperiosteal abscess forms most commonly on the medial wall of the orbit adjacent to the lamina papyracea.

Orbital cellulitis and intra-orbital abscesses may cause blindness due to direct compression of the optic nerve, occlusion of the retinal artery or inflammation of the optic nerve.

Orbital complications may precede, and hence coexist with, intracranial complications. There should therefore be a high degree of suspicion of intracranial sepsis where an orbital complication is found.

INTRACRANIAL

Intracranial complications of sinusitis occur less frequently in children than in adults and include:

- Meningitis
- Encephalitis
- Extradural abscess
- Subdural abscess
- Cerebral abscess
- Venous sinus thrombosis

OSSEOUS

Bony complications account for 5–10% of all complications and usually complicate frontal sinusitis. As such, their occurrence is generally confined to adolescents and adults, and they were discussed in Chapter 6, (Rhinology section).

- Osteomyelitis
- Pott's puffy tumour

HISTORY AND EXAMINATION

Acute sinusitis generally follows a viral URTI or common cold. The diagnosis should be suspected when there is a worsening of symptoms after a period over which it would be expected that the symptoms of a cold would abate (approximately 5 days) or a persistence of symptoms over a period of 10 days. Typical symptoms of acute sinusitis in children are: nasal obstruction, purulent nasal discharge, facial pressure/pain and cough.

Three out of the following should lead to a suspicion of acute bacterial sinusitis:

- Purulent discharge
- Severe local pain
- Temperature >38 °C
- A deterioration following milder symptoms (or 'double sickening')
- Elevated ESR/CRP

Children tend to experience less facial pain than do adults, but an absence of pain certainly does not exclude the diagnosis. The presence of severe pain, especially frontal pain, should alert the clinician to the possibility of an intracranial complication.

Initial examination should assess the general condition of the child, including temperature, to immediately identify those children with systemic sepsis requiring urgent treatment. Severe sepsis may occur with an identified focus of infection and should be suspected if two or more of the following are present:

- Core temperature <36°C or >38.5°C
- Tachycardia
- Altered mental state (lethargy, sleepiness, irritability, decreased level of consciousness)
- Reduced peripheral circulation (identified by prolonged capillary refill time)

If these are present, a diagnosis of systemic sepsis should be considered and urgent action taken to manage this with the appropriate clinical teams.

Many children will not tolerate nasal endoscopy, although this is certainly possible in older children and teenagers and will often show pus in the region of the sinus ostia. Otherwise, anterior rhinoscopy can be carried out. Often the most useful tool for this purpose is an otoscope rather than the traditional head mirror/light and speculum, which children generally find uncomfortable and intimidating.

Examination should then proceed to consider the presence of complications. If orbital complications are suspected, the eye should be assessed for the following (if possible):

- Oedema of overlying skin
- Proptosis and/or displacement of the globe
- Chemosis (conjunctival oedema and/or erythema)
- Restricted ocular movements (ophthalmoplegia)
- Colour vision
- Visual acuity
- Pupillary reflexes

Children with pre-septal cellulitis present with oedema and erythema of the eyelids in the absence of any of the other signs associated with orbital infection. In general they also have much less systemic upset compared to children with post-septal infection. Children with post-septal infection tend to be more systemically unwell and are often pyrexial. The presence of proptosis, globe displacement or restricted ocular movements indicate significant post-septal infection, but the absence of these signs does not exclude the diagnosis. A subperiosteal abscess, if large enough, may displace the globe infero-laterally (Figure 21.1). Reduced visual acuity, which is preceded by loss of colour vision, is a sign of optic nerve compression and indicates imminent visual loss. An afferent pupillary defect is indicative of visual loss and is an ominous sign. The presence of bilateral signs should raise concerns of cavernous sinus thrombosis.

From a pragmatic, practical point of view, while in some cases it is obvious, the distinction between pre-septal and post-septal infection is sometimes difficult, and the key issue on assessment is to distinguish between those children who require imaging and those who can be treated medically (see Investigations section).

The presence of intracranial complications should be suspected when children have severe persistent headache or reduced consciousness level,

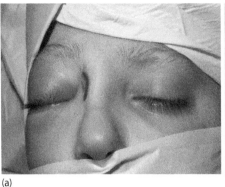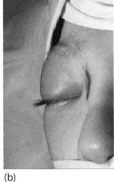

(a)   (b)

Figure 21.1 **(a)** Right periorbital oedema and erythema in an 11-year-old boy with a radiologically confirmed right subperiosteal abscess. **(b)** External approach to drainage of a medially placed subperiosteal abscess. (Image courtesy of M-L Montague, Royal Hospital for Sick Children, Edinburgh.)

or when they are more obtunded or unwell than might be expected in a child with a sinus infection. Often these signs can be very subtle in practice. The diagnosis of intracranial sepsis due to sinus infection is very often delayed in clinical practice, and maintaining a high level of suspicion, and investigating appropriately, is important in the assessment of children. Where intracranial complications are suspected, the child should be assessed for the following:

- Level of consciousness
- The presence of any focal neurological deficit
- Meningism (e.g. neck stiffness)

INVESTIGATIONS

INVESTIGATIONS FOR ACUTE SINUSITIS

Very few investigations are required to confirm the diagnosis of acute sinusitis, which is, in most cases, a clinical one. Imaging studies, whether plain x-ray, computed tomography (CT) or magnetic resonance imaging (MRI), have no role to play in the diagnosis of acute sinusitis, as the high rate of incidental findings of mucosal thickening and sinus opacification render these modalities meaningless in this context.

INVESTIGATIONS FOR SUSPECTED COMPLICATIONS

When orbital complications are suspected, the most useful and practical investigation is a CT scan of the orbits with contrast (Figure 21.2). Intracranial complications may also be detected using CT scanning, although MRI is likely to have greater sensitivity in detecting subtler intracranial complications. The disadvantages of MRI scanning are that it is more time-consuming and younger children not infrequently require sedation or general anaesthesia. Furthermore, CT scanning

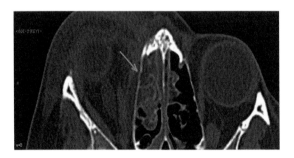

Figure 21.2 Contrast CT scan of the child in Figure 21.1 showing a large right medial subperiosteal abscess and a defect in the lamina papyracea (green arrow). Image courtesy of M-L Montague, Royal Hospital for Sick Children, Edinburgh.

will give useful information regarding bony anatomy should surgery be required. It therefore seems reasonable to investigate initially with a contrast-enhanced CT scan and proceed to MRI where this provides incomplete information or there is persisting clinical concern.

Where there is a suspected complication, pus should be obtained for culture and sensitivity prior to antibiotic administration, if possible. In these children, on admission, blood should be taken for FBC, CRP and blood cultures.

MANAGEMENT

MANAGEMENT OF ACUTE SINUSITIS

In children with uncomplicated acute bacterial sinusitis, empirical treatment with a broad spectrum antibiotic with activity against the likely causative organisms is reasonable. The first choice would be amoxicillin in a dose appropriate to the patient's age and/or weight for a period of 7 days. In cases of allergy to penicillin then erythromycin or doxycycline for a period of 7 days is recommended. Where there is no improvement after 48 hours of treatment with a first line antibiotic then amoxicillin-clavulanate for 7 days or azithromycin for 3 days is recommended.

A topical nasal steroid spray may provide some modest improvement in symptoms. The onset of benefit from using sprays of this type is somewhat delayed, however. A nasal steroid spray would be worthwhile considering in children with more prolonged symptoms.

Topical nasal decongestants provide noticeable symptomatic relief but are only licensed in children over the age of 12 and should not be used for protracted periods (more than 10 days), as prolonged use may cause rhinitis medicamentosa.

Antipyrexials and analgesics (paracetamol and non-steroidal anti-inflammatory drugs (NSAIDs) such as Ibuprofen) are recommended for symptomatic relief.

Oral decongestants have no role in the management of acute sinusitis.

MANAGEMENT OF COMPLICATIONS

Orbital

The optimal management of suspected orbital sepsis relies on early diagnosis, the establishment of an appropriate treatment plan and regular, attentive review of the patient's progress. This is best achieved by a multidisciplinary approach. A multidisciplinary team (MDT) comprising otolaryngology, ophthalmology and paediatrics allows a comprehensive and safe approach to the assessment and management of this condition. Children with clinical signs of orbital infection should be urgently assessed by senior clinicians in otolaryngology and ophthalmology, as a minimum.

Although distinction is made between pre- and post-septal infection, in practice this can be difficult to distinguish, especially in younger children. Therefore, a significant majority of children will require admission for medical treatment, even when immediate imaging and surgery is not required. Whether or not imaging is required immediately, all children should be started on medical treatment consisting of intravenous antibiotics (a third-generation cephalosporin and metronidazole is recommended) as well as a topical nasal decongestant, such as Xylometazoline 0.05%.

The critical decision in most children admitted with orbital infection is when imaging should be carried out. The flow chart in Figure 21.3 illustrates the decision-making process.

When a subperiosteal abscess is found on imaging, surgery should be considered. Small abscesses may be effectively treated medically and surgery avoided. This relies on a complete absence of signs suggesting any impending visual impairment, such as loss of colour vision or reduced visual acuity, and close monitoring with surgical intervention at the first sign of any deterioration.

When surgery is required this may be carried out externally via a Lynch–Howarth incision or endoscopically using endoscopic sinus surgery techniques. The goal of surgery is to drain the collection of pus, decompress the orbit, drain the concomitant sinusitis and obtain material for culture if this has not been possible before. The decision as to

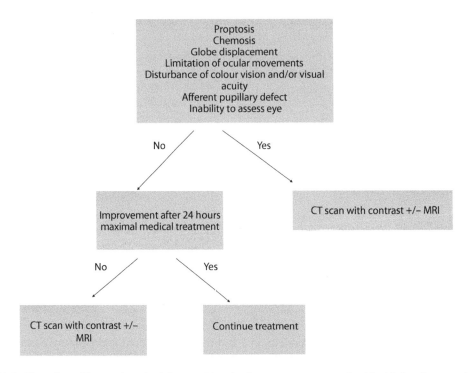

Figure 21.3 Flow chart illustrating decision-making in the management of orbital infections and, in particular, when to consider imaging.

which approach to take will ultimately depend on the experience and preference of the surgeon and the location of the abscess. While an endoscopic approach has the advantage of avoiding a facial scar, endoscopic surgery in a child with acute sinusitis is technically challenging because of bleeding and limited access. Hence, it can only really be recommended for experienced endoscopic sinus surgeons. Endoscopic techniques are less successful when dealing with abscesses not confined to the medial wall of the orbit. If there is extension of the abscess within the orbit beyond the medial wall, an open technique should be considered (Figure 21.4). Clinicians should be mindful of the fact that this is a potentially sight-threatening condition, and open drainage is, in most surgeons' hands, the safest and most reliable approach.

Intracranial

Intracranial complications require a combined approach involving otolaryngology and neurosurgery. As a general rule, management consists of neurosurgical management of the intracranial

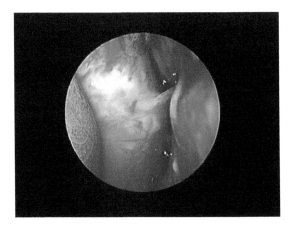

Figure 21.4 Intraoperative view during open drainage of the right subperiosteal abscess in the child in Figures 21.1 and 21.2. Note the mesentery of the anterior ethmoidal artery clearly defined superiorly and the bead of pus traversing the lamina from the ethmoid sinuses. External ethmoidectomy and middle meatal antrostomy with lavage of the maxillary sinus were carried out after drainage of the subperiosteal abscess. Image courtesy of M-L Montague, Royal Hospital for Sick Children, Edinburgh.

aspect of the disease with maximal medical management of the sinus disease, combined with surgical drainage of the affected sinuses, including external frontal trephine if necessary.

CAVERNOUS SINUS THROMBOSIS

Cavernous sinus thrombosis is a rare complication of sinus infection but still has a high mortality rate. The principles of management are the use of high-dose intravenous antibiotics and surgical drainage of the affected paranasal sinuses. The use of anticoagulation is a controversial issue, and there is no evidence to support or refute its use. The use of anticoagulants is best considered on a case-by-case basis and after discussion with colleagues in neurosurgery and neurology.

KEY LEARNING POINTS

- Viral upper respiratory infections are very common in children.
- Suspect sinusitis when symptoms worsen after 5 days or persist for longer than 10 days.
- Maintain a high level of suspicion for acute sepsis in children.
- Where an orbital abscess is suspected, the imaging modality of choice is CT scanning with contrast.
- Maintain a high level of suspicion for intracranial complications, especially in children with orbital complications.

FURTHER READING

Fokkens WJ, Lund VJ, Mullol J et al. European position paper on rhinosinusitis and nasal polyps *Rhinology* 2012 Mar; 50(1):1–12.

National Institute for Health and Care Excellence. Clinical knowledge summaries: sinusitis, 2017. https://cks.nice.org.uk/sinusitis

Wald ER, Applegate KE, Bordley C, Darrow DH, Glode MP, Michael Marcy S, Nelson CE, Rosenfeld RM, Shaikh N, Smith MJ, Williams PV, Weinberg ST. Clinical practice guideline for the diagnosis and management of acute bacterial sinusitis in children aged 1 to 18 years. *Pediatrics* 2013;132(1): e262–e280. Available from: pediatrics.aappublications.org/content/132/1/e262.

Acute tonsillitis

PETER J ROBB

INTRODUCTION

Acute sore throat is a common symptom that each year in the UK accounts for about 35 million days lost through time off school or work. The estimated cost to the NHS is £100m annually. In the USA, it is estimated that acute sore throat accounts for 1–2% of all outpatient attendances.

The peak incidence is between the ages of 5 and 15 years, with symptoms of pain, fever, systemic malaise and sometimes dehydration, vomiting and tender, enlarged cervical lymph nodes. Typically, in this age group, each episode will result in two days' absence from school.

In the published literature, the term 'sore throat' is unhelpfully used interchangeably with acute pharyngitis, acute tonsillitis, tonsillopharyngitis and bacterial pharyngitis.

The most common bacterial organism, group A beta-haemolytic streptococcus (GABHS), has a wide reported range of between 5% and 36% of episodes of acute tonsillitis, making diagnosis of streptococcal infection clinically difficult. Of infective sore throats, 50–80% are of viral origin, with 1–10% of these caused by Epstein–Barr virus (EBV); the remainder are caused by common upper respiratory viruses. GABHS, staphylococci, pneumococcus and haemophilus account for more than 75% of bacteria isolated from tonsils during acute tonsillitis. Rarely, secondary syphilis, gonorrhoea, lymphoma or squamous carcinoma may present as atypical tonsillitis.

The progression of acute tonsillitis to recurrent acute or chronic tonsillitis is likely to be due to biofilm formation within the tonsils; tonsilloliths represent low grade biofilm infection within the tonsillar crypts.

HISTORY AND EXAMINATION

History should confirm acute onset of sore throat and associated malaise, fever (typically >38°C) and enlarged tender cervical glands. Referred otalgia is common. In adults, smoking and alcohol intake are relevant. Enquire about symptoms of gastro-oesophageal reflux as a cause of sore throat.

Examining the patient, assess general hydration and temperature, and confirm or exclude trismus. Examine the ears to exclude a local cause of otalgia

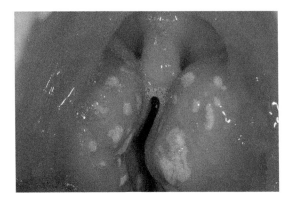

Figure 22.1 Acute tonsillitis with redness and swelling of the tonsils and the surrounding area. The white spots on the tonsil surface correspond to the lymphatic follicles – hence, the term *follicular tonsillitis*.

or associated acute otitis media, more prevalent in children. Examine the mouth – the tonsils will be red and inflamed, usually with an associated whitish exudate (Figure 22.1). Examine the neck for enlarged, palpable cervical lymph nodes (typically levels IIa and III).

In the context of an acute infection, asymmetry of the tonsils is likely to indicate peritonsillar abscess formation (quinsy) (Figure 22.2). In the absence of fever or acute onset, consider other causes for asymmetry, including neoplasm or parapharyngeal space mass pushing the tonsil medially. In EBV infection ('glandular fever'), the tonsils are often markedly enlarged, sometimes enough to cause stertor and incipient airway compromise. They are red and 'beefy' in appearance, and there is associated marked, tender enlargement of lymph nodes and often more generalised lymphadenopathy (Figure 22.3). If EBV infection is suspected, examine the abdomen for hepatic and splenic enlargement and tenderness.

The Centor scoring system cannot be relied upon for precise diagnosis and is not validated in those under 3 years of age; it is instead a tool to

aid decision-making in the prescribing of antibiotics for bacterial infection. The modified Centor scoring system includes bacteriological throat swab, which is not recommended in UK guidance (Table 22.1).

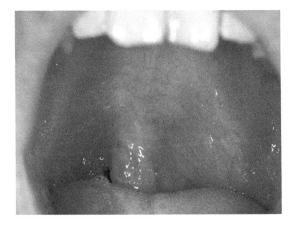

Figure 22.2 Left peritonsillar abscess (*quinsy*) in a 13-year-old female with typical swelling, redness and protrusion of the tonsil, faucial arch and palate. The uvula is pushed towards the right side.

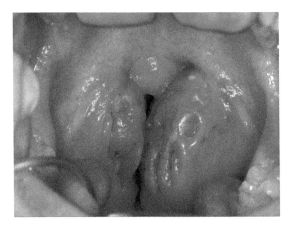

Figure 22.3 Significant enlargement of the tonsils in a 12-year-old boy with infectious mononucleosis. He presented with upper airway obstruction failing to resolve with supportive care and steroids and necessitating tonsillectomy.

Table 22.1 Modified Centor (McIsaac) scoring system

3–14 years	+1
15–44 years	0
45 years and older	−1
Exudate or swelling on tonsils	+1
Tender/swollen anterior cervical lymph nodes	+1
Fever >38°C	+1
Cough absent	+1
Cough present	0

<2 – no antibiotics or throat culture

2–3 – throat culture. Antibiotic if culture positive

>3 – empiric antibiotics

INVESTIGATIONS

No routine investigations are recommended for acute tonsillitis, pending response to appropriate treatment.

If EBV infection is suspected, full blood count, liver function tests and clotting screen are recommended.

The monospot (heterophile antibody) test is commonly used to confirm EBV infection. While up to 92% sensitive and 100% specific, it is much less sensitive in the first 2 weeks of infection, after the acute infection has resolved and in younger children. This test is frequently negative in the presence of clinically diagnosed EBV infection. The monospot test is considered 'not very useful' by the US Centers for Disease Control. Where the diagnosis is in doubt, specific EBV serology is reliable, both for recent (IgM) and past (IgG) EBV infection.

Throat culture swabs are unreliable and not recommended, as they produce a positive GABHS culture in 40% of asymptomatic carriers. Bacterial colonisation of the crypts with biofilm formation means that usual bacteriological techniques will not produce representative results. Culture swab might be appropriate with a clinical diagnosis of bacterial tonsillitis and a negative rapid streptococcal antigen test (RSAT) result.

In contrast to US guidance and practice elsewhere in Europe, current UK guidance (1999; updated in 2010) does not recommend RSAT (or rapid strep test, RST), although the test is fast (10 minutes) and cheap (£1). The test is 95–100% specific for streptococci (sensitivity 65–80%). The test cannot exclude asymptomatic carriage, but in an individual with acute sore throat and a clinical diagnosis of bacterial tonsillitis, a positive RSAT aids decision-making for antibiotic prescribing.

Newer techniques, utilising a finger-prick blood test to measure a biomarker (human neutrophil lipocalin, or HNL), are in development and are likely to be available for clinical use within a few years. This test delivers a rapid detection result within 10 minutes, confirming bacterial rather than viral infection and permitting an informed decision on antibiotic prescribing. This type of biomarker test would make the need for a throat swab or RSAT redundant.

DIFFERENTIAL DIAGNOSIS

As discussed previously, differentiation between viral and bacterial throat infection is the most common dilemma, with the latter being an indication for antibiotics.

In atypical presentation with sore throat, consider unusual infective agents (e.g. syphilis, HIV). Vesicular ulceration can be associated with herpes infections. Stomatitis with recurrent infection indicates possible PFAPA syndrome (periodic fever, aphthous stomatitis, pharyngitis, cervical adenitis).

Inflammation in association with tonsil ulceration, while sometimes aphthous, warrants further investigation, including excision biopsy if the ulceration does not rapidly resolve. Consider squamous carcinoma, particularly in adults with relevant risk factors.

Consider lymphoma in the absence of symptoms of infection with an asymmetrically enlarged non-ulcerated tonsil and associated or generalised lymphadenopathy. Enquire about systemic 'B' signs. HPV associated tonsillar malignancy can present as atypical unilateral enlargement with infection.

In children with an acute fever, sore throat, dysphagia for saliva and stridor, consider bacterial epiglottitis, although it is now uncommon in children in the UK since introduction of the haemophilus influenzae b (Hib) vaccine (see Chapter 24, Acute Epiglottitis section).

MANAGEMENT

Acute tonsillitis is managed initially with oral fluids, rest, anaesthetic mouthwashes or sprays, and simple analgesics. Advise regular oral paracetamol. In 2016, UK guidance reduced the dose schedule of paracetamol from 15 mg/kg QDS to an age-based instead of a weight-based dosage. Paracetamol and ibuprofen (5 mg/kg QDS) on an alternating schedule is generally an effective analgesic combination. If necessary, these can be administered as liquid preparations. Aspirin must never be given to children under the age of 18 years.

Where stronger analgesia is required, oral codeine (30–60 mg QDS prn) can be added for adults over the age of 18 years. For children, oral morphine solution at 1 mg/kg QDS prn is effective analgesia but has no anti-pyretic effect. (Oramorph® 10 mg/5 mL liquid morphine sulfate solution is *not* a controlled drug within the UK Misuse of Drugs Regulations.)

A single oral dose of dexamethasone produces rapid reduction in pain. (Adults up to 4 mg as a single dose or QDS for 24 hours in EBV infection. Children 10–100 mcg in a single dose or two divided doses.) In EBV infections, dexamethasone is helpful in reducing swelling and inflammation of the tonsils and improving swallowing and airway obstruction.

In clinically definite or proven bacterial tonsillitis, antibiotics in children under the age of 18 years reduce fever and pain, shortening the duration of illness by one day, but more importantly, reducing the risk of sequelae and complications.

A UK study of emergency department attendees with tonsillitis reported that 80% were prescribed antibiotics, with 66% being given penicillin V (phenoxymethyl penicillin), but 25% were given a range of other broad-spectrum antibiotics, including amoxicillin and co-amoxiclav. In a questionnaire study of specialists and GPs across seven European countries, 63% prescribed amoxicillin for acute tonsillopharyngitis [*sic*].

Recommended antibiotic treatment is penicillin V at the appropriate dose (adults 500 mg QDS; children 62.5–500 mg QDS, dependent on age) for 10 days. In those allergic to penicillin, a macrolide (either azithromycin or clarithromycin) is preferred to erythromycin, which commonly produces unpleasant and sometimes significant abdominal pain and diarrhoea. Azithromycin has the advantage of a once-daily dose for 3 days only, improving patient concordance. A macrolide antibiotic is appropriate for those with both tonsillitis and acute otitis media.

If ampicillin, amoxicillin or co-amoxiclav is prescribed for tonsillitis due to EBV infection, 90% of patients will develop a generalised, sometimes severe and usually clinically significant skin rash.

Antibiotics are unlikely to be effective in the management of chronic or recurrent tonsillitis. These are likely to represent low-grade biofilm infection of the tonsils, unresponsive to antibiotics in therapeutic doses.

Data from the 2005 UK National Prospective Tonsillectomy Audit indicates that those who have four sore throats each year can expect a further 2.5 days of sore throat every 6 months. Where episodes of recurrent tonsillitis meet local guidance criteria for surgical treatment, tonsillectomy (as a day case procedure where appropriate) is recommended.

COMPLICATIONS

During the period 2010–2011 in the UK, there were 61,000 admissions to hospital for the management of tonsillitis. These generally were to deliver parenteral fluid replacement and effective analgesia and to manage complications, mostly abscess formation. Death is a rare but recognised complication of acute tonsillitis.

Peritonsillar abscess (usually unilateral) can generally be drained using topical anaesthesia in older children and adolescents, followed by supportive intravenous antibiotics and fluids. Peroral needle aspiration and incision and drainage using topical anaesthesia are often not tolerated by younger children, and the management provided is primarily supportive (see Chapter 23).

Suppurative lymphadenitis, retropharyngeal or parapharyngeal abscess may require imaging (ultrasound, CT and/or MRI) and, if not responding to appropriate parenteral antibiotic treatment, surgical drainage.

Acute otitis media is a common complication in younger children, possibly accounting for the high prevalence of broad-spectrum antibiotic prescribing in primary care (see Chapter 20).

In developed countries, chorea, scarlet fever, rheumatic fever and glomerulonephritis are rare complications.

Upper airway obstruction, particularly during acute EBV infection, can be improved with parenteral dexamethasone. Airway support without acute surgical intervention can usually be achieved using a nasopharyngeal airway(s).

For those with guttate psoriasis, acute streptococcal tonsillitis can precipitate severe exacerbation. In others, it may trigger the onset of generalised psoriasis, due to a complex interaction of HLA-type, skin-homing T-cells and streptococcal super antigen.

In PFAPA syndrome, acute stomatitis complicates the discomfort of acute tonsillitis.

Bleeding in haemorrhagic tonsillitis can be managed with topical anaesthesia and silver nitrate cautery and/or with a short course of oral tranexamic acid at a dose of 15 mg/kg TDS for 3 days.

Following political pressure in the UK to reduce healthcare expenditure between 1991 and 2011, the tonsillectomy rate, already lower than in the USA and many other European countries, fell by 44%. During the same period the admission rate for tonsillitis rose by 310%. The complications of tonsillitis, including peritonsillar abscess (quinsy), parapharyngeal abscess and retropharyngeal abscess, are serious and potentially life-threatening. During the same period, the rate of admission for quinsy rose by 31%, and for retro- and parapharyngeal abscess by 39%.

This study concluded that during 1991–2011, there had been a 14% increase in hospital bed day usage from tonsillitis and complications of infection with no net financial saving resulting from the reduction in the rate of elective tonsillectomy.

Those recovering from EBV infection should be advised against physical activity and contact sports for up to 6 weeks following resolution of the acute infection because of the small (1:500–1:1000) risk of splenic rupture. Hepatitis, meningitis, encephalitis, lower motor neurone facial palsy, Guillain–Barré syndrome and pneumonia are uncommon (1:100) complications. More commonly, post-viral fatigue and frequent, recurrent tonsillitis with persistently enlarged tonsils follow acute EBV infection, sometimes without a history of recurrent tonsillitis prior to the EBV infection.

CONCLUSION

Acute bacterial tonsillitis is common and usually managed in primary care with symptomatic and supportive measures, simple analgesics and, where appropriate, suitable oral antibiotics. Acute tonsillitis can be difficult to distinguish clinically from viral pharyngitis.

In the UK, restricted access to surgery for recurrent tonsillitis (and possibly changes in antibiotic prescribing in primary care) has led to a rise in admissions to hospital for management of tonsillitis and potentially serious complications of this infection.

KEY LEARNING POINTS

- The Centor scoring systems cannot be relied upon for precise diagnosis of tonsillitis.
- Throat swabs are clinically unhelpful in the diagnosis of bacterial tonsillitis. Newer rapid detection biomarker tests for bacterial infection are likely to supersede traditional tests (including RSAT) to inform antibiotic prescribing.
- The monospot test for EBV is less reliable in young children and in adults during the first 2 weeks of this infection.
- Consider malignancy or unusual infective causes in atypical clinical presentations of sore throat and tonsillitis.
- Avoid prescribing ampicillin or its derivatives. Prescribe penicillin V at full doses as first-line antibiotic therapy. Consider azithromycin or clarithromycin for those penicillin-allergic or where there is associated acute otitis media.
- In the UK, as tonsillectomy has been restricted, admissions to secondary care for tonsillitis and its complications have risen dramatically, with additional financial burden to the healthcare system.

FURTHER READING

Bird JH, Biggs TC, King EV. Controversies in the management of acute tonsillitis: an evidence-based review. *Clinical Otolaryngology*. 2014; 39: 368–74.

Kanji K, Saatci D, Rao GG, Khanna P, Bassett P, Williams B, Khan M. Antibiotics for tonsillitis: should the emergency department emulate general practice? *Journal of Clinical Pathology*. 2016 Jun 29: jclinpath-2016.

Lau AS, Upile NS, Wilkie MD, Leong SC, Swift AC. The rising rate of admissions for tonsillitis and neck space abscesses in England, 1991–2011. *Annals of the Royal College of Surgeons of England*. 2014; 96: 307–10.

National Institute for Health and Clinical Excellence. *Guideline 69*. Prescribing of antibiotics for self-limiting respiratory tract infections in adults and children in primary care. 2008. www.nice.org.uk.

Philips and Diagnostics Development win European Union 'Horizon Prize – Better Use of Antibiotics' for the rapid detection of bacterial infection on Philips' Minicare I-20 platform. www.philips.com/a-w/about/news/archive/standard/news/press/2017/20170207-philips-and-diagnostics-development-win-european-union-horizon-prize-better-use-of-antibiotics.html. *Accessed July 3 2017*.

Schams SC, Goldman RD. Steroids as adjuvant treatment of sore throat in acute bacterial pharyngitis. *Canadian Family Physician*. 2012; 58: 52–4.

Scottish Intercollegiate Guidelines Network (SIGN). *Guideline 117*. Management of sore throat and indications for tonsillectomy. 2010. www.sign.ac.uk/sign-117-management-of-sore-throat-and-indications-for-tonsillectomy.html

Stelter K. Tonsillitis and sore throat in children. *GMS Current topics in Otorhinolaryngology – Head and Neck Surgery*. 2014; 13: 5–24.

Stoodley P, deBeer D, Longwell M, Nistico L, Hall-Stoodley L, Wenig B, Krespi YP. Tonsillolith: not just a stone but a living biofilm. *Otolaryngology – Head and Neck Surgery*. 2009; 141: (3) 316–21.

Woo JH, Kim ST, Kang IG, Lee JH, Heung EC, Kim DY. Comparison of tonsillar biofilms between patients with recurrent tonsillitis and a control group. *Acta Oto-Laryngologica*. 2012; 132: (10) 1115–20.

Vijayashree MS, Viswantha B, Sambamurthy BN. Clinical and bacteriological study of acute tonsillitis. *IOSR Journal of Dental and Medical Sciences*. 2014; 13: 37–43.

23

Paediatric deep neck space infections

MARY-LOUISE MONTAGUE

INTRODUCTION

Deep neck space infection (DNSI) is defined as infection within the potential spaces and fascial planes of the neck. DNSIs are commonly seen in both children and adults, but the presentation, progression and treatment in these two groups can differ greatly. They are of clinical significance because of their potentially life-threatening complications, including the spread of infection to adjacent vital structures and airway compromise.

The focus of this chapter is on the commonest DNSIs occurring in children, including peritonsillar abscess (PTA), parapharyngeal abscess (PPA) and retropharyngeal abscess (RPA). The relevant anatomy, clinical presentation, diagnostic investigations, treatment options and potential complications are discussed.

ANATOMY OF THE NECK SPACES

A thorough knowledge of the anatomy of the deep neck spaces is a prerequisite to understanding infection within them, the complications that may develop if infection progresses, the interpretation of cross-sectional imaging and the surgical drainage procedures that may be required in their management.

The deep neck spaces are potential spaces between the deep fascial layers of the neck that may be broadly classified into three groups based on their relationship to the hyoid bone. They comprise those that involve the entire length of the neck, those that are superior to the hyoid (the suprahyoid spaces) and those that are infrahyoid (Table 23.1).

The two major fascial layers in the neck are the superficial cervical and deep cervical fascia.

Table 23.1 Classification of neck spaces according to their relationship to the hyoid bone

Entire length of neck	Suprahyoid	Infrahyoid
Superficial neck space	Submental space	Pretracheal space
Deep neck spaces	Submandibular space (comprising	
• Retropharyngeal	sublingual and submaxillary spaces)	
space	Peritonsillar space	
• Carotid space	Parotid space	
• Danger space of	Parapharyngeal space	
Gillette	Masticator space	
Prevertebral space		

The superficial cervical fascia encloses platysma and surrounds the neck. The deep cervical fascia is divided into three layers – the superficial layer or investing fascia, the middle (pretracheal) layer and the deep (prevertebral) layer. The carotid sheath consists of fascia from all three deep layers and surrounds the common carotid artery, internal jugular vein and vagus nerve.

Of primary importance for DNSIs in children are the peritonsillar, parapharyngeal, retropharyngeal and submandibular spaces.

The peritonsillar space is bound by the capsule of the tonsil medially, the superior constrictor muscle laterally and the tonsillar pillars anteriorly and posteriorly. A PTA may extend through the superior constrictor muscle into the parapharyngeal space.

The parapharyngeal space is bound by the petrous portion of the temporal bone superiorly, the superior constrictor muscle medially, the pterygoid muscles, mandible and parotid gland laterally and the hyoid bone inferiorly (Figure 23.1). It is divided into anterior (pre-styloid) and posterior (post-styloid) compartments by the styloid process. The pre-styloid compartment contains connective tissue, fat, the internal maxillary artery and maxillary nerve. The post-styloid compartment contains the contents of the carotid sheath and cranial nerves IX, X, XI and XII.

The retropharyngeal space is bound anteriorly by the posterior pharyngeal wall, posteriorly by the alar fascia and superiorly by the skull base. Its inferior extent is the superior mediastinum at the level of T2, where the middle and deep cervical

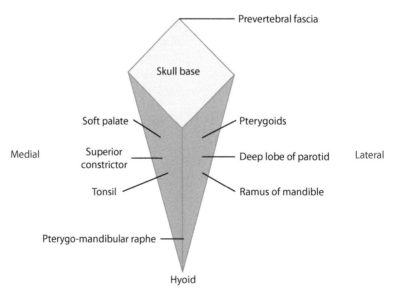

Figure 23.1 Schematic diagram showing the anatomical relations of the parapharyngeal space.

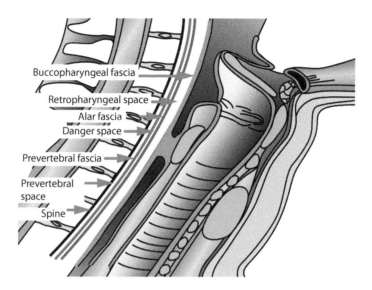

Figure 23.2 The anatomy of the danger space and its relationship to the retropharyngeal space in sagittal section.

fascial layers fuse. It communicates laterally with the parapharyngeal space and may drain into the prevertebral space.

The danger space is also worthy of mention, just posterior to the retropharyngeal space lying between the alar fascia and the prevertebral fascia and extending from the skull base into the posterior mediastinum down to the level of the diaphragm, creating a potential pathway for widespread infection (Figure 23.2). Infection in this space presents initially in an almost identical fashion to retropharyngeal space infection.

The submandibular space is divided into the sublingual and submaxillary spaces above and below the mylohyoid muscle, respectively.

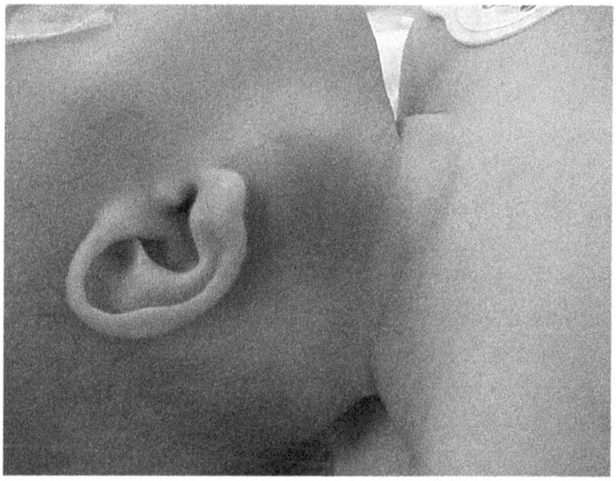

PATHOPHYSIOLOGY

Cervical lymphadenitis is a common source of paediatric deep neck space infections. It is associated with a variety of head and neck infections, and although it is usually viral in aetiology in children, suppuration usually implies bacterial infection. Bacterial infection within a cervical lymph node may progress to cause local cellulitis and abscess (Figure 23.3).

Figure 23.3 Infant with an acute cervical lymph node abscess.

PTA or quinsy usually follows acute tonsillitis and is more common in adolescents and young adults than in children. PPA generally occurs as a complication of peritonsillar infection. RPA in children is caused by suppuration within retropharyngeal lymph nodes following respiratory infections with drainage from the nose, sinuses and pharynx. RPA is seen predominantly in children under the age of 5 years, as these lymph nodes have usually regressed in older children.

Ludwig's angina refers to a rapidly progressive polymicrobial cellulitis of the submandibular space (sublingual and submaxillary spaces) with potentially life-threatening airway compromise. Submandibular space infection is usually from an odontogenic source and is much less common in children compared to adults, since it originates from periapical abscesses of the second or third mandibular molars. It can also occur as a complication of peritonsillar or parapharyngeal infection.

Other potential sources of infection to be considered in children include oropharyngeal trauma, foreign body ingestion (of sharp foreign bodies in particular with resultant pharyngeal perforation), surgical instrumentation (e.g. rigid oesophagoscopy), branchial cleft anomalies and thyroglossal duct cysts.

HISTORY AND EXAMINATION

The presenting symptoms and signs of neck space infection are dependent on the location and contents of the affected neck space. It must also be borne in mind that infection can extend into adjacent neck spaces.

A detailed history should establish the child's age and the duration of illness. Seek a history of preceding coryzal illness or sore throat. Enquire about symptoms involving the airway. If there is neck swelling, determine if there has been a change in its size or consistency. Symptoms of fever, pain, odynophagia, and restricted neck movement should also be sought.

Prior antibiotic therapy, risk factors for MRSA, recent travel and a possible immunocompromised state may also be relevant.

Clinical examination should include careful inspection of the oral cavity, including the floor of mouth, teeth, gums and oropharynx, looking for a possible source of cervical lymphadenitis and for any potential for airway compromise. Inspect the neck for asymmetry and neck swelling and determine if midline or lateral. Give attention to any discolouration of the overlying skin and the presence of a sinus or fistula, the latter being of particular relevance when there is a

history of recurrent PPA. Palpate for tenderness, consistency and mobility. It is important to note that DNSI in children may present with malaise, fever, neck pain and torticollis in the absence of visible or palpable neck swelling and associated erythema.

Odynophagia and trismus are typical of PTA and PPA. Sublingual space infection can be rapidly progressive with incipient airway obstruction. Cranial neuropathies may help provide localising information. In some children the infection is so rapidly progressive that they may present with significant sepsis.

Table 23.2 summarises the symptoms and signs of the common DNSIs in children.

INVESTIGATIONS

Following a thorough history and clinical examination, laboratory blood testing and diagnostic imaging studies may be required, especially prior to surgical intervention but also to chart clinical progress in those children managed conservatively.

No investigations are required for PTA, its diagnosis being primarily clinical based on examination of the pharynx with the characteristic fluctuant, enlarged tonsil and contralateral deviation of the uvula.

LABORATORY BLOOD TESTS

It is important to obtain a full blood count with differential count, urea and electrolytes and C-reactive protein (CRP). A leukocytosis is typical. Monitoring the CRP aids in determining progression of infection over time. Blood cultures should also be done at presentation. In cases of sepsis where disseminated intravascular coagulation is suspected, a coagulation screen should be obtained.

IMAGING

Ultrasound (US) can be helpful in discriminating between abscess formation and inflammatory lymphadenitis. Whilst a useful non-invasive first

Table 23.2 Clinical presentation of DNSIs in children

Neck space location	Symptoms	Signs
Peritonsillar	Fever Sore throat Dysphagia Odynophagia Drooling Ear pain	Muffled 'hot potato' voice Trismus Uvula displaced to contralateral side Ipsilateral bulging of the palatine arch Inferomedial displacement of ipsilateral tonsil Ipsilateral cervical lymphadenopathy
Parapharyngeal (*Pre-styloid*)	Fever Sore throat Odynophagia	Trismus Displacement of tonsil anteromedially External swelling behind angle of jaw Torticollis

Parapharyngeal
(*Post-styloid*)
	Similar to pre-styloid but more
	    subtle
		Bulge of pharynx behind posterior pillar
		Swelling of parotid region
		Torticollis
		Carotid sheath complications may be
		    present:
		    • Internal jugular vein thrombosis
		    • Carotid aneurysm
		    • Horner's syndrome
		    • IX–XII neuropathies

Retropharyngeal	Fever Irritability Dysphagia Odynophagia Neck pain Noisy breathing/snoring	Unilateral swelling of posterior pharyngeal wall Nuchal rigidity Hoarse/soft voice occasionally Progressive airway obstruction

Submandibular
(*Ludwig's angina*)
	Fever
	Odynophagia
	Drooling
	Toothache
		Sublingual space infection
		    • Floor of mouth swelling
		    • Tongue displacement
		Submaxillary space infection
		    • Brawny tender non-fluctuant swelling
		      below chin
		    • Trismus
		    • Stridor

mode of assessment for children with superficial neck space infection, it does not provide sufficient anatomical detail or information about deep extent in DNSI.

Contrast-enhanced computed tomography (CT) is the imaging modality of choice for DNSI, delineating the extent of an abscess more accurately, confirming spread into adjacent areas and detecting the presence of complications such as venous thrombosis and mediastinitis. It has the added advantage of a fast scan acquisition time, avoiding the need for general anaesthesia in young children. The classic CT appearance of an abscess is an area of low attenuation with a rim of contrast enhancement, surrounded by soft tissue swelling (Figures 23.4 and 23.5). It is important to image the chest up to the aortic arch to exclude mediastinal extension of RPA.

Magnetic resonance imaging (MRI) is also an option but is generally not the imaging modality of first choice in young children, as general

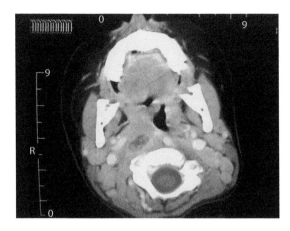

Figure 23.4 Axial contrast CT neck demonstrating a right parapharyngeal abscess in a 6-year-old child.

anaesthesia is usually required. Magnetic resonance angiography (MRA) is used to evaluate potential vascular complications.

A lateral neck radiograph may be requested if RPA is suspected and may show widening of the retropharyngeal space, defined as greater than 7 mm at the level of C2 or greater than 14 mm at the level of C6 in children younger than 14 years of age from the anterior surface of the vertebrae to the posterior border of the airway if positive. The radiograph must be taken with the child's neck held in extension and at the end of inspiration to avoid the possibility of false positive widening of the retropharyngeal space, but this may be difficult to achieve in a young, uncooperative or sick child.

MICROBIOLOGY

The types of bacteria found in paediatric DNSIs may vary regionally, but Group A beta-haemolytic streptococcus (GABHS), *Staphylococcus aureus* and anaerobes are the most commonly isolated bacteria in paediatric deep neck abscess cultures. GABHS has been reported to be rising in incidence and contributing to an overall increase in the number of neck abscesses. Many infections are in fact polymicrobial, containing Gram-positive, Gram-negative and anaerobic organisms. This differs from the adult population in whom the sources are more often odontogenic pathogens such as *Streptococcus viridans* and *Staphylococci* and anaerobes such as *Peptostreptococcus*.

MANAGEMENT

At presentation the first priority must be to recognise and manage immediate or impending obstruction of the paediatric airway. Care must

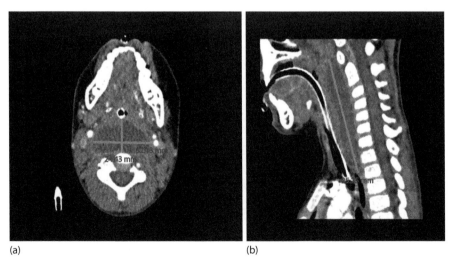

(a)   (b)

Figure 23.5 Axial (a) and sagittal (b) contrast CT neck and thorax demonstrating a large retropharyngeal abscess in a 5-year-old girl.

be taken when intubating a child with a suspected retropharyngeal abscess to avoid possible rupture of the abscess and aspiration of its contents. Tracheostomy is rarely required.

After detailed clinical assessment, the principles of management of DNSI in children include early antibiotic therapy and drainage of the abscess if required.

MEDICAL MANAGEMENT

Intravenous antibiotics are the mainstay of treatment of PTA in young children who are not sufficiently cooperative to permit needle aspiration or incision and drainage. Studies have shown that the use of a single dose of intravenous steroids in addition to antibiotics may help to reduce symptoms and speed recovery.

In both PPA and RPA, high-dose broad-spectrum intravenous antibiotic therapy including anaerobic cover is routinely administered at the outset. The choice of antibiotic therapy will be influenced by local microbiology guidance, the condition of the child and prior antibiotic treatment. Amoxicillin/clavulanic acid (co-Amoxiclav) is frequently used, with the combination of a cephalosporin with flucloxacillin or with clindamycin being alternatives. The duration of intravenous antibiotic therapy is really a clinical judgement, with resolution of fever, fall in white cell count

and CRP, and improved neck mobility being commonly used markers for a response.

It has been shown that small abscesses less than 2.5 cm in size in clinically stable children can be managed effectively with high-dose intravenous antibiotic therapy alone and may not require surgical drainage. Those children who fail to respond quickly to antibiotics are more likely to require surgery to achieve resolution.

SURGICAL MANAGEMENT

Surgical drainage is warranted if there is evidence of airway compromise, septicaemia, development of complications, extension of infection inferiorly or to adjacent neck spaces, or no clinical response to initial intravenous antibiotics after 48 hours.

Needle aspiration or incision and drainage under local anaesthesia in older children and adolescents and acute quinsy tonsillectomy under general anaesthesia are all acceptable surgical treatments for acute PTA, with little difference between them in terms of effectiveness and recurrence rates. Interval tonsillectomy is usually carried out if there is a background of chronic or recurrent tonsillitis or a previous history of PTA.

Transoral drainage is safe for RPA and PPA medial to the great vessels (Figure 23.6). Transcervical drainage is reserved for abscesses lateral to the carotid artery. Pus samples are sent for culture and

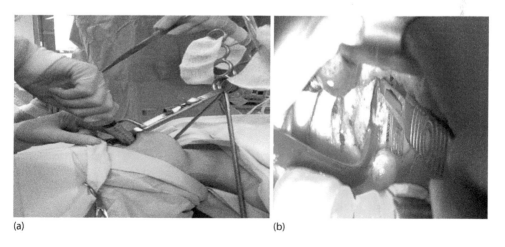

(a)   (b)

Figure 23.6 Intraoperative (a) per-oral aspiration of the large retropharyngeal abscess in Figure 23.5, followed by (b) per-oral incision and drainage.

sensitivity after surgical drainage to inform ongoing antibiotic treatment. Following transcervical drainage, a drain is left in situ to prevent re-accumulation. Whilst formal incision and drainage is the commonest surgical management in children, ultrasound-guided needle aspiration or catheter placement for unilocular abscesses have become gradually more popular in adults, and may have a role in older children or adolescents in an attempt to avoid surgery.

Postoperative airway control with prolonged intubation or a tracheostomy are rarely required after drainage of a retropharyngeal abscess in children.

The management of Ludwig's angina is considered separately in Chapter 8, as it occurs more commonly in adults.

COMPLICATIONS

Complications of DNSIs are fortunately rare but can be associated with significant morbidity and mortality.

Delayed diagnosis or treatment of DNSI may result in local, regional or systemic complications, including upper airway obstruction, mediastinitis, internal jugular vein thrombophlebitis, cranial neuropathies, cervical osteomyelitis, meningitis, sepsis and death. Carotid artery rupture may also result from an unresolved abscess. Lemierre's syndrome is an occlusive septic thrombophlebitis of the internal jugular vein due to spread of infection into the carotid space. It is associated with metastatic foci of infection, most commonly to the lungs. Treatment requires prolonged antibiotic therapy, and anticoagulation is indicated if there is evidence of thrombus progression or septic emboli.

CONCLUSION

The child with suspected DNSI should be approached in a systematic way. Early diagnosis, rapid assessment of the airway and early targeted antibiotic therapy are key to avoiding morbidity and mortality. A clear knowledge of the anatomical fascial planes of the neck is imperative to understanding how DNSIs present and propagate through the different neck spaces. Medical and surgical modalities are viable management options, and may complement each other in an individualised management plan.

KEY LEARNING POINTS

- Impending airway obstruction is the first management priority in children with DNSI.
- Contrast-enhanced computed tomography (CT) is the gold standard for diagnosis and surgical planning. Ultrasound is a less invasive alternative and may be equally effective in certain cases.
- Medical therapy with high-dose intravenous antibiotics may be a viable alternative to surgical drainage in some children, especially for small deep space neck abscesses in older children, without airway compromise or complications.
- Needle aspiration may be as effective as open surgical drainage in smaller, uncomplicated DNSIs with abscess formation.
- Surgical drainage is indicated for DNSIs associated with airway compromise or complications or if unresponsive to 48 hours of intravenous antibiotic therapy.
- Complications of DNSIs are uncommon but carry severe sequelae.

FURTHER READING

Carbone PN, Capra GC, Brigger MT. Antibiotic therapy for pediatric deep neck abscess: a systematic review. *Int J Pediatr Otorhinolaryngol* 2012; 76:1647–1653

Lawrence R, Bateman N. Controversies in the management of deep neck space infection in children: an evidence-based review. *Clin Otolaryngol* 2017; 42:156–163

Novis S, Pritchett C, Thorne M, Sun G. Pediatric deep neck space infections in U.S. children. 2000–2009. *Int J of Pediatr Otorhinolaryngol* 2014; 78:832–836

Standring S, Berkovitz B. *Neck*, in *Gray's Anatomy: The Anatomical Basis of Clinical Practice*, S. Standring, Editor. 2005, Elsevier: Edinburgh. 531–566

Wong DK, Brown C, Mills N, Spielmann P, Neeff M. To drain or not to drain – Management of pediatric deep neck abscesses: a case control study. *Int J Pediatr Otorhinolaryngol* 2012; 76:1810–1813

24

Acute airway conditions

PANAGIOTIS ASIMAKOPOULOS AND MARY-LOUISE MONTAGUE

INTRODUCTION

The otolaryngologist may encounter paediatric airway emergencies presenting with acute airway obstruction. This chapter addresses the emergency safe principles of paediatric airway assessment and immediate management in a multidisciplinary team setting with emergency department doctors, anaesthetists and paediatricians, with a focus on croup (laryngotracheobronchitis), bacterial tracheitis, epiglottitis, foreign body aspiration and blunt and penetrating trauma to the upper airway. Thermal and chemical burns are also discussed.

ANATOMY AND PHYSIOLOGY

The narrowest part of the infant airway is the subglottis, in contrast to the glottis in adults. Poiseuille's Law dictates that the resistance to flow is inversely proportional to the fourth power of the radius, meaning that a 1 mm reduction in the calibre of a 3 mm subglottic airway increases the resistance to airflow by at least five times. As neonates have a large surface area to weight ratio, their basal metabolic rate and energy requirement to maintain temperature homeostasis is higher than adults. They therefore have a higher oxygen requirement and, as their lung capacity is also smaller, they are less tolerant to long apnoeic periods. Children are at higher risk of foreign body aspiration compared to adults because of their tendency to place objects in their mouths, lack of posterior dentition and uninhibited inspirations when crying or laughing. Children are less prone to airway injury because their larynx is relatively high in the neck and is protected by the mandible and sternum. Laryngeal fractures are uncommon, due to the increased elasticity of the laryngeal and tracheal cartilages. Significant airway oedema can still occur, however, in the absence of fractures.

EMERGENCY AIRWAY ASSESSMENT AND MANAGEMENT

In the immediate emergency setting, often in the resuscitation room of the emergency department, a rapid assessment (primary survey) of the airway and breathing should be performed adopting an 'ABCD' approach according to APLS principles. The presence of stridor should alert the clinician to start immediate medical management. The child should not be disturbed by intravenous cannulation or upsetting examinations such as fibreoptic laryngoscopy. Initial medical treatment should include high flow oxygen and nebulised adrenaline. Airway adjuncts such as oropharyngeal, nasopharyngeal or laryngeal mask airways should be considered in the deteriorating child. Impending complete upper airway obstruction in a child requires the airway to be secured with an endotracheal tube or rarely with a surgical tracheostomy.

HISTORY AND EXAMINATION

A thorough history should be taken from the child's parents once the airway is considered stable. The onset and duration of stridor should be quantified. Any recent upper respiratory tract infections or contacts with them should be noted, as they can predispose to infectious causes of upper airway obstruction. Previous episodes of stridor or stertor, quality of cry and voice, coughing, choking and cyanotic episodes, reduced exercise tolerance, feeding difficulties and faltering growth are important, as they can indicate underlying airway pathology. A history of previous intubation should also be sought.

Key points in the airway examination include listening carefully for upper airway noise such as stridor or stertor. If stridor is present, it is important to determine whether it is inspiratory, biphasic or expiratory. Associated colour changes such as pallor or cyanosis should also be noted. The respiratory rate should be recorded, and the

child's voice, cry or cough should also be assessed. Tracheal tug, sternal and intercostal or subcostal recession are signs of respiratory distress and increased work of breathing. Chest auscultation is a vital part of the examination. Auscultation with the bell of the stethoscope placed near the patient's mouth can be useful in detecting soft stridor.

Early signs of respiratory failure include tachypnoea progressing to bradypnoea and tachycardia. Further clinical deterioration will result in bradycardia and increased work of breathing, which will then progress to fatigue and decreased work of breathing. Cyanosis and altered level of consciousness are ominous signs of respiratory arrest.

A history of rapidly progressive sore throat associated with stridor, dysphagia, drooling, muffled voice and incomplete immunisation history is suggestive of acute epiglottitis. The child will be in acute distress, febrile, drooling and sitting in the classic 'tripod position'. A prodromal viral illness followed by a seal-like barking cough with stridor and sternal or intercostal recession that worsens when the child is agitated is characteristic of croup. Children with bacterial tracheitis may have symptoms consistent with a croup-like illness but will deteriorate suddenly after 2 to 7 days of medical treatment. They typically present with fever, toxic appearance and persistent painful cough with biphasic stridor.

Sudden onset of choking and coughing while playing or eating is classically described by parents of children with foreign body (FB) aspiration. Children witnessed by adults to insert toys or other FBs in their mouth should always raise the suspicion of FB aspiration. Even in the absence of such witnessed episodes, non-specific symptoms such as coughing, wheezing and shortness of breath can be suggestive of FB aspiration. Signs on clinical examination may include stridor, unilaterally decreased breath sounds, localised wheezing or obstructive hyper-inflation.

Typical mechanisms of injury in children with airway trauma include 'clothesline' injuries sustained during sports, following a motor accident or from accidental or intentional hanging. Examination findings include stridor, dysphonia, neck haematoma, bruising, tenderness and crepitus. A mechanism of injury that is inconsistent with examination findings should alert to the possibility of non-accidental injury.

In the case of caustic ingestion, it is important to identify the type of corrosive agent, time of ingestion and associated symptoms that might suggest laryngeal (stridor, dysphonia), oesophageal (dysphagia, drooling) or gastric injury (abdominal pain, haematemesis). Children may have evidence of oral burns, such as lip and tongue oedema or oral cavity ulceration. It is important to remember, however, that symptoms of caustic ingestion do not predict the presence or severity of oesophageal injury. Alkali agents are colourless, odourless liquids that are more likely to cause injury to the proximal upper aerodigestive tract and penetrate the submucosa and muscularis, resulting in perforation. Acidic liquids have a bitter taste, decreasing their volume of ingestion, and they are less likely to penetrate the submucosa, resulting in a lower risk of oesophageal perforation. Children with significant thermal burns of the head and neck are at risk of associated inhalation burns, particularly if there has been closed-space smoke exposure for longer than 10 minutes or any altered level of consciousness. They may present with stridor, dysphonia, soot in their face or mouth, and singed nasal hairs.

INVESTIGATIONS

The clinician must balance the benefit of the potential diagnostic value of a plain radiograph or computerised tomography (CT) against the risk of delaying treatment by moving the child into a radiology department without resuscitation facilities. As a rule, the airway should be stabilised or secured first.

Plain chest x-rays can be useful in localising radiopaque foreign bodies (Figure 24.1). Most aspirated foreign bodies are in fact radiolucent, and therefore only 16% of them are diagnosed on x-rays. False negative rates of up to 30% are reported. In cases of suspected radiolucent foreign bodies, inspiratory and expiratory chest radiographs may show air-trapping or mediastinal shift due to a ball-valving effect. Consolidation on chest

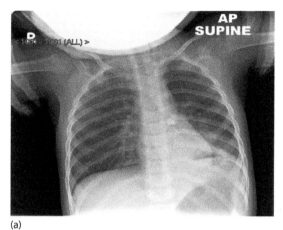

(a)

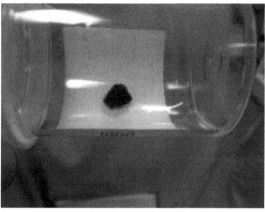

(b)

Figure 24.1 (a) Plain CXR demonstrating an aspirated radiopaque foreign body in the left main bronchus of a 22-month-old child; (b) The small stone that was subsequently removed at rigid bronchoscopy.

x-ray caused by bronchiectasis, lung abscess and empyema is a late sign of FB aspiration.

A lateral neck radiograph may aid in the diagnosis of epiglottitis by showing the characteristic 'thumbprint' sign. The classical finding of the subglottic 'steeple sign' on an anterior-posterior neck or chest radiograph can be helpful in confirming a diagnosis of croup (Figure 24.2). This is not always present, however, and the role of radiographs in such cases is mainly to exclude alternative diagnoses.

CT has a role in laryngeal trauma. In cases of blunt injury to the neck, CT can be helpful in delineating cartilaginous fractures of the larynx

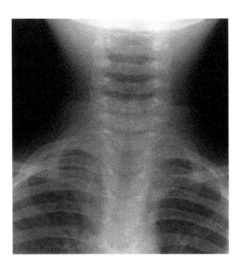

Figure 24.2 CXR demonstrating the steeple sign caused by subglottic oedema and narrowing in a case of severe croup.

or tracheal rings. CT angiography can be useful in determining vascular injury in children with penetrating neck trauma.

Laboratory studies can be helpful in establishing leukocytosis in acute epiglottitis or bacterial tracheitis. Blood cultures and sensitivities can also be crucial in guiding antibiotic therapy. As mentioned earlier, blood samples should always be taken after the airway has been stabilised or secured. Nasopharyngeal aspirates or swabs may be sent for viral culture. Parainfluenza virus type 1 is the agent most commonly identified in cases of croup.

Direct visualisation of the airway is the gold standard investigation when managing paediatric airway emergencies. As instrumentation of the upper airway will upset the child and can potentially cause laryngospasm, it should be performed in the controlled environment of the operating theatre in the presence of an experienced paediatric anaesthetist.

DIFFERENTIAL DIAGNOSIS

The differential diagnoses in children presenting with paediatric airway emergencies are summarised in Table 24.1.

MANAGEMENT

ACUTE EPIGLOTTITIS

This is fortunately now rare in children in the UK, owing to the success of the *Haemophilus influenzae* type b (Hib) vaccine, and most cases now occur in adults. The onset and progression of symptoms in children is usually rapid. Initial management comprises administration of oxygen, nebulised adrenaline, and oral or parenteral corticosteroids. Definitive management includes securing the airway, preferably by intubation in the operating theatre with an experienced paediatric anaesthetist. A swab for culture and sensitivities from the epiglottis should be taken at the time of direct laryngoscopy and intubation to guide antibiotic treatment. Intubation is frequently challenging in children with epiglottitis, and if the degree of supraglottic oedema is such that standard intubation is not feasible, then the otolaryngologist may do so by passing an endotracheal tube under direct vision over a Hopkin's telescope (Figure 24.3). If this is not possible, cricothyroidotomy or tracheostomy may be necessary. The latter should only be performed if the child is in extremis.

Systemic antibiotics should be administrated to the intubated child as per local resistance protocols. Empiric treatment regimens should cover common pathogens such as *Haemophilus influenzae*, *Streptococcus pneumonia*, *Staphylococcus aureus*, and MRSA. Trial of extubation should be considered after 72 hours of antibiotic treatment.

CROUP

Management of croup will depend on the severity of the condition. Mild croup (cough without stridor or sternal recession at rest) can be managed with oral or nebulised corticosteroids. In moderate croup (cough with stridor and sternal recession at rest), give humidified oxygen to keep the oxygen saturations above 93%; nebulised adrenaline should be added to corticosteroids. Resolution of stridor and sternal or intercostal recession should occur within 10 to 30 minutes. The child should be reassessed hourly and, if responding to this treatment regimen, they can be safely discharged home

Table 24.1 Differential diagnoses in children with acute upper airway obstruction

Condition	History	Signs	Investigations
Croup	Usually 6 months to 4 years of age, preceding URTI, cough typically worse at night and increased with agitation	Barking, seal-like cough, stridor, chest wall or sternal in-drawing	Usually clinical diagnosis, subglottic narrowing ('steeple sign') on chest x-ray
Epiglottitis	Fever, sore throat, dysphonia, drooling, dysphagia, incomplete immunisation history	Stridor, dyspnoea, toxic child in 'tripod position'	Usually clinical diagnosis, supraglottic 'thumb print sign' on lateral x-ray, raised inflammatory markers
Bacterial tracheitis	Sudden deterioration after 2–7 days of a mild to moderate croup-like viral illness	Toxic appearance, painful cough, poor response to nebulised adrenaline	Erythematous tracheal mucosa with thick, purulent secretions on bronchoscopy, raised inflammatory markers
Peritonsillar abscess	Gradual onset, fever, dysphagia, drooling, unilateral cervical adenopathy	Oedematous peritonsillar area, tonsillar displacement and uvular deviation, occasionally stertor	Raised inflammatory markers
Retropharyngeal abscess	Gradual onset, fever, dysphagia, drooling, unilateral cervical adenopathy	Usually none, occasionally stridor, posterior pharyngeal wall oedema, neck stiffness	Retroflexion of cervical vertebrae and posterior pharyngeal oedema on lateral x-ray
Foreign body aspiration	Sudden onset choking and coughing, history suggestive of FB aspiration, no preceding viral illness	Asymptomatic, stridor, unilaterally decreased breath sounds, localised wheezing or obstructive hyper-inflation	Usually not radio-opaque, direct visualisation, and removal in theatre confirms diagnosis
Anaphylaxis	Rapid onset stridor, dysphagia, previous history of similar episodes or allergy	Urticarial rash, facial, tongue or pharyngeal oedema	Allergy testing (RAST/skin prick) at later stage

after 4 hours of observation. Severe croup (cough with stridor and sternal recession at rest associated with agitation or lethargy) should be treated with 100% oxygen, nebulised, or parenteral corticosteroids and nebulised adrenaline, and senior anaesthetic help should be sought early.

Corticosteroids are the mainstay of treatment in croup. A systematic review has shown that they reduce the need for adrenaline in children by 10%, reduce the average length of hospital stay by 12 hours, and reduce admissions or return visits by 50%. The usual treatment regime is a single oral dose of 0.6 mg/kg dexamethasone with a treatment effect within 2 hours and further beneficial effects noted up to 10 hours later. Evidence now suggests that lower dexamethasone doses of 0.15 mg/kg can be used in croup. Children with severe hypoxia might benefit from inhaled budesonide (2 mg single dose) as their intestinal and tissue perfusion can be impaired. Nebulised budesonide is also an appropriate alternative in children with persistent vomiting or respiratory distress, which

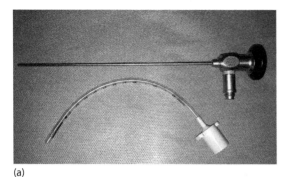

(a)

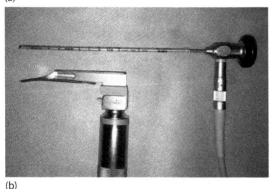

(b)

Figure 24.3 Technique for difficult intubation using a size 3.0 endotracheal tube **(a)** placed over a 2.7 mm 0° Hopkins telescope and introduced using a paediatric straight blade Miller laryngoscope **(b)**.

can make oral administration difficult. As croup symptoms will resolve within 3 days of onset, and the anti-inflammatory effects of dexamethasone last between 2 to 4 days, a second dose is unlikely to be necessary in most children.

The benefits of nebulised adrenaline are maintained for at least 1 hour and usually diminish 2 hours later. 2.5 mL of 1 in 1000 adrenaline diluted with 2.5 mL normal saline is administered to children under 1 year and 5 mL of 1 in 1000 adrenaline undiluted to children over 1 year. This can be repeated after 30 minutes, if necessary, and the child transferred to high dependency or PICU. In children who fail to respond to combination treatment of corticosteroids and adrenaline, a differential diagnosis of foreign body aspiration or bacterial tracheitis should always be considered.

Children with pre-existing narrowing of the upper airway (e.g. subglottic stenosis) and children with Down syndrome are prone to more severe croup, and their admission should be considered even with mild symptoms.

BACTERIAL TRACHEITIS

Although bacterial tracheitis is a rare condition, it has become an increasingly more prevalent infectious cause of acute upper airway obstruction in children since corticosteroids are now used to manage croup successfully, and *Haemophilus influenzae* b vaccine has decreased the incidence of acute epiglottitis. Bronchoscopy will confirm the diagnosis with diffuse inflammation and pseudo membranes extending from the true vocal folds to the trachea and possibly to the mainstem bronchi. Bacterial swabs should be taken at the time to guide antimicrobial treatment. *Staphylococcus aureus* is the most common pathogen, followed by group A *Streptococcus* and *Haemophilus influenzae*. The child should remain intubated for a minimum of 4–5 days to facilitate humidification and repeat tracheal aspiration.

FOREIGN BODY ASPIRATION

Management of the airway in children with FB aspiration depends on the severity of the obstruction. In the unconscious child, endotracheal intubation should be performed urgently unless the FB can be seen in the upper airway and can be easily removed. If intubation and ventilation are not possible due to extensive laryngeal oedema or difficult anatomy, cricothyroidotomy or surgical tracheostomy should be performed.

Definitive treatment should be provided once the airway is secured or deemed stable. Both flexible and rigid bronchoscopy are appropriate methods for removal of foreign bodies. Initial assessment with flexible bronchoscopy has been found to have a success rate greater than 90%. It is therefore reasonable to perform flexible bronchoscopy initially to confirm the diagnosis and attempt removal of the foreign body. Indications for initial assessment with rigid bronchoscopy include stridor, asphyxia, radio-opaque object seen on x-ray, witnessed FB aspiration with unilateral decreased air entry, localised wheezing, obstructive hyper-inflation or atelectasis. Failed attempts with flexible bronchoscopy is also an indication for rigid bronchoscopy. The latter has the advantage of securing the airway while providing a lumen for endotracheal ventilation and instrumentation to allow removal of the FB.

Suspension laryngoscopy using an age-appropriate Parson's laryngoscope (Figure 24.4) with optical forceps (Figure 24.5) is the method of choice for FB removal in infants with small

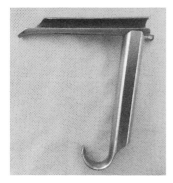

Figure 24.4 Storz Parson's laryngoscope, available in sizes 1–4. Note its straight blade and side split, allowing safe and straight passage of a telescope or rigid ventilating bronchoscope through the laryngeal inlet without local tissue damage or bending of the telescope.

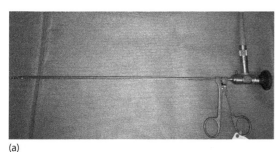

(a)

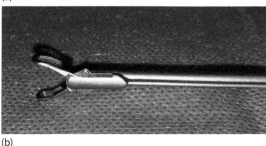

(b)

Figure 24.5 (a) Optical forceps for removal of aspirated FBs; (b) Close-up view showing detail of peanut grasping forceps.

airways. A fine suction catheter is used to remove secretions and deliver adrenaline to decongest the inflamed or oedematous airway mucosa.

Spontaneous ventilation is the preferred method of anaesthesia, using an inhalation induction followed by application of a metered dose of lignocaine spray to the vocal cords and nasopharyngeal tube insufflation. Maintenance of anaesthesia is with either gas or total intravenous anaesthesia (TIVA). Ventilation can also be provided via the ventilation circuit on an age-appropriate ventilating bronchoscope during FB retrieval (Figure 24.6). Good communication with an experienced paediatric anaesthetist and theatre staff is vital in this 'shared airway' situation. Surgery is rarely indicated in cases of repeated failed bronchoscopy attempts. In such cases thoracotomy may be

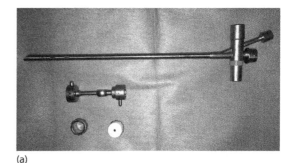

(a)

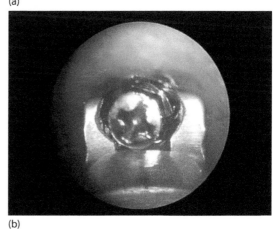

(b)

Figure 24.6 (a) Storz rigid ventilating bronchoscope with distal fenestrations to permit distal oxygenation; (b) The endoscopic view afforded during removal of a metal screw from the right main bronchus of a 6-year-old boy using the Storz ventilating bronchoscope and optical forceps.

necessary, and close liaison with thoracic surgeons would be appropriate.

LARYNGEAL TRAUMA

Children with blunt or penetrating neck injuries should be assessed as per the APLS protocol. Cervical spine injuries must be excluded, and if the airway needs to be secured, in-line traction must be used during intubation. Once the airway has been secured, direct laryngoscopy under general anaesthesia will allow assessment of the degree of laryngeal injury. Penetrating neck injuries must be explored in the operating theatre. Injuries to the great vessels should ideally be repaired with a vascular surgeon present. Children with grade 1 (mild laryngeal oedema, no fracture) and grade 2 laryngeal injuries (laryngeal oedema with mucosal disruption, no exposed cartilage, undisplaced thyroid cartilage fracture) can be managed conservatively with corticosteroids. Grade 3 (severe laryngeal oedema, displaced thyroid cartilage fracture, fixed cord) and grade 4 laryngeal injuries (multiple fracture lines) require open surgical exploration with a covering tracheostomy. Stents can be used in laryngeal trauma involving the anterior commissure or multiple displaced fractures.

UPPER AIRWAY BURNS

Thermal burns should be managed in a specialised burns unit. Nebulised adrenaline can be used to manage children with minor laryngeal mucosal burns and no airway compromise. Severe burns require direct laryngoscopy under anaesthetic to assess the airway. Intubation should be avoided if the mucosal burns are in direct contact with the endotracheal tube. In such cases tracheostomy is the ideal method of securing the airway.

Children presenting with ingestion of caustic agents who are symptomatic, or have evidence of oropharyngeal burns, should undergo upper endoscopy ideally between 12 and 24 hours following the ingestion. Performing endoscopy too early may not show the full extent of the caustic injury and, if it is performed after 48 hours, the risk of perforation is increased. Early flexible oesophagogastro-duodenoscopy has historically been the mainstay of emergency assessment of

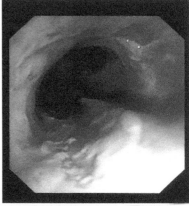

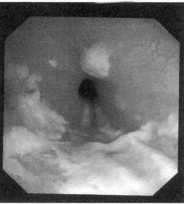

Figure 24.7 Caustic burns of the oesophagus and just above cricopharyngeus seen at flexible upper GI endoscopy 12 hours after ingestion of oven cleaner by a 2-year-old girl. The airway was spared. Image courtesy of Dr Paul Henderson, Consultant Paediatric Gastroenterologist, Royal Hospital for Sick Children, Edinburgh.

caustic injuries (Figure 24.7). The major disadvantage of endoscopy, however, is the limitation in predicting the depth of corrosive damage, which can lead to unnecessary resections and life-long devastating functional outcomes.

COMPLICATIONS

The most serious complication from any upper airway emergency in children is the obvious threat to life from respiratory arrest and asphyxiation. Additionally, sharp objects or foreign bodies that cause surrounding tissue inflammation (e.g. iron tablets, potassium chloride tablets, button batteries and caustic agents) can result in significant complications (e.g. ulceration, perforation, stenosis, tracheo-oesophageal fistula) and should be removed on an urgent basis.

Children with caustic ingestion are at risk of stricture formation 1 to 2 months following injury. Alkaline agents cause oesophageal strictures leading to dysphagia, while acidic agents cause pyloric strictures leading to symptoms of gastric outlet obstruction. Noncircumferential oesophageal injuries are at low risk for stricture formation. Follow-up in these cases can be with imaging (e.g. contrast swallow) or endoscopy performed on an as-required basis (Figure 24.8). In contrast, circumferential oesophageal injuries are at high risk of developing strictures frequently requiring endoscopic dilation.

CONCLUSION

Otolaryngologists must be able to promptly recognise paediatric acute upper airway obstruction and initiate immediate management. Early diagnosis and establishment of a definitive management plan will improve patient outcomes. Working as part of a multidisciplinary team with paediatric anaesthetists, paediatricians and emergency department staff is of paramount importance.

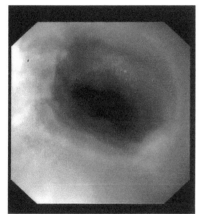
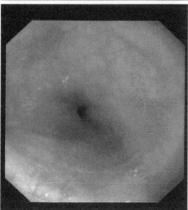

Figure 24.8 Follow-up endoscopy of the child in Figure 24.7 6 days later, showing the improved appearance of the oesophagus and cricopharyngeus. Image courtesy of Dr Paul Henderson, Consultant Paediatric Gastroenterologist, Royal Hospital for Sick Children, Edinburgh.

KEY LEARNING POINTS

- Airway emergencies in children can be caused by infective conditions (e.g. epiglottitis, croup, bacterial tracheitis), foreign body aspiration, trauma (blunt and penetrating) and burns (thermal and chemical).
- Rapid assessment and management of the airway takes place in the resuscitation room by an otolaryngologist, paediatricians and anaesthetists.
- The child should not be disturbed with intravenous cannulas or upsetting examinations such as nasendoscopy.
- Imaging can be helpful in paediatric airway emergencies but should be deferred until the airway has been stabilised or secured.
- Direct visualisation of the airway is the gold standard investigation when managing paediatric airway emergencies and should be performed in the controlled environment of the operating theatre with an experienced paediatric anaesthetist present.

FURTHER READING

Bjornson C, Johnson D. BMJ Best Practice. Croup. 2017. bestpractice.bmj.com/topics/en-gb/681

Chatterjee AB. BMJ Best Medical Practice. Foreign body aspiration. 2017. bestpractice.bmj.com/topics/en-gb/653

Chirica M, Bonavina L, Kelly MD, Sarfati E, Cattan P. Caustic ingestion. *Lancet*. 2017; 389(10083): 2041–2052.

Kurowski JA, Kay M. Caustic ingestions and foreign bodies ingestions in pediatric patients. *Pediatr Clin North Am*. 2017; 64:(3) 507–524.

Shah RK, Acevedo JL. BMJ Best Practice. Epiglottitis. 2017. bestpractice.bmj.com/topics/en-gb/452

25

Foreign bodies

ROHIT GOHIL AND MARY-LOUISE MONTAGUE

INTRODUCTION

It is very much accepted that as children develop an awareness of their surrounding environment and once their pincer grasp has been mastered at around the age of 9 months, they commonly place foreign bodies in their ears, noses and mouths. If retained, the otolaryngologist is often called upon for retrieval. This risk may arise sooner if the child has older siblings. Foreign body (FB) ingestion is most common in children aged 3 years or younger. Children aged 2–5 years have the highest incidence of nasal FBs. Aural FBs have been demonstrated to be more common up to 7–8 years of age.[1,2] FB insertion can occur beyond this age and may be associated with other underlying developmental and psychological conditions. Multiple FBs and recurrent events are not unusual in children.

Vegetable matter and coins remain the most common FBs, but anything that can be placed in the ears, nose, or mouth is a potential hazard. The management of FBs in children varies depending on the nature of the foreign body, the site of insertion, other associated symptoms and background history. This chapter discusses in greater detail the significance of different FBs and their management in the ear, nose and oropharynx in children. Paediatric airway FBs are considered separately in Chapter 24 (Acute Airway Conditions).

HISTORY AND EXAMINATION

Once a child attends hospital, an initial history should be taken from the parent/carer. It must be established if insertion or ingestion of a FB was witnessed or not. In the latter case, the child may simply report what they have recently done to their parent. The timeline of FB insertion or ingestion should be established, and thereafter, the exact nature of the foreign body must be determined. Sometimes a proactive parent may bring an example of the foreign body in question. Any symptoms of choking or coughing, or a cyanotic episode, should alert to the possibility of an airway foreign body and should be managed as such. Dysphagia may be a prominent feature of ingested FBs. Interestingly, cough and wheeze may also be prominent symptoms of an ingested solid FB (e.g. a coin) in a small child, especially if there is any delay in presentation or diagnosis, this usually being secondary to compression and oedema of the airway anterior to an impacted cricopharyngeal or upper oesophageal FB.

With respect to aural and nasal FBs, symptoms of pain, discharge or associated bleeding should be enquired after, as well as previous attempts at removal by the carers themselves or by previous referring physicians. This will help to predict the child's likely compliance with further examination. You should ask if this is the child's first presentation with a FB, or whether they have presented repeatedly. Thereafter, a systemic enquiry into the child's general health should be sought.

Examination of the child will be dependent on their compliance and every effort should be made with the parents and child to build confidence and rapport early in the assessment. A FB in the ear or nose can be assessed simply using a well-illuminated otoscope with the child positioned on the parent's lap, with the parent 'hugging' the child's arms with one arm and the other holding the head to the chest. Examine both ears and both sides of the nose even when there is only a report of a unilateral FB, as contralateral FBs are a surprise find on occasion.

The oral cavity and oropharynx should be examined gently using a wooden tongue depressor if permitted. Hypopharyngeal and oesophageal FBs cannot be visualised; however, palpation of the neck for pain, surgical emphysema and assessment of range of neck movement is prudent.

INVESTIGATIONS

Imaging of children with FBs inserted into the ear or nose is of little value.

Radiopaque ingested FBs can be seen on a chest radiograph (Figure 25.1) or on a lateral soft tissue neck x-ray (Figure 25.2), giving an indication of the level of impaction.

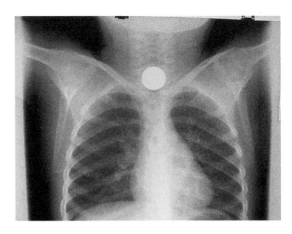

Figure 25.1 PA chest radiograph demonstrating a round radiopaque FB impacted at cricopharyngeus, typical of an ingested coin.

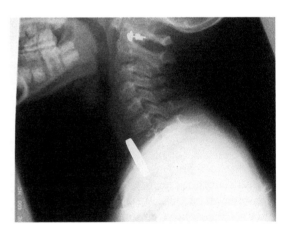

Figure 25.2 Lateral soft tissue neck x-ray confirming the coin in Figure 25.1 is within the upper oesophagus behind and separate from the airway anteriorly.

The most common ingested FB is a coin, with more than half of ingested FBs being metallic. When a circular radiopaque impacted foreign body is seen on a chest radiograph, it is important not to assume that it is a coin. A careful search should be made for the double density or 'halo' sign typical of a button battery and absent for coins on PA chest radiographs – a crucial discriminator when considering immediate management for unwitnessed ingestions (Figure 25.3).[3] In addition a 'step-off' is seen on a lateral x-ray view in the case of button batteries but not for coins.

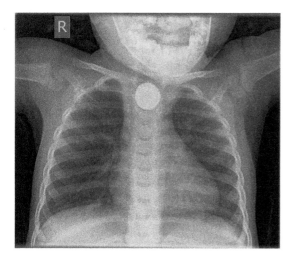

Figure 25.3 PA chest radiograph revealing a button battery lodged in the upper oesophagus. Note the classic 'halo' sign or 'double density' in the opacity, the interface between the anode and cathode components of the cell, affording differentiation from an ingested coin.

A handheld metal detector (HHMD) may be deployed to identify the location of an ingested FB in the gastrointestinal tract. The xiphisternum is used as a landmark, with any signal detected above it indicating that the ingested FB is potentially located in the oesophagus. Any signal detected below the xiphisternum indicates that the FB is located distal to the oesophagus and will most probably pass spontaneously through the gastrointestinal tract. The overall sensitivity of the HHMD is 95–100% with a specificity of 82–93% for detecting the location of metallic objects.[4]

In older children, fish bones can lodge in the oro- or hypopharynx, leading to significant discomfort. They have a tendency to become deeply embedded in the base of the tongue or piriform fossa. They will most often be non-radiopaque. Adolescents may tolerate visualisation with a laryngeal mirror or a fine fibrescope passed endonasally.

NATURE OF DIFFERENT FOREIGN BODIES

The main distinction to be made is whether a FB is inorganic (inert), organic or a button battery.

INORGANIC FOREIGN BODIES

Inorganic FBs are typically plastic or metal and, in children, commonly include items such as beads and other craft materials, and small parts from toys. By virtue of being inert they pose less of a short-term risk to the patient whilst they are in situ. They are often asymptomatic initially and may be discovered incidentally. Their removal can be delayed to a more convenient time depending on where the foreign body is and how symptomatic the child is. However, given time, these foreign bodies will pose their own risks by serving as a focus for infection and by causing chronic trauma to the mucosal surfaces.

ORGANIC FOREIGN BODIES

Organic FBs include food, rubber, wood and sponge. They tend to react more easily with the native mucosa, especially in nasal insertions. They may produce earlier symptoms and can be associated with additional symptoms of pain, blockage, discharge and bleeding. Peas, beans and nuts are among the more common organic FBs. They generally need to be removed sooner.

BUTTON BATTERIES

Button batteries warrant specific attention as they are potentially so damaging, regardless of whether they are ingested or inserted. They are both small and powerful and are used in a number of household appliances and toys. They come in a variety of sizes, from 9 mm to 30 mm in diameter. Larger batteries are more likely to impact upon ingestion and cause damage. 20 mm diameter batteries are associated with the most severe outcomes, with smaller diameters being more likely to pass naturally.[5,6]

A variance in battery voltage has been demonstrated between 1.5 V and 3.0 V, with the latter being associated with poorer outcomes in animals and humans. Lithium batteries are associated with greater morbidities, but manganese, silver and mercury varieties are also in use.

Button batteries are biologically unsealed and therefore readily discharge their alkaline contents in moist environments. Damage mechanisms are thought to include direct mucosal caustic injury, pressure necrosis, damage from an electrolytic current and absorption of toxic substances. Complications such as mucosal damage or caustic burns will occur within minutes to 2 hours. This is followed by risks of tympanic membrane, septal or oesophageal perforation, mediastinitis, tracheo-oesophageal fistula formation, oesophageal stricturing and aorto-oesophageal fistula with rapid fatal haemorrhage.

Therefore, all suspected ingested, aural and nasal button batteries should be emergently examined and ingested batteries removed immediately under general anaesthesia. Ingested button batteries may require input from other specialties such as paediatric or cardiothoracic surgery and they should be alerted and mobilised to the operating theatre promptly.[7]

MANAGEMENT

GENERAL PRINCIPLES

Careful attention to detail is required for removal of any FB. Good visualization, use of appropriate instruments (Figure 25.4) and careful retrieval should assist in removal with the minimum of injury to the surrounding tissues.

The best modality for removal of the FB will depend on a number of factors, including the age and clinical condition of the child; the type, size and shape of the FB; its anatomical location; and operator experience.

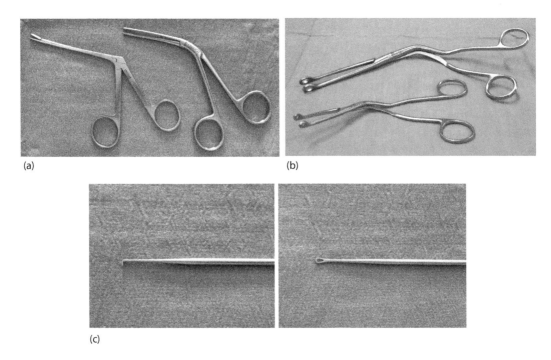

(a)

(b)

(c)

Figure 25.4 ENT instruments commonly used to remove FBs in children. (a) Alligator forceps (left) and Hartmann forceps (right). Alligator forceps have a distal joint and serrations useful for removal of small, irregularly shaped FBs in the ear and nose. Hartmann forceps have a proximal joint, allowing removal of larger FBs, and are especially useful in the nose and ear. (b) Magill forceps – useful for the removal of hypopharyngeal and proximal oesophageal FBs. They may also be used for appropriately shaped laryngeal FBs. (c) Angled probe (left) and Jobson–Horne probe (right) – useful in the management of aural FBs.

FOREIGN BODIES IN THE EAR

Aural FBs (Figure 25.5) may be referred as the sole presenting complaint or may be an incidental finding. Children with chronic ear infections tend to place FBs such as tissue or cotton wool in their ears more often.

Once the diagnosis is established, the FB should be removed in a timely fashion. As discussed earlier, the removal of an inorganic FB from the external auditory canal need not be emergent. Methods described include the use of a headlight and probe or suitable forceps to remove laterally placed and readily apparent FBs. Syringing a FB out of the ear canal is also described, more usually being undertaken by a nurse trained in the procedure and in the absence of contraindications to ear syringing. Instrumentation in unskilled hands is associated with canal trauma and tympanic membrane perforation.[8]

It is the authors' preference to remove FBs from the deeper medial ear canal using an ENT microscope, a fine suction tip and a Jobson–Horne probe.

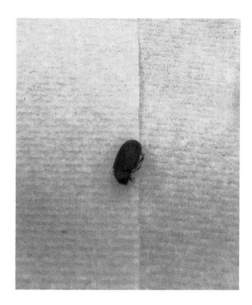

Figure 25.6 **A 7-year-old girl on a camping holiday presented to the emergency department with the sensation of something moving in her ear. This common beetle was removed with suction after it had been immersed in oil. Photo courtesy of Dr C Wright, RHSC, Edinburgh.**

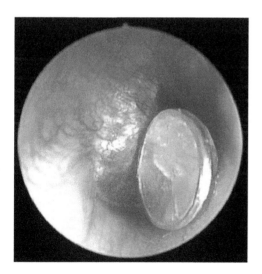

Figure 25.5 Intraoperative otoendoscopic view of a FB within the right external auditory canal. In this case, a large craft gemstone is lodged medially against the tympanic membrane.

In this way the ear can be adequately examined, any wax cleared without trauma and the FB removed with ease either with suction or by passing the probe around and behind it, thus drawing it out. Some children may not tolerate awake instrumentation of the ear and they will require a short day-case procedure under general anaesthesia to remove the FB. The contralateral ear should also be formally examined.

A live insect in the external auditory canal can cause massive anguish to children and adults alike. Once diagnosed, the insect can be drowned using preparations of olive oil, methylated spirit or lignocaine. Once killed, the insect can be suctioned out[9] (Figure 25.6).

FOREIGN BODIES IN THE NOSE

A FB in the nose can present acutely following a witnessed insertion, or a child may be referred to

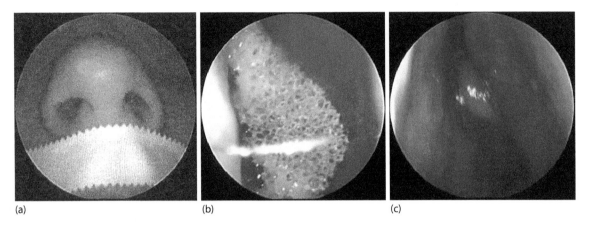

(a) (b) (c)

Figure 25.7 **(a)** Characteristic right-sided vestibulitis secondary to nasal FB and associated chronic nasal discharge. **(b)** Intraoperative nasendoscopic view of offending FB – in this case, a fragment of sponge. **(c)** Evidence of previous FB impaction with irritation of the inferior turbinate (left), nasal septum (right) and mucopus posteriorly. Photos courtesy of Dr A Williamson, RHSC, Edinburgh.

the ENT clinic with a chronic offensive unilateral nasal discharge. In the latter situation there may be evidence of unilateral vestibulitis on external examination (Figure 25.7). The offensive discharge is so overwhelming that, characteristically, parents report that they find it difficult to cuddle their child. Nasal FBs may also present with unilateral nasal blockage and intermittent epistaxis.

The site of impaction is usually between the anterior septum and inferior turbinate. The inhalation of a nasal FB is a known risk, yet uncommon. It is more likely to occur in the neurologically impaired child with an uncoordinated swallow reflex. The child is more likely to spit it out or swallow the object.

Once diagnosed, the FB should be removed in a timely manner. A parental kiss manoeuvre may be used to move a nasal FB anteriorly or even expel it. This is performed by asking the parent to perform a short, sharp blow into the child's mouth as they hold them. They may try to cover the unaffected nostril also. The insufflation of air causes reflex closure of the child's glottis and the air exits through the nostril(s) only.[10]

Repeated attempts at nasal FB removal are likely to be successively more difficult, and the object may become more deeply lodged. Therefore, careful planning is important to maximise the likelihood of removal on the first attempt. In a cooperative child, a headlight and an appropriate choice of

instrument can be used to remove the FB. Young children rarely tolerate stretching of the nasal alae with a Thudichum's speculum, the FB generally being exposed by turning the tip of the nose up gently with the thumb of the non-dominant hand. With parental consent, a younger child may be swaddled in a blanket and the head held by another healthcare professional to facilitate removal of the FB. Failing this, examination and removal under general anaesthesia is warranted. Care must be taken to examine the contralateral nasal cavity.

When removal of a nasal button battery is required, it is particularly important not to irrigate the nasal cavities, in order to avoid spreading alkaline content that may have leaked out.

INGESTED FOREIGN BODIES

As previously mentioned, ingestion of FBs occurs more in younger children aged 3 years and under. We must reiterate that a choking and cyanotic episode should alert the physician to a potential inhaled foreign body and should be managed as such.

Ingested FBs predominantly impact at the level of cricopharyngeus, this being the narrowest segment of the oesophagus. Other sites include at the level of the aortic arch, the left main bronchus and the gastro-oesophageal junction. They may impact at the supraglottic or glottic level, causing immediate airway compromise and a high risk of fatality – notable objects being whole grapes and unchewed pieces of hot dog. In these cases the management of choking in children should be observed in line with guidance from the UK Resuscitation Council.

A single finger-sweep manoeuvre should only be used if a FB is visible in the mouth of a choking child who is, or becomes, unconscious. Blind or repeated finger-sweeps should be avoided as they risk cranial or caudal displacement of the object more deeply into the pharynx and may cause injury (Figure 25.8).

Once diagnosed, the FB should be removed emergently under general anaesthesia. The pharynx should be examined formally before rigid oesophagoscopy is performed and the object retrieved. If impacted more distally, the FB may be removed more safely via gastroscopy and the paediatric surgical team should be notified of the child and involved in their care.

Soft oesophageal food boluses tend to be unusual in children. If there is a strong suspicion of an impacted food bolus in a child, then rigid or flexible oesophagoscopy is recommended to remove it, depending on the site, within 24 hours of the impaction, to reduce the incidence of complications.

Sharp FBs in the paediatric population are also, thankfully, rare; however, if the history and any imaging is suggestive of this, the child should be examined under general anaesthesia and the object removed emergently within 12 hours (Figures 25.9 and 25.10). Optical forceps and a Hopkins telescope

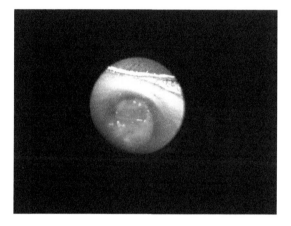

Figure 25.9 An ingested FB impacted at the level of the cricopharyngeal sphincter in a 2-year-old girl.

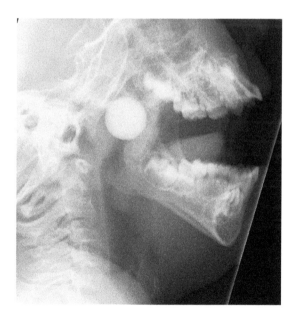

Figure 25.8 Lateral plain x-ray illustrating a FB within the nasopharynx. This child was witnessed placing a marble in their mouth. Finger-sweeps performed by a parent displaced the marble superiorly into the nasopharynx. It is held by the soft palate anteriorly and the adenoid pad posteriorly. Removal under general anaesthesia was required with the airway secured.

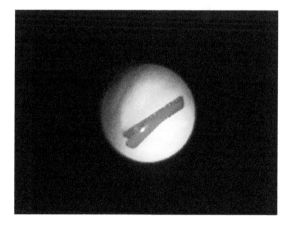

Figure 25.10 A hard, sharp, red plastic hair clasp was removed carefully using optical forceps deployed via a paediatric rigid oesophagoscope.

deployed via a rigid paediatric oesophagascope afford an optimal view and safer FB removal for sharp oesophageal FBs. The level of impaction may require the additional expertise of a paediatric surgeon.

A button battery lodged in the oesophagus of a child must be removed *immediately*. Serious burns can occur in 2 hours. Removal must not be delayed even if the child has eaten recently. Endoscopic removal with forward-grasping or coin forceps is preferred, affording direct visualisation of tissue injury. After removal, the mucosa surrounding the battery should be inspected carefully to determine the extent, depth, and location of tissue damage, specifically looking for evidence of perforation. If there is no evidence of perforation, the United States National Battery Ingestion Hotline (NBIH) Button Battery Ingestion Triage and Treatment Guideline recommends irrigation of the injured areas with 50–150 mL of 0.25% sterile acetic acid (obtained from the hospital pharmacy) and suction of excess fluid and debris through the endoscope.

The child should be observed closely after removal for the development of early or delayed complications.

KEY LEARNING POINTS

- Foreign body insertion/ingestion is very common in the paediatric population.
- The nature of the foreign body should be established in the history.
- Button batteries can cause massive and potentially fatal injury in a short period. They should be removed emergently.
- Inorganic foreign bodies in the ear can be removed at a more convenient time.
- A child with persistent offensive unilateral nasal discharge should be presumed to have a nasal foreign body until proved otherwise.
- Ingested foreign bodies usually impact at the level of cricopharyngeus and should be removed emergently.
- Depending on the level and nature of oesophageal foreign body impaction, the input of the paediatric or cardiothoracic surgeon should be sought.

REFERENCES

1. Heim SW, Maughan KL. Foreign bodies in the ear, nose and throat. *Am Fam Physician*. 2007; 76(8): 1185–1189.
2. Ansley JF, Cunningham MJ. Treatment of aural foreign bodies in children. *Pediatrics*. 1998; 101: 638–641.
3. Maves MD, Lloyd TV, Carithers JS. Radiographic identification of ingested disc batteries. *Pediatr Radiol*. 1986; 16: 154–156.
4. Lee JB, Ahmad S, Gale CP et al. Detection of coins ingested by children using a hand-held metal detector: a systematic review. *Emerg Med J*. 2005; 22: 839–844.
5. Litovitz TL, Schmitz RN. Ingestion of cylindrical and button batteries: an analysis of 2382 cases. *Pediatrics*. 1992; 89: 747–757.
6. Litovitz T, Whitaker N, Clarke L, White NC, Marsolek M. Emerging battery-ingestion hazard: clinical implications. *Pediatrics*. 2010; 125: 1168–1177.
7. Gohil R, Culshaw J, Jackson P, Singh S. Accidental button battery ingestion presenting as croup. *J Laryngol Otol*. 2014; 128: 292–295.
8. Davies PH, Bengar JR. Foreign bodies in the nose and ear: a review of techniques for removal in the emergency department. *Emerg Med J*. 2000; 17: 91–94.
9. Votey S, Dudley JP. Emergency ear, nose and throat procedures. *Emerg Med Clin North Am*. 1989; 7: 117–154.
10. Handbook of Non Drug Intervention (HANDI) Project Team. Mother's kiss for nasal foreign bodies. *Aust Fam Physician*. 2013; 42: 288–289.

FURTHER READING

Carney SA, Patel N, Clarke R. Foreign bodies in the ear and aerodigestive tract. Chapter 92, pp.1184–1193. *Scott-Brown's Otorhinolaryngology, Head and Neck Surgery*. 7th Edition, vol.1. 2008, Edward Arnold Publishers, Ltd.

Maconochie I, Bingham B, Skellett S. Paediatric Basic Life Support. 2015 Guidelines. Resuscitation Council (UK). www.resus.org.uk /resuscitation-guidelines/paediatric-basic-life -support/#choking. Accessed 20 July 2017.

National Battery Ingestion Hotline (NBIH). Button Battery Ingestion Triage and Treatment Guideline. www.poison.org/battery/guideline. Accessed 20 July 2017.

26

Paediatric post-tonsillectomy and post-adenoidectomy haemorrhage

SALIL SOOD, MARY-LOUISE MONTAGUE AND RAVI SHARMA

INTRODUCTION

Tonsillectomy, adenoidectomy and adenotonsillectomy are among the most common surgical procedures performed in children. They may be complicated by post-operative haemorrhage, which is a potentially life-threatening emergency because of the potential for airway obstruction and hypovolaemic shock. Bleeding, even if apparently minor initially, should be considered seriously in children, as a small 'herald' bleed may be the precursor to a larger later bleeding episode, often within 24 hours. Particular caution is also required in children, as the bleeding is more often occult, with children tending to swallow blood rather than spit it out. Consequently, the blood loss is usually greater than estimated at presentation.

CLASSIFICATION

Post-tonsillectomy haemorrhage is classified as either primary (occurring within the first 24 hours of surgery, and usually at the time of surgery or in the immediate post-operative period) or secondary (greater than 24 hours after surgery).

EPIDEMIOLOGY

The true rate of post-operative haemorrhage is difficult to estimate due to variation in reporting, with minor bleeding sometimes not recorded. The overall post-tonsillectomy haemorrhage rate in the UK has been shown to be 3.3%, which is similar to other reports. The bleeding rate shows seasonal variation being higher during winter months. Operative technique would also appear to influence bleeding rates, with the 2004 UK National Prospective Tonsillectomy Audit showing that patients undergoing tonsillectomy with diathermy had an increased rate of post-operative secondary haemorrhage compared with those who had dissection and haemostasis without diathermy. The relative risk of post-operative haemorrhage was 2–3 times greater for diathermy techniques.

PATHOPHYSIOLOGY

It is well recognised that the tonsils have a very rich vascular supply, provided by five external carotid artery branches. The lower tonsillar pole receives its supply from the dorsal lingual artery, the ascending palatine artery from the facial artery, and the tonsillar branch of the facial artery. The upper tonsillar pole receives its supply from the ascending pharyngeal artery and the lesser palatine artery. The tonsillar branch of the facial artery is the largest vessel. Meticulous haemostasis is thus of great importance in avoiding primary haemorrhage.

Following surgery, the normal healing process commences, with fibrin clot formation in the tonsillar fossae within 24 hours. By the fifth post-operative day, the fibrin clot has proliferated and has the appearances of a thick, whitish slough. Mucosa from the periphery of the wound begins to grow inward, and the slough begins to separate from the underlying tissue after around 1 week. Complete wound healing takes approximately 2 weeks.

Secondary haemorrhage tends to occur about 5–10 days after tonsillectomy, when the fibrin clot sloughs off. It is normally secondary to infection of the tonsillar fossae. Adequate post-operative analgesia is essential to improve swallowing, preventing stasis and, in turn, minimising the secondary haemorrhage rate.

Table 26.1 APLS approach to assessment of shock in children

A	Airway: patency
B	Breathing: respiratory rate
C	Circulation: heart rate, CRT <3 secs, urine output 0.5 mL/kg/hr, blood pressure
D	Disability: mental status, AVPU (alert, responds to voice, pain, unresponsive)

ASSESSMENT

INITIAL ASSESSMENT

Rapid initial assessment is required in the child presenting with post-tonsillectomy haemorrhage, as they may require prompt operative intervention. The APLS primary survey approach to assessing the child's airway and haemodynamic stability (Table 26.1) and commencing fluid resuscitation takes precedence over a detailed history and examination initially.

Once the child is stable and there is no evidence of continued bleeding, a more detailed history and examination can be carried out.

HISTORY AND EXAMINATION

The pertinent points to cover in the history are the timing of surgery and technique used, the analgesia provided and taken by the child, intercurrent illnesses – especially upper respiratory tract infection – and any relevant past medical and family history, including any clues that may point to a possible bleeding disorder. Make an estimate of blood loss by enquiring about haemoptysis and haematemesis, its duration and frequency.

Examination of the child presenting with post-operative haemorrhage should be approached in a calm and reassuring yet efficient manner. On arrival oxygen saturation, heart rate, respiratory rate, blood pressure and temperature should all be recorded (Table 26.2). Signs of shock, including depressed mental state, lethargy, tachycardia, prolonged capillary refill time to more than

Table 26.2 Normal vital signs in children (APLS values)

	Infant	1–2 years	2–5 years	5–12 years	Adolescent
Heart rate (bpm)	110–160	100–150	95–140	80–120	60–90
Respiratory rate (rpm)	30–40	25–35	25–30	20–25	14–18
Blood pressure systolic mmHg	80–90	85–95	85–100	90–100	100–140
Temperature		35–37°C			36–37.5°C
Saturations			94–98%		

3 seconds, pallor and cool peripheries, indicate that major blood loss has already occurred. Be wary of any child who is very quiet and withdrawn or drowsy, as this may be secondary to reduced cerebral perfusion and signal the development of hypovolaemic shock. Changes in heart rate should be observed for closely, and in particular, be vigilant for an increasing tachycardia as a sign of persistent bleeding (Figure 26.1).

Interestingly, normotension may be a falsely reassuring sign in the bleeding child, as children vasoconstrict to maintain their blood pressure (compensated shock). Hypotension usually occurs late and is a worrying pre-terminal sign.

Look at the oropharynx within the limits of cooperation of the child for signs of active bleeding or a clot in the tonsillar fossae. If unable to visualise the oropharynx, an audible gurgling sound in the throat during respiration, or repeated swallowing, may be a clue to active bleeding in the absence of overt bleeding from the mouth. It is also imperative to be vigilant for signs of imminent airway obstruction in a child who is choking or gagging with a reduced oxygen

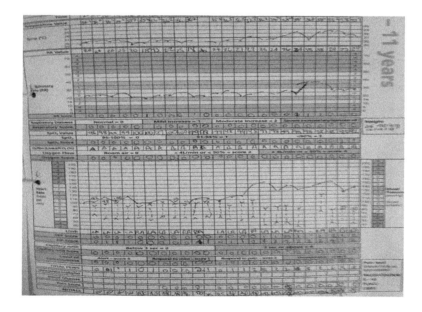

Figure 26.1 Paediatric Early Warning Score (PEWS) chart showing a rising heart rate alongside an increasing respiratory rate after admission to the ward with post-tonsillectomy haemorrhage that had appeared to stop spontaneously.

saturation, difficulty breathing or signs of respiratory distress.

INVESTIGATIONS

A full blood count (FBC) should be requested to assess a baseline haemoglobin level, but it is important to be aware that this may not be representative of the actual degree of blood loss. This also permits confirmation of a normal platelet count. Urea and electrolyte estimation will allow an assessment of the degree of dehydration, and a coagulation screen is essential to assess coagulation pathways. Blood should also be sampled for group and save in the stable child in whom bleeding has stopped, but a cross-match should be requested for children with signs of hypovolaemic shock at presentation or in those who become unstable.

In a child with signs of shock, blood should also be taken for blood gas (including lactate, haemoglobin and ionised calcium) and a capillary blood glucose done, in addition to the laboratory tests.

A von Willebrand's screen should be considered if repeated episodes of bleeding occur, in order to detect a previously unrecognised coagulopathy.

MANAGEMENT

RESUSCITATION

The basic principles in the first-line management of post-tonsillectomy and post-adenoidectomy haemorrhage in children are to:

- Summon help.
- Protect the airway – sit the child upright or place them in the lateral decubitus position.
- Administer high-flow oxygen through a face mask with a reservoir or, if needed, via high-flow nasal cannulae.
- Avoid unnecessary or excessive suctioning.
- Secure early intravenous access for intravenous fluid resuscitation.

Preparations are then made to place a second IV line. Waiting for EMLA cream is acceptable in a stable child. If IV access cannot be obtained, intraosseous (IO) access is a viable alternative in the child with signs of shock. In children an initial 20 mL/kg bolus of crystalloid is administered in 10 mL/kg aliquots, with rapid assessment between aliquots to correct physiological parameters. This can be repeated if required, followed by further ABC assessment of the child. If the child remains haemodynamically unstable, normovolaemia may be achieved with the transfusion of blood. Arrangements should be made simultaneously to transfer the child to the operating theatre.

Bleeding is alarming for most parents and frightening for the child concerned, so it is wise to readmit all children presenting with secondary haemorrhage even if it appears to have stopped spontaneously and the child is stable, as close monitoring is required.

PRIMARY HAEMORRHAGE

Primary haemorrhage is usually brisk. Children should be returned to the operating theatre promptly after an intravenous infusion has been set up, and resuscitation commenced if required. A second anaesthetic can be hazardous because of the greater risks of hypoxia and aspiration and should ideally be administered by an experienced anaesthetist. The bleeding source is localised and controlled using diathermy or ligatures, or occasionally by sewing the anterior and posterior pillars over a gauze swab for 24 hours, with the latter being a last resort in light of the potential risk of inhalation or ingestion of the swab.

SECONDARY HAEMORRHAGE

The management of young children with secondary post-tonsillectomy bleeding differs from that of adolescents and adults in that they rarely tolerate trials of topical cautery under local anaesthesia or the application of pressure to the bleeding site in the tonsillar fossa with a gauze swab. Similarly, children do not tolerate dilute hydrogen peroxide gargles well, and these should be used with caution in any case.

The haemorrhage and associated infection frequently settle with intravenous antibiotic therapy (usually co-amoxiclav), but examination and surgical control under general anaesthesia with a rapid sequence induction is generally recommended for children who have signs of ongoing active bleeding or any signs of clinical deterioration. An experienced anaesthetist is vital, as airway management can prove difficult in an actively bleeding child positioned supine.

In theatre, good lighting is essential. Clot is evacuated from the tonsillar fossa of the bleeding side and direct pressure applied laterally onto the tonsillar fossa with gauze wrapped around the end of forceps. The addition of 1:10,000 adrenaline to the gauze may be helpful. Surgical arrest of bleeding is usually achieved with bipolar diathermy or ligatures. An adjunct in the management of post-tonsillectomy bleeding may include the administration of tranexamic acid, which has been shown to reduce the need for transfusion in surgical patients. Of note, however, is that there is no benefit to be gained from using tranexamic acid to reduce intraoperative bleeding during adenotonsillectomy in children.

Post-operatively, it is important to monitor the child closely in a well-lit ward area within view of nursing staff or in a paediatric high-dependency unit with regular observation of vital signs. The haemoglobin should be remeasured. A minimum haemoglobin of 8 g/dL is acceptable, provided there is no further bleeding. Such a child will require oral iron supplementation post-operatively for up to 6 weeks. IV antibiotics are administered and converted to the oral route when oral intake is re-established, facilitated by adequate analgesia, usually without ongoing prescription of a nonsteroidal anti-inflammatory drug (NSAID). Significant blood loss may necessitate blood transfusion, but if prompt measures are taken, this should not be required routinely.

POST-ADENOIDECTOMY HAEMORRHAGE

Post-adenoidectomy haemorrhage is less common than post-tonsillectomy haemorrhage but is nonetheless a serious complication. Careful inspection of the nasopharynx immediately before adenoidectomy and adenoidectomy performed under visual control with a mirror or endoscope is helpful to prevent direct injury to any aberrant arteries (Figure 26.2). A steady drip from the nose will

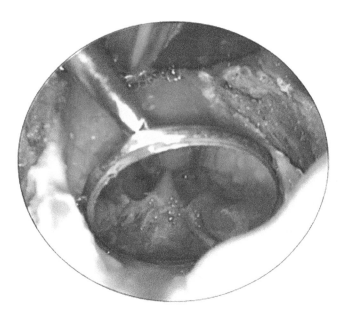

Figure 26.2 Indirect view of the nasopharynx provided by a mirror during coblation adenoidectomy.

be apparent when haemorrhage follows removal of the adenoids in an awake child sitting upright, but this may not be the case for a sleeping child, in whom the blood is more often swallowed silently, to be vomited later.

The principles of management of post-adenoidectomy haemorrhage are, in general, the same as those for post-tonsillectomy haemorrhage. Use of adrenaline-soaked gauze swabs and suction monopolar diathermy under general anaesthesia are the main techniques used to arrest post-adenoidectomy bleeding. Rarely, a postnasal pack may be required to be left for 24–48 hours to tamponade and stop the haemorrhage, this necessitating admission to the paediatric intensive care unit with the child intubated.

In all cases of primary and secondary tonsillar haemorrhage and adenoid haemorrhage returned to theatre, it is wise to pass a nasogastric tube before emergence from general anaesthesia to empty the child's stomach of old swallowed blood.

COMPLICATIONS

Death due to post-operative haemorrhage is, fortunately, very rare (0.0007%). However, a greater proportion of children may experience morbidity from hospital readmission, blood transfusion or further surgery to arrest ongoing haemorrhage.

KEY LEARNING POINTS

- Post-tonsillectomy haemorrhage is the commonest and most dangerous complication after tonsillectomy and must be recognised and managed without delay in children.
- It may be difficult to measure blood loss, as bleeding may occur over several hours and large amounts of blood may be swallowed.
- Tachycardia, tachypnoea, delayed capillary refill and decreased urine output are early indicators of hypovolaemic shock,

whereas hypotension and altered consciousness level are late signs of hypovolaemia, with decompensated shock.

- As a general rule, a child who is bleeding should be taken to theatre as soon as possible. However, the child must be resuscitated before induction of anaesthesia to avoid cardiovascular collapse.
- Important anaesthetic considerations in a child who is bleeding after tonsillectomy include the potential for hypovolaemic shock, pulmonary aspiration (of regurgitated swallowed blood or post-operative oral intake), difficult intubation due to blood obscuring the view, or oedema from previous airway instrumentation and surgery.

FURTHER READING

Bhattacharyya N. Rapid communication: the risk of additional post-tonsillectomy bleeding after the first bleeding episode. *Laryngoscope* 2015; 125:354–355.

Lowe D, van der Meulen J. National Prospective Tonsillectomy Audit. Tonsillectomy technique as a risk factor for postoperative haemorrhage. *Lancet* 2004; 364:697–702.

Leaper D, Whitaker I. The child in shock. Chapter 6. In *Advanced Paediatric Life Support: A Practical Approach to Emergencies*, 6th Edition. Edited by Martin Samuels and Sue Wieteska. Published 2016 by John Wiley & Sons, Ltd.

Brum MR, Miura MS, Castro SF et al. Tranexamic acid in adenotonsillectomy in children: double blind randomized clinical trial. *Int J Pediatric Otorhinolaryngol* 2012; 76(10): 1401–1405.

De Luca Canto G, Pacheco-Pereira C, Aydinoz S et al. Adenotonsillectomy complications: a meta analysis. *Paediatrics* 2015; 136:702–718.

27

Paediatric epistaxis

JAIME DOODY AND HELENA ROWLEY

INTRODUCTION

Epistaxis in the paediatric population is exceedingly common. Fortunately, cases of acute paediatric epistaxis are rarely severe, with most being self-limiting and managed with simple first-aid measures in the community setting.

Usually, the role of the otolaryngologist is to treat children with recurrent epistaxis in the outpatient setting, but their expertise may on occasion be called upon for children presenting to the emergency department with acute, refractory epistaxis that cannot be controlled with simple measures such as tamponade.

There is usually no underlying pathology; however, the clinician must remain vigilant for the few serious local and systemic conditions that it can be associated with. The treatment required for acute paediatric epistaxis is very much dependent on the severity, anatomical site and underlying cause of the bleed. The treatment algorithm adopts a 'step ladder' approach, with treatment steps only escalating when less invasive measures fail.

ANATOMY

One of the main reasons the nose is so susceptible to epistaxis is its rich blood supply from both the internal and external carotid arteries. The lateral nasal wall is supplied by the anterior ethmoidal, sphenopalatine, posterior lateral nasal and the ascending and greater palatine arteries. Most epistaxis originates from the nasal septum. The superior part of the septum is supplied by the anterior and posterior ethmoidal arteries, which are both branches of the internal carotid artery. The inferior part of the septum is supplied by the superior labial, sphenopalatine and greater palatine arteries, all of which are branches of the external carotid artery. These arteries anastomose to form Kiesselbach's plexus – otherwise

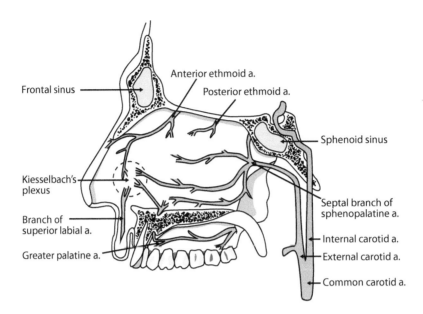

Figure 27.1 The blood supply of the nasal septum from branches of the internal and external carotid arteries.

known as 'Little's area' – located anteroinferiorly on the nasal septum (Figure 27.1). This is covered by a thin layer of mucosa that is especially vulnerable to trauma and inflammation. The venous drainage of the nose is via the anterior facial, sphenopalatine and ethmoidal veins. The ethmoidal vein is of clinical significance, as it drains into the cavernous sinus (via the ophthalmic vein), allowing intracranial spread of infection originating in the nose, which is a consideration when nasal packing is required.

EPIDEMIOLOGY

Epistaxis affects 30% of children under the age of 5 years and over 50% of children aged 5 years and older.[1] Epistaxis is seen more commonly in males than females.[2] It is rare in children under the age of 2 years and in this age group usually has an identifiable underlying cause.

CLASSIFICATION

Epistaxis can be classified either aetiologically or anatomically. The aetiological classification divides epistaxis into either 'primary/idiopathic', with no identifiable underlying cause, or 'secondary' epistaxis, which occurs as a result of a systemic condition. Primary or idiopathic epistaxis makes up over 90% of cases. Anatomically speaking, epistaxis can be divided into 'anterior' or 'posterior'. The anatomical site of the bleeding source is very important when choosing a treatment modality, as posterior epistaxis is far more difficult to treat and usually requires more invasive measures.

HISTORY AND EXAMINATION

A good history is key to determining whether epistaxis is idiopathic or secondary in nature. A detailed description of the nature of the bleeding (severity, frequency, duration, originating side) as well as asking targeted questions aimed at uncovering an undiagnosed bleeding disorder (unexplained bruising, prolonged bleeding, family history of bleeding disorder) are very important. Associated symptoms such as unilateral nasal obstruction, diplopia, facial swelling or headache are of particular importance, especially in the male adolescent cohort, as juvenile nasopharyngeal angiofibroma (JNA), although rare, can present with these symptoms.

Physical examination is also of vital importance. In the child presenting with acute severe epistaxis to the emergency department, resuscitation and first-aid measures will take priority. Once adequate control of bleeding has been obtained, the child can be examined in a stepwise fashion in the same way as the child presenting with recurrent epistaxis in the absence of active bleeding.

On inspection, look for signs of anaemia (pale conjunctiva, blanched palmar creases, etc.) and possible bleeding disorders (bruising, telangiectasia, bleeding gums). Given that the vast majority of children present with anterior nosebleeds, anterior rhinoscopy is the next step of the exam. Use a headlight and Thudichum's or Killian nasal speculum with fine Zoellner suction to thoroughly examine the anterior nose, looking for engorged vessels or a possible bleeding point. In very young children, anterior rhinoscopy may be performed using a well-illuminated otoscope (Figure 27.2). If no obvious bleeding point is seen, light agitation of the nasal septum using a cotton tipped swab is appropriate and can reveal occult bleeding points. If no bleeding point or obvious vessel is seen, flexible nasendoscopy (FNE) or rigid endoscopy using an appropriate topical decongestant with local anaesthetic (e.g. co-phenylcaine) is warranted, if tolerated. Endoscopy is also an essential diagnostic procedure in any male presenting with unilateral epistaxis or where JNA is a concern.

INVESTIGATIONS

In acute epistaxis that responds quickly to basic first-aid measures, blood tests such as a full blood count, (if looking for a suspected anaemia), or coagulation studies may be ordered at the clinician's discretion but need not be ordered routinely. In children presenting with acute severe epistaxis, urgent blood testing to include full blood count, coagulation studies and a group and save or cross-match should be performed. If a bleeding disorder is confirmed on blood testing, an urgent haematology opinion is necessary in order to treat a correctable abnormality with blood factors or platelets.

DIFFERENTIAL DIAGNOSIS

The vast majority of paediatric epistaxis occurs for no obvious reason. Little's area is the most common site for bleeding for several postulated reasons. Firstly, it is the anastomotic site of the internal and external carotid arteries and is highly vascular. Secondly, the mucosa overlying the plexus is thin and is susceptible to damage due to the drying effects of the adjacent nasal airflow. Lastly, this area is also vulnerable to physical damage, be it self-inflicted digital trauma or external blunt trauma. When the mucosa is breached in this area, it leads to crusting and irritation, which leads to further digital trauma of the area by the child.

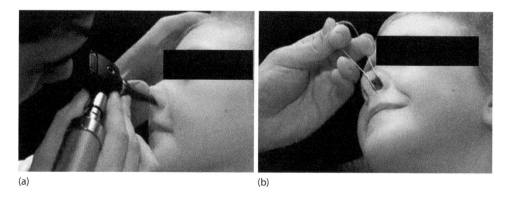

(a)   (b)

Figure 27.2 Anterior rhinoscopy exposing the anterior nasal septum using (a) a well-illuminated otoscope and (b) a Thudichum's nasal speculum.

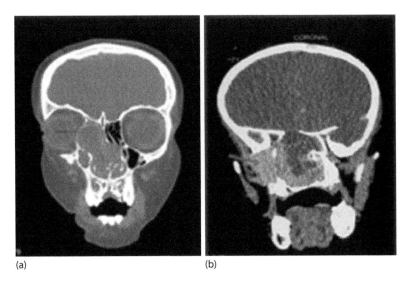

(a) (b)

Figure 27.3 Coronal CT scans showing a right sided JNA in an adolescent male with expansion of the lesion into the right orbit (a) and local invasion into the skull base and the right pterygopalatine fossa (b).

It has been suggested that *Staphylococcus aureus* may play a role in the pathogenesis of idiopathic epistaxis by causing a low-grade inflammation that promotes angioneogenesis, thus increasing the local blood supply and rendering the area more prone to spontaneous bleeding.[3] There is also an increased incidence of epistaxis during winter months, which has been attributed to an increase in upper respiratory tract infections, dehumidification of the nasal passages by domestic central heating, and alteration in nasal blood flow due to fluctuations in ambient temperature upon moving from hot to cold environments.[4]

Allergic rhinitis is a predisposing factor in paediatric epistaxis due to the increased inflammation and friability of the nasal mucosa. It has also been shown that intranasal steroid therapy can cause epistaxis. Less than 10% of paediatric patients presenting with recurrent epistaxis are found to have a coagulopathy, but it appears that younger patients with persistent epistaxis are more likely to have an underlying bleeding disorder.[5] The main predictor of a child presenting with recurrent epistaxis having an underlying coagulopathy is family history, with traditionally recognised signs such as easy bruising and bleeding gingiva having little predictive value in diagnosing a coagulopathy.[6]

Epistaxis is often the telltale symptom in paediatric patients diagnosed with hereditary haemorrhagic telangiectasia (HHT) and can often help in the diagnosis of this uncommon condition.[7] Adolescent males presenting with recurrent epistaxis are a particular cohort that warrant special attention due to their predilection for the exclusive development of JNA. JNA has a peak incidence in the second decade,[8] and this benign tumour should be excluded in all male paediatric patients presenting with unilateral nasal obstruction and dramatic unexplained epistaxis.

Other neoplastic tumours causing mass effects and epistaxis are rare entities in the paediatric population. When a unilateral nasal mass is suspected or confirmed in a child or adolescent presenting with epistaxis, cross-sectional imaging is imperative before embarking on biopsy or excision for histology (Figure 27.3).

MANAGEMENT

The child presenting with acute, severe epistaxis should be managed according to the ABCDE approach for resuscitation with a parallel attempt to arrest the epistaxis. Fortunately, most children with acute epistaxis have spontaneous anterior bleeding in the absence of a compromised airway or haemodynamic instability. Nonetheless, general appearance, airway stability, haemodynamic and mental status should be assessed rapidly at initial presentation. Airway intervention and/or fluid resuscitation may be indicated in children with respiratory instability or haemorrhagic shock.

Active bleeding usually responds to simple compression, but other measures, including cautery, application of a haemostatic agent, nasal packing or surgical intervention, may be required.

SIMPLE COMPRESSION

Bleeding may be controlled in the first instance with tamponade (or 'pinching of the nose') with the child sitting upright and leaning forward for 10 to 15 minutes (Figure 27.4). Some children may permit pledgets soaked in topical local anaesthetic and vasoconstrictor to be placed intranasally,

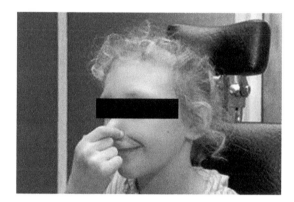

Figure 27.4 Demonstration of the correct method for anterior nasal compression as the first step in management of epistaxis.

followed by further tamponade. This is often enough to arrest an acute anterior bleed.

NASAL CAUTERY

The approach is then similar to that for managing a stable child in the absence of bleeding. The clinician should use a headlight, nasal speculum and suction to examine the anterior nose in an attempt to locate a bleeding point. If an anterior bleeding point is found – usually in the vicinity of Little's area – chemical cautery with silver nitrate may be attempted (Figure 27.5). 75% silver nitrate is preferable to the 95% preparation, as it is more effective and causes less pain. It is recommended that only one side of the nasal septum is cauterised at a time, to reduce the chance of septal perforation. Do not apply silver nitrate without being somewhat certain that you are addressing a likely bleeding point, as it can cause adverse effects and non-judicial use can be detrimental.

If the bleeding point is more posterior, FNE or rigid endoscopy may be performed, if tolerated. If the child is not a suitable candidate for FNE or silver nitrate cautery under local anaesthesia, or the suspected bleeding point is too far posterior, proceeding to examination under general anaesthesia with possible chemical or electrocautery is entirely appropriate.

HAEMOSTATIC AGENTS

Newer topical haemostatic agents, such as the gelatin-thrombin matrix sealant Floseal, are starting to show benefit in the treatment of adult

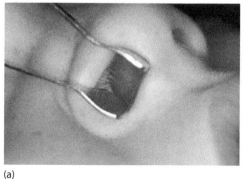

(a)

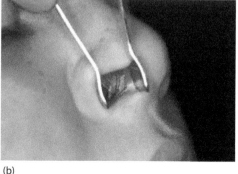

(b)

Figure 27.5 Prominent vessels on Little's area before cautery (a) and the appearance after cautery (b).

epistaxis,[9] but no large-scale study has been done to show their efficacy in the paediatric population.

NASAL PACKING

In the very rare instance of uncontrollable or posterior paediatric epistaxis, nasal packing may be required, preceded by the application of topical anaesthesia and vasoconstrictor. In the case of brisk anterior bleeding, a prefabricated nasal tampon (e.g. Merocel) may be placed along the floor of the nasal cavity and expanded with 10 mL of normal saline. This will require removal in 1 to 5 days.

Absorbable nasal packs made of gelatin (e.g. Gelfoam or Nasopore), cellulose (e.g. Surgicel) or an alginate dressing are easier to place in children and do not require subsequent removal. They are preferred when minimal pressure is required for bleeding control or when standard nasal packs may traumatise the nasal mucosa, causing more bleeding (e.g. children with bleeding disorders) (Figure 27.6). After anterior nasal packing is placed, the oropharynx should be examined to confirm adequate haemostasis.

For posterior epistaxis, the modern method for nasal packing involves the placement under general anaesthesia of an inflatable tamponading single or double balloon catheter (Figure 27.7). These balloons can be left in situ for up to 48 hours, but antibiotic cover must be provided to reduce the risk of intracranial spread of possible infection. Once the balloon(s) is/are removed, the child should be observed for an appropriate amount of time and discharged accordingly.

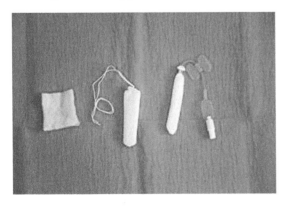

Figure 27.6 A selection of commercially available anterior nasal packs suitable for use in children.

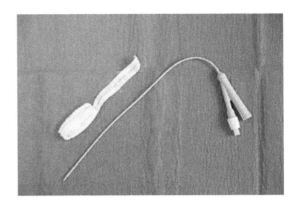

Figure 27.7 Foley catheter and BIPP packing are often used as an alternative to commercially available balloon catheters.

SURGICAL INTERVENTION

If all of the above measures fail, or if the child rebleeds after removal of an indwelling pack and there is no correctable bleeding disorder present, examination under anaesthesia with ligation of the anterior ethmoid and/or sphenopalatine arteries may be necessary, but it is rarely required in children. Transantral internal maxillary artery ligation is contraindicated in children because of the risk of injury to the unerupted dentition.

Selective embolisation of the internal maxillary artery has been reported to be successful in cases of intractable epistaxis unresponsive to other treatments and can also be useful in controlling bleeding secondary to JNA prior to surgical excision, the detail of which is beyond the scope of this chapter (Figure 27.8).

PREVENTION OF RECURRENT EPISODES

Prior to discharge, educate the parent or care-giver and, if appropriate, the child or young person, in first-aid measures such as direct digital tamponade in the event of recurrence of an acute bleed. Education to prevent recurrent episodesshould also include advice about prevention of local trauma by discouraging nose-picking, humidification, topical nasal lubricants and antiseptic cream/ointment. Medical management of co-existing allergic rhinitis should also be optimised.

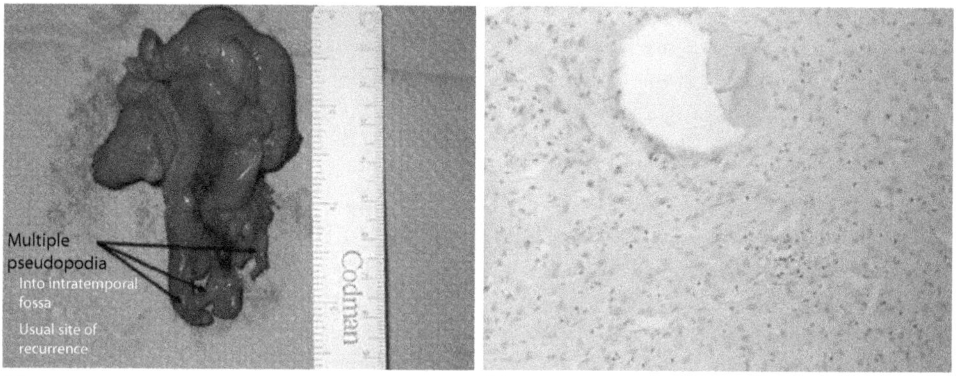

(a)   (b)

Figure 27.8 Excised juvenile nasopharyngeal angiofibroma with pseudopodia-like projections (a) and the diagnostic histopathology of fibrous tissue stroma with vascular spaces (b).

KEY LEARNING POINTS

- Most cases of paediatric epistaxis are idiopathic and anterior.
- Most cases of paediatric epistaxis respond to simple compression and/or topical vasoconstrictor.
- Cautery, haemostatic agents or nasal packing may be required if active bleeding does not respond to compression.
- Do not forget to screen for a family history of bleeding disorders.
- Beware of juvenile nasopharyngeal angiofibroma in the adolescent male.
- Arterial ligation and embolization are rarely required in children.

REFERENCES

1. Petruson B. Epistaxis in childhood. *Rhinology*. 1979; 17(2): 83–90.
2. Sengupta A, Maity K, Ghosh D, Basak B, Das SK, Basuet D. A study on role of nasal endoscopy for diagnosis and management of epistaxis. *J Indian Med Assoc*. 2010; 108(9): 597–598.
3. Montague M-L, Whymark A, Howatson A, Kubba H. The pathology of visible blood vessels on the nasal septum in children with epistaxis. *Int J Pediatr Otorhinolaryngol*. 2011; 75(8): 1032–1034.
4. Nunez DA, McClymont LG, Evans RA. Epistaxis: a study of the relationship with weather. *Clin Otolaryngol Allied Sci*. 1990; 15(1): 49–51.
5. Elden L, M Reinders, Witmer C. Predictors of bleeding disorders in children with epistaxis: value of preoperative tests and clinical screening. *Int J Pediatr Otorhinolaryngol*. 2012; 76(6): 767–771.
6. Sandoval C, Dong S, Visintainer Paul, Ozkaynak MF, Jayabose S. Clinical and laboratory features of 178 children with recurrent epistaxis. *J Pediatr Hematol Oncol*. 2002; 24(1): 47–49.
7. Folz BJ, Zoll B, Alfke H, Toussaint A, Maier RF, Werner JA. Manifestations of hereditary hemorrhagic telangiectasia in children and adolescents. *Eur Arch Otorhinolaryngol*. 2006; 263(1): 53–61.
8. Barnes L, Eveson JW, Reichart P, Sidransky D (Eds): World Health Organization Classification of Tumours. Pathology and Genetics of Head and Neck Tumours. IARC Press: Lyon 2005.

9. Côté D, Barber B, Diamond C, Wright E. FloSeal hemostatic matrix in persistent epistaxis: prospective clinical trial. *J Otolaryngol Head Neck Surg.* 2010; 39(3): 304–308.

Patel N, Maddalozzo J, Billings KR. An update on management of pediatric epistaxis. *Int J Pediatr Otorhinolaryngol.* 2014; 78(8): 1400–1404.

Qureishi A, Burton MJ. Interventions for recurrent idiopathic epistaxis (nosebleeds) in children. *Cochrane Database Syst Rev.* 2012, Issue 9. Art. No.: CD004461.

FURTHER READING

Clarke R. Epistaxis in children. In *Scott-Brown's Otorhinolaryngology, Head and Neck Surgery* 7th Edition. CRC Press, Apr 2008, 1063–1069.

28

ENT trauma in children

KATE STEPHENSON

INTRODUCTION

Ear, nose and throat (ENT) injuries are relatively common in children. However, major trauma to the head and neck region is, thankfully, rare. The mechanisms of trauma are different to those of adults and vary according to age of the child and geographical area. Special considerations relate to the care of the child with an ENT injury. Prompt tailored management is necessary to limit the morbidity and, in rare cases, mortality associated with ENT injuries.

AETIOLOGY

Younger children are more likely to suffer certain types of accidental injury, such as falls and foreign body injuries. Injuries in school-age children may often result from sporting activities, whereas the risk of interpersonal violence is increased in older children and adolescents. Children are also at particular risk of head and neck injury in pedestrian vehicle accidents, due to their height relative to the moving vehicle. Lack of proper restraint for child passengers involved in a road traffic accident may also increase the risk of injury.

PREVENTION

Prevention of ENT trauma in children can occur in several settings. Use of protective equipment within sport, road and traffic safety measures and correct vehicular restraints are all associated with risk reduction. Safety measures within the home are particularly important for the younger child.

SPECIAL CONSIDERATIONS

DIAGNOSIS

Full diagnosis of an injury may be delayed in the younger child who may not be able to articulate their symptoms. Careful observation and a tailored examination may be required. For example, a facial nerve weakness may be more difficult to assess in the child who cannot follow commands. External injuries may be readily identified, in comparison to 'concealed' injuries, such as a septal haematoma or traumatic perforation of the tympanic membrane. Minor non-life-threatening ENT injuries may also be masked in the context of polytrauma and may be detected in the secondary survey.

TREATMENT

In contrast to adults, the treatment of ENT-related injuries in children is not likely to be possible under local anaesthesia. Procedures such as drainage of an auricular haematoma, suturing of a facial laceration or nasal manipulation will all likely require a general anaesthetic.

PERINATAL TRAUMA

A history of difficult vaginal delivery with significant traction on the neck is associated with injury. Instrumental delivery, paralysis with the use of forceps, can result in lacerations or bruising to the face, nose or pinna. Vaginal delivery is also associated with anterior nasal septal deviations, many of which improve spontaneously.[1] Unilateral and bilateral vocal cord paralysis may also result from stretching and irritation of the recurrent laryngeal nerves. Intracranial, eye and other peripheral nerve injuries are also recognised birth traumas.[2]

NON-ACCIDENTAL INJURY

Non-accidental injury (NAI) warrants separate consideration, as it may commonly involve the head and neck region. Pharyngeal perforations have been found to be a frequent abusive ENT injury, predominantly affecting infants. A large proportion of these children have additional injuries, many of which involve the external ear (e.g. burns, abrasions, lacerations and resultant auricular deformity).

Fabricated and induced injury (FII), formerly known as Munchausen's syndrome by proxy, is defined as creation or exaggeration of illness or injury in a child by a caregiver. This may result in unnecessary investigations or medical interventions.

The majority of ENT presentations of FII involve an ear-related complaint, such as haemorrhage from the ear or chronic otorrhoea.[3] FII represents a form of child abuse and, although rare, should be considered in cases which are particularly chronic, recurrent and perplexing and do not respond to treatment as expected. Figure 28.1 summarises these key points.

Suspicion of NAI or FII should lead to a full evaluation and prompt involvement of child protection staff with a view to introduction of safeguarding measures. Early recognition and intervention is critical to prevent repetition and progression of abuse.

THE SERIOUSLY OR MULTIPLY INJURED CHILD

Advanced paediatric and trauma life support principles should be applied to the seriously or multiply injured child. A structured approach is applied to assessment and management of the patient. The primary survey should identify and treat life-threatening problems as they are identified, and in a major trauma setting can be summarised as <C>ABC. This describes the order of the survey and resuscitation, from control of catastrophic external haemorrhage (<C>), to airway with cervical spine control (A), breathing (B) and circulation (C).

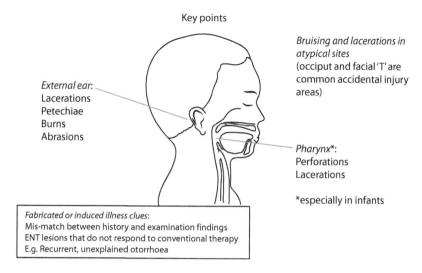

Key points

External ear:
Lacerations
Petechiae
Burns
Abrasions

Bruising and lacerations in
atypical sites
(occiput and facial 'T' are
common accidental injury
areas)

Pharynx*:
Perforations
Lacerations

*especially in infants

Fabricated or induced illness clues:
Mis-match between history and examination findings
ENT lesions that do not respond to conventional therapy
E.g. Recurrent, unexplained otorrhoea

Figure 28.1 Non-accidental ENT injuries in children.

TRAUMA TO THE EAR AND TEMPORAL BONE

Injuries of the outer, middle and inner ear may occur in isolation or in combination. The pinna is particularly vulnerable to isolated injury, given its exposed position. Middle and inner ear injuries are associated with high-energy injuries and may occur in the context of polytrauma. Bilateral and accidental ear injuries in the infant are very rare and should raise concern regarding non-accidental injury[4] (Figure 28.2).

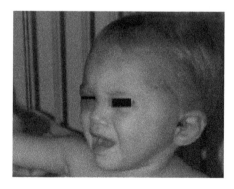

Figure 28.2 Ear bruising typically seen in cases of NAI. VJ Palusci, D Nazer, P Brennan. In *Diagnosis of Non-Accidental Injury: Illustrated Clinical Cases* (Case 74), CRC Press, 2015.

HAEMATOMA OF THE PINNA

Disruption of the tissue planes of the pinna typically results from shearing forces such as those occurring in rugby and wrestling injuries. Chronic seroma formation has also been observed in paediatric wheelchair users, due to repetitive friction of the pinna on the wheelchair headrest. Bleeding and haematoma formation occurs in the potential space between the cartilage of the pinna and the covering perichondrium, which is normally tightly applied and covered by thin, compact layers of connective tissue and skin (Figure 28.3).

Two principal complications may result from an auricular haematoma. Devascularisation of the auricular cartilage can occur, causing cartilage necrosis and deformation of the pinna - a 'cauliflower ear'. Superinfection of the haematoma leads to perichondritis and potential abscess formation; this increases the risk of cartilage loss and deformation.

Treatment

An auricular haematoma should be drained as soon as possible and measures taken to prevent re-accumulation. Simple aspiration and use of compressive bandaging is usually insufficient. This drainage requires general anaesthesia in the child. Surgical measures to re-appose the tissue layers include use of mattress sutures and an 'invasive

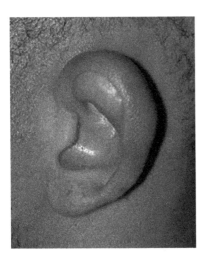

Figure 28.3 Auricular haematoma of the scaphoid fossa and triangular fossa of the left ear. J. Loock. Haematoma auris. In J. Gleeson (ed.) *Scott-Brown's Otorhinolaryngology, Head and Neck Surgery,* 7th edition, CRC Press, 2008 (Figure 236m.1 (a)).

dressing' – a bolster or splint secured through the pinna.[5,6]

Many clinicians would recommend prophylactic antibiotic treatment to guard against superinfection. Should perichondritis be present, prompt, high-dose, targeted antibiotics are required.

AURICULAR LACERATIONS

Minor auricular lacerations may be managed with adhesive dressings such as 'butterfly stitches' (Steri-Strips™). The principles governing management include preservation of the contours of the pinna, coverage of auricular cartilage and prevention of secondary infection. Depending on the severity of the injury and local policies, these may be managed by the emergency department, ENT or plastic surgery. Repair by suturing and skin grafting may be necessary under general anaesthesia.

TRAUMATIC TYMPANIC MEMBRANE PERFORATION

Traumatic perforation of the tympanic membrane may rarely occur as a result of penetrating trauma and is typically associated with foreign body insertion (e.g. cotton bud misuse). In children, barotrauma causing rupture of the tympanic membrane typically results from a slap-like blow over the external auditory meatus. Blast and diving-related barotrauma are far rarer causes in the paediatric population. Symptoms and signs of a traumatic perforation include otalgia, bloody otorrhoea and sudden onset of conductive hearing loss.

Examination

A traumatic perforation commonly involves the pars tensa, is irregular in shape and may involve a significant area of the tympanic membrane. Bleeding into the external auditory canal often limits visualisation without the aid of microscopy and microsuction, which may be difficult in the younger child.

Investigation and management

An audiological assessment is advisable to gauge the presence and degree of hearing loss. A conductive loss greater than 30–40 dB raises the concern of ossicular injury. The patient should be advised to keep the ear dry. The use of ototoxic topical treatments and syringing of the ear should be avoided. In children, conservative treatment and active observation is recommended, as the majority of traumatic perforations will heal within approximately 2 months. Surgical repair of the tympanic membrane may be considered should a perforation persist. The timing of repair should be guided by the age of the child and the contralateral ear state.

TEMPORAL BONE INJURY

The diagnosis, investigation and management of paediatric temporal bone injuries mirrors that of adults and is covered in detail in Chapter 16, Ear Trauma.

TRAUMA TO OTOLOGIC IMPLANTS

Implants used within paediatric ENT surgery may also be vulnerable to trauma, particularly from falls and sporting activities. These implants may be osseointegrated (e.g. a bone-anchored hearing aid) or non-osseointegrated (e.g. cochlear implant). Several cases of trauma to bone-anchored hearing aids have been reported; significant complications are, fortunately, very rare.[7] Good fixation of cochlear implant internal components is recommended in paediatric patients due to the increased risk of minor head trauma and thin overlying soft tissue. The internal magnetic component within the receiver-stimulator package of a cochlear implant may be liable to displacement either as a result of trauma or from strong magnetic traction.[8,9] This may be replaced and secured surgically.

NASAL TRAUMA

NASAL BONE FRACTURE

Like the auricle, the nose is a prominent facial feature and is particularly vulnerable to injury. Fractures of the nasal bones in older children mirror those of adults; however, bony fractures in younger children are rarer due to the soft and compliant external nose, which is relatively less projected.

Examination

A nasal bone fracture is typically a clinical diagnosis and is supported by a change in shape, i.e. deviation or depression of the nose from its normal appearance (Figure 28.4). If this is masked by initial soft tissue swelling, an interval examination should be performed 4–5 days after the injury. Crepitus may be felt on palpation of the nasal bones. Careful palpation of the full facial skeleton should be performed so that fractures of the orbitoethmoid complex, zygoma and maxilla do not go undetected. It is also important not to overlook cerebrospinal fluid rhinorrhoea and anosmia which can result from base of skull fractures.

Investigation and management

Plain radiographs do not play a role in the assessment of paediatric nasal fractures. If significant craniofacial fractures are suspected, CT scanning is the investigation of choice.

Controversy surrounds the best management of neonatal nasal deformity. Significant deviations of the nose and septum have been observed to improve within the first days of life. Nasal obstruction may cause significant airway and feeding problems in the neonate. Closed manipulation of the nasal septum and cases of limited septoplasty have been described.[10]

Undisplaced nasal fractures do not require specific treatment. Optimal treatment of displaced nasal fractures is vital to prevent a resultant deformity that may impact on facial growth. As with adults, manipulation of the deformed nose should be performed in the first 7–10 days following injury. Management of cartilaginous deformity is usually delayed until later adolescence so that nasal growth is not disrupted.

SEPTAL HAEMATOMA

Children are particularly vulnerable to development of a nasal septal haematoma, a collection of blood between the anterior cartilaginous septum and its covering mucoperichondrium. This may be uni- or bilateral and causes the principal symptom of nasal obstruction (Figure 28.5). It can occur without any external abnormality and may not be associated with epistaxis. Any child with a history of nasal trauma should undergo anterior rhinoscopy to check for a haematoma. No other investigations are required.

Management

As with an auricular haematoma, a septal haematoma needs expedient management to avoid the complications of superinfection, abscess formation, cartilage deformation (Figure 28.6) and a saddle deformity of the nasal dorsum. Septal haematomas have a higher risk of progression to abscess formation, given the microbiological environment of the nasal cavity. Furthermore, midfacial infection may lead to significant morbidity and even mortality as a result of septic spread; cavernous sinus thrombosis and intracranial infection can occur.

In a child, the haematoma should be drained under general anaesthesia via a hemitransfixion incision and measures taken to prevent

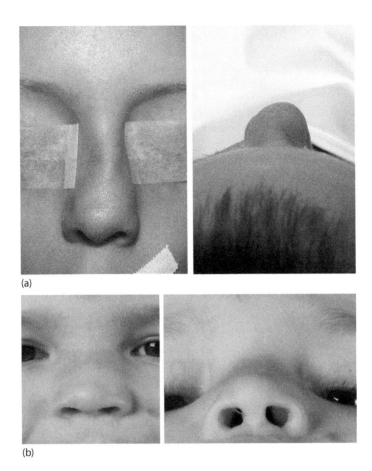

Figure 28.4 **(a)** C-shaped nasal deformity seen in older children with nasal fractures (left – frontal view; right – view on examination from above and behind). **(b)** Splaying of the nasal bones over the frontal process of the maxilla more commonly seen in younger children (left – frontal view, right – skyline view). Images courtesy of Dr M-L Montague, RHSC, Edinburgh.

recurrence. In children, septal transfixion sutures are recommended rather than nasal packing. A broad-spectrum antibiotic should be given for 5 days.

TRAUMATIC EPISTAXIS

In children, two particular circumstances are more likely and warrant emphasis. Anterior epistaxis is likely to be related to digital trauma (nose-picking) or foreign body insertion.

Brisk and intermittent epistaxis following trauma to the nose is often from the anterior ethmoidal artery or its branches (e.g. rupture of a high septal vessel). The bleeding point can be sought endonasally and cauterised; otherwise, anterior ethmoidal artery ligation may be required in severe cases. This requires an external approach. The anterior ethmoidal artery is not amenable to embolisation, given its origin from the internal carotid circulation and relation to the ophthalmic artery.

TRAUMA TO THE NECK

PENETRATING

Penetrating neck injuries are rare in children. They may be accidental or non-accidental, either by assault or self-inflicted. Stabbing, penetrating missile and animal attack (e.g. dog bite) injury

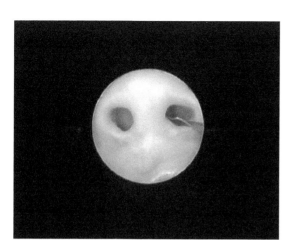

Figure 28.5 Unilateral septal haematoma causing right nasal obstruction. Image courtesy of Dr M-L Montague, RHSC, Edinburgh.

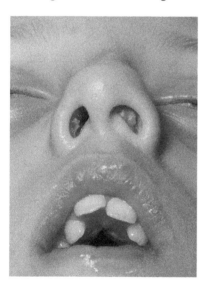

Figure 28.6 A thickened fibrotic nasal septum in a young boy – the result of an untreated septal haematoma. Image courtesy of Dr M-L Montague, RHSC, Edinburgh.

may occur. These injuries may be life-threatening; a recent series describes a mortality rate of 40%.[11]

Injury is classified according to the area of the neck penetrated. Zone 1 extends from the thoracic inlet to the level of the cricoid cartilage, zone 2 lies between the cricoid cartilage and angle of the mandible, and zone 3 lies above the level of the angle of the mandible (Figure 28.7). The management

of these cases should follow both APLS and ATLS principles. It is uncommon for penetrating neck injury to be associated with cervical spine injury; however, this is very much dependent on the mechanism of injury and must be considered.

The management of penetrating neck trauma is similar to that of adults. Whilst optimal management is controversial, a policy of selective investigation and surgical exploration has evolved that is guided by the clinical presentation and haemodynamic stability of the patient. Examination and investigation should not only focus on vascular injury but also cover neurological, laryngopharyngeal and oesophageal trauma. In particular, vascular injuries in zone 3 may be managed by embolization. Intrathoracic injuries should also be considered in cases of zone 1 trauma.

Blunt

Like penetrating cervical trauma, blunt neck injury is rarely encountered in children. Significant morbidity and mortality may result due to the risk of laryngotracheal disruption. Vascular and oesophageal trauma may also occur. A high index of suspicion may be required to detect an injury, and a proactive policy for investigation should be employed. Trauma to the paediatric airway is covered in Chapter 24.

SOFT TISSUE INJURY OF THE HEAD AND NECK

Oral and palatal injuries are particularly common in children and typically relate to falls with a foreign body in the mouth. Trauma to the tongue, soft palate or pharynx commonly results.[12]

The principles of management typically mirror those of adults; however, as previously stated, the need for a general anaesthetic for debridement and suturing is significantly greater. Minor injuries may be treated conservatively and heal rapidly. Particular caution should be taken with significant injuries of the palate, which may result in an oronasal fistula. Development of thrombosis or pseudoaneurysm of the internal carotid artery is also a rare but significant concern.

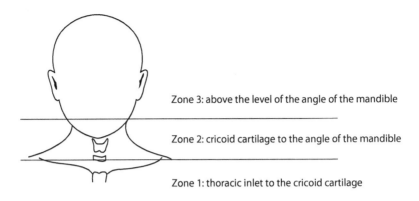

Zone 3: above the level of the angle of the mandible

Zone 2: cricoid cartilage to the angle of the mandible

Zone 1: thoracic inlet to the cricoid cartilage

Figure 28.7 Classification of penetrating neck trauma by area.

KEY LEARNING POINTS

- Minor ENT injury is common in children. Major injuries are, fortunately, rare but are associated with significant morbidity and mortality.
- Non-accidental injury in children commonly involves the ENT region. External ear injuries and pharyngeal injuries in infants are particular manifestations.
- Management of major trauma should follow ATLS and APLS principles. Control of catastrophic external haemorrhage and airway management are the first priorities with cervical spine control.
- The diagnosis of ENT injuries may be delayed in the multiply injured child.
- Special considerations relate to the diagnosis and management of ENT injuries in a child; general anaesthesia may be required for imaging, examination and/or intervention.

REFERENCES

1. H Kawalski, P Śpiewak. How septum deformations in newborns occur. *Int J Pediatr Otorhinolaryngol* 1998; 44: 23–30.
2. C Hughes, EH Harley, G Milmoe, R Bala, A Martorella. Birth trauma in the head and neck. *Arch Otolaryngol Head Neck Surg* 1999; 125: 193–199.
3. M Alicandri-Ciufelli, V Moretti, M Ruberto, D Monzani, L Chiarini, L Presutti. Otolaryngology fantastica: the ear, nose, and throat manifestations of Munchausen's syndrome. *Laryngoscope* 2012; 122: 51–57.
4. BD Steele, PO Brennan. A prospective survey of patients with presumed accidental ear injury presenting to a paediatric accident and emergency department. *Emerg Med J* 2002; 19: 226–228.
5. WC Giles, KC Iverson, JD King, FC Hill, EA Woody, AL Bouknight. Incision and drainage followed by mattress suture repair of auricular hematoma. *Laryngoscope* 2007; 117: 2097–2099.

6. K Kakarala, DA Kieff. Bolsterless management for recurrent auricular hematomata. *Laryngoscope* 2012; 122: 1235–1237.

7. A-L McDermott, J Barraclough, AP Reid. Unusual complication following trauma to a bone-anchored hearing aid: case report and literature review. *J Laryngol Otol* 2009; 123: 348–350.

8. JM Yun, MW Colburn, PJ Antonelli. Cochlear implant magnet displacement with minor head trauma. *Otolaryngol – Head Neck Surg* 2005; 133: 275–277.

9. JI Mickelson, FK Kozak. Magnet dislodgement in cochlear implantation: correction utilizing a lasso technique. *Int J Pediatr Otorhinolaryngol* 2008; 72: 1071–1076.

10. AJ Emami, L Brodsky, M Pizzuto. Neonatal septoplasty: case report and review of the literature. *Int J Pediatr Otorhinolaryngol* 1996; 35: 271–275.

11. MK Kim, R Buckman, W Szeremeta. Penetrating neck trauma in children: an urban hospital's experience. *Otolaryngol – Head Neck Surg* 2000; 123: 439–443.

12. D Radkowski, TJ McGill, GB Healy, DT Jones. Penetrating trauma of the oropharynx in children. *Laryngoscope* 1993; 103: 991–994.

FURTHER READING

JC Oosthuizen. Paediatric blunt laryngeal trauma: a review. *Int J Otolaryngol.* Vol. 2011, Article ID 183047.

M Samuel, S Wietska (eds.), *Advanced Paediatric Life Support*, 6th edition, Wiley Blackwell, 2016.

MS Yilmaz, M Guven, G Kayabasoglu, AF Varli. Efficacy of closed reduction for nasal fractures in children. *Br J Oral Maxillofac Surg.* 2013; 51(8): e256–e258.

N Alshaikh, S Lo. Nasal septal abscess in children: from diagnosis to management and prevention. *Int J Pediatr Otorhinolaryngol.* 2011; 75: 737–744.

P Rees, A Al-Hussaini, S Maguire. Child abuse and fabricated or induced illness in the ENT setting: a systematic review. *Clin Otolaryngol.* 2017; 42(4): 783–804.

WL Biffl, EE Moore, DH Rehse, PJ Offner, RJ Franciose, JM Burch. Selective management of penetrating neck trauma based on cervical level of injury. *Am J Surg.* 1997; 174: 678–682.

Index

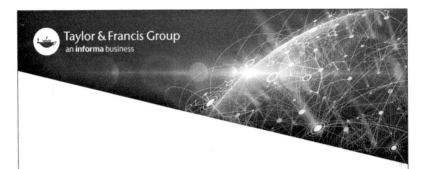